National Safety Council

First Aid and CPR

Infants and Children

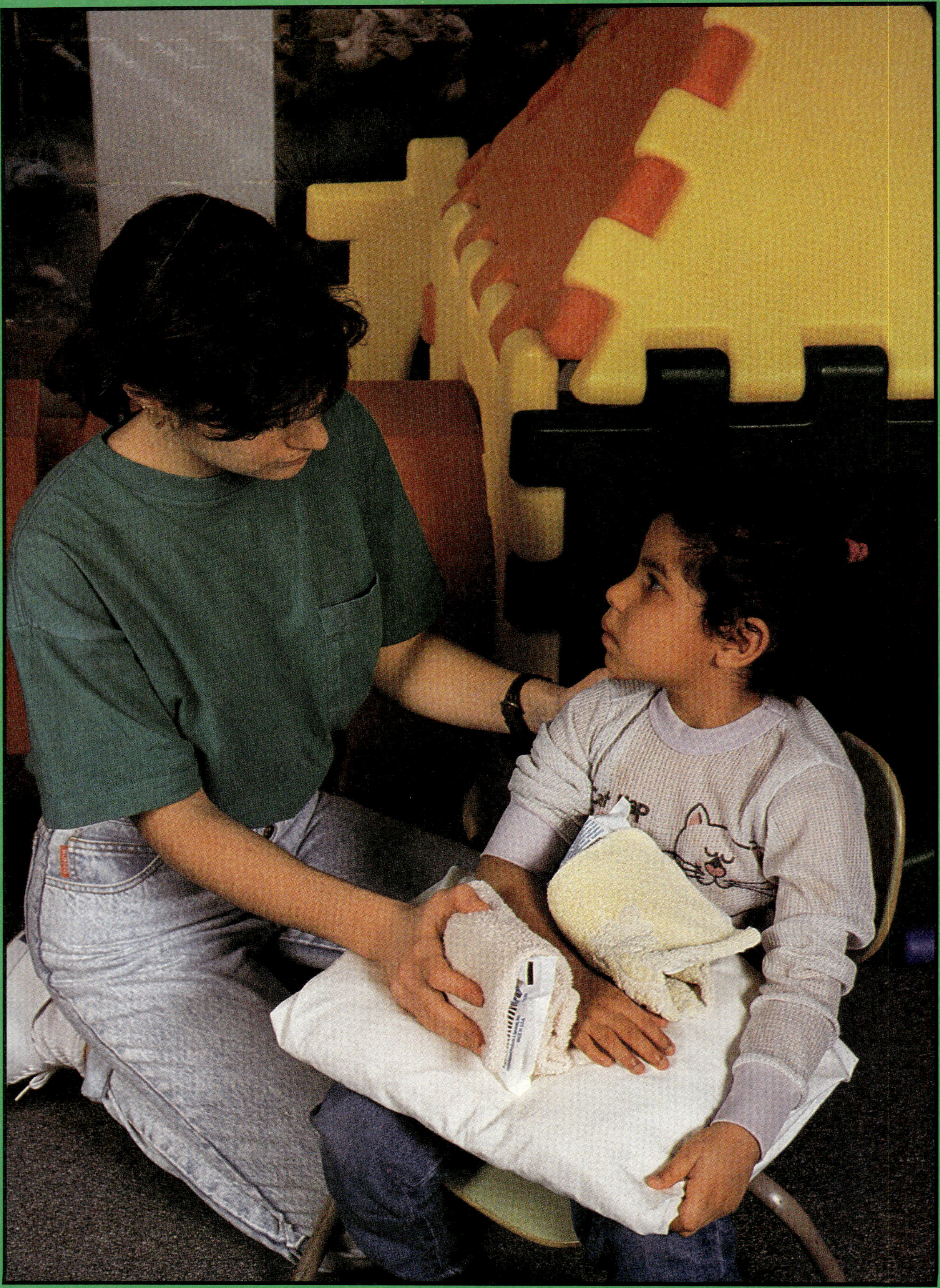

National Safety Council

First Aid and CPR

Infants and Children

Second Edition

Editorial, Sales, and Customer Service Offices
Jones and Bartlett Publishers
40 Tall Pine Drive
Sudbury, MA 01776
(508) 443-5000
(800) 832-0034

Jones and Bartlett Publishers International
7 Melrose Terrace
London W6 7RL
England

The first aid and CPR procedures in this book are based on the most current recommendations of responsible medical sources. The National Safety Council and the publisher, however, make no guarantee as to, and assume no responsibility for, the correctness, sufficiency or completeness of such information or recommendations. Other or additional safety measures may be required under particular circumstances.

Library of Congress Cataloging-in-Publication Data

First aid and CPR : infants and children / National Safety Council.—2nd ed.
p. cm.
Includes index.
ISBN 0-86720-833-3
1. Pediatric emergencies. 2. First aid in illness and injury. 3. CPR (First aid) for children. 4. CPR (First aid) for infants. I. National Safety Council.
RJ370.F57 1994
618.92′0025—dc20

93-35537
CIP

We would like to thank the following programs for their cooperation with the photographs:

Action for Boston Community Development, Inc./South End Head Start Program
Charlestown, Massachusetts Head Start/Day Care Program

We would also like to thank the children and teachers who so generously posed for us.

Vice President and Publisher ■ Clayton E. Jones
Assistant Editor ■ Heather Stratton
Production Editor ■ Anne Noonan
Typesetter ■ NK Graphics
Illustrator ■ Dave Young
Principal Photographer ■ Frank Siteman
Cover Designer ■ Hannus Design Associates
Printer and Binder ■ Semline, Inc.

Printed in the United States of America
96 10 9 8 7 6 5 4 3

Table of Contents

Acknowledgments

Principal Authors

Stephanie L. O'Neill, B.S., R.N.*
O'Neill-Page, Inc.
Belmont, MA

Constance Q. Page, B.A., R.N.*
O'Neill-Page, Inc.
Belmont, MA

Alton L. Thygerson, Ph.D.
Brigham Young University
Provo, UT

Reviewers

The National Safety Council would like to thank the following individuals for their efforts in reviewing the complete manuscript or selected chapters of this text.

Deborah Z. Altschuler
National Pediculosis Association
Newton, MA

Margaret Anderson
Pfizer Central Research Division
Groton, CT

Carol Bufton
Minnesota Safety Council
St. Paul, MN

Phipps Y. Cohe
SIDS Alliance
Columbia, MD

Ann Coley
Sumter Area Technical College
Sumter, SC

Richard Cooper
SEMTA
Rye, NH

Susan Denton
Central Florida Safety Council
Orlando, FL

Betty Jane Evans
Dade County Citizens Safety Council
Miami, FL

Linda Gosselin
MECTA
Millbury, MA

Barbara Jacobs
Boston Head Start, ABCD, Inc.
Boston, MA

Claudella Jones
The National Institute for Burn Medicine
Ann Arbor, MI

Sandra Lewis
Sandra Lewis Training Associates
So. Easton, MA

Barbara Miller
First Response
Laguna Nigel, CA

Cindy Pasquarello
Joslin Diabetic Center
Boston, MA

Jodi Rupe
Texas Safety Association
Austin, TX

R. Lorraine Samuel
Cambridge School Department
Cambridge, MA

Barbara Seabolt
Comprehensive Health and Safety Education
Farmington, MI

Linda Softley
Massachusetts Poison Control Center
Boston, MA

Rose Ann Soloway
National Capital Poison Center
Washington, DC

Judy Walker
Harvard University Child Care
Cambridge, MA

John Ward
North Alabama Chapter National Safety Council
Birmingham, AL

Kathleen Zents
Safety & Health Council of Western Missouri & Kansas
Kansas City, MO

*Stephanie O'Neill and Constance Page are founders of O'Neill-Page, Inc., a Massachusetts-based company dedicated to the delivery of quality pediatric first aid, health, and safety training to child care providers and parents.

Welcome Message

Congratulations on your decision to enroll in the National Safety Council first aid and CPR program for infants and children.

This course is unique in that it focuses on the first aid training needs and responsibilities of child care providers. Your up-to-date first aid knowledge can help you respond appropriately and confidently to an emergency situation and might help save a life.

Protecting life and promoting health have been the National Safety Council's only mission since 1913.

On behalf of the National Safety Council, as well as our local safety councils and training agencies, I hope that you enjoy learning about first aid and CPR and wish you success in your training program.

Sincerely,

Gerard F. Scannell, President
National Safety Council

1

Introduction

■ Size of the Injury Problem ■ Need for Injury Prevention Education ■
■ Need for First Aid Training ■ Legal Aspects of First Aid ■

Size of the Injury Problem

In the United States injuries are the leading health problem in children over the age of 1 year. Injuries cause more deaths to children than all diseases combined and are the leading cause of disability.

Each year an estimated 600,000 children are hospitalized for injuries, and almost 16 million are seen in emergency medical facilities for treatment.

The Centers for Disease Control estimates that more than 30,000 children suffer permanent disabilities from injuries each year. These disabilities have an enormous, adverse impact on the children's development and future productivity, and severely strain the financial and emotional resources of their families.

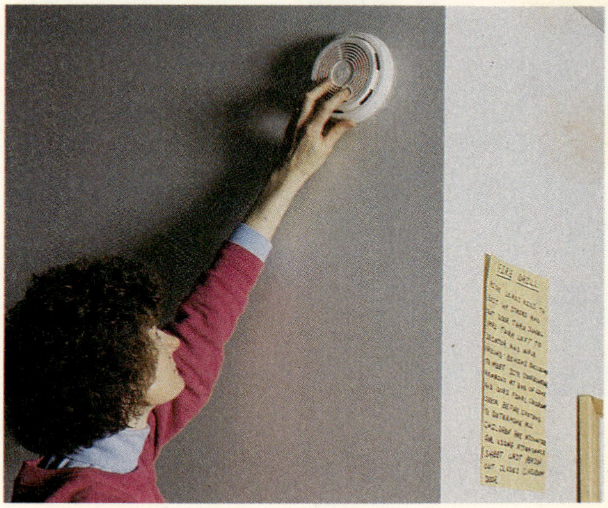

Need for Injury Prevention Education

Unintentional injuries are often mistakenly referred to as accidents because they occur unexpectedly and seem uncontrollable. In fact, however, many injuries are predictable and preventable. Consider: an injury resulting from a child's swallowing a cleaning product could likely have been prevented with proper storage. An injury resulting from a child's falling down an open flight of stairs could likely have been prevented by a doorway gate.

Public education and awareness programs have had a positive impact on the reduction of childhood injuries and deaths. Thousands more could be avoided every year through currently available prevention strategies. For instance:

- The reduction of driving speed limits, the enactment of state seat belt laws and child safety restraint laws, and the efforts to reduce drunk driving have all contributed to the reduction of car-related injuries and death.
- Public awareness concerning the use of smoke detectors has reduced injuries and deaths that result from home fires.
- Product safety testing on juvenile products has significantly reduced injuries in young children.
- The proper use of bicycle helmets has reduced the severity of head injuries.
- Educational programs for preschool and elementary school children concerning fire prevention, poison prevention, motor vehicle restraints, and water safety have all contributed to a decrease in the numbers of injuries in children.

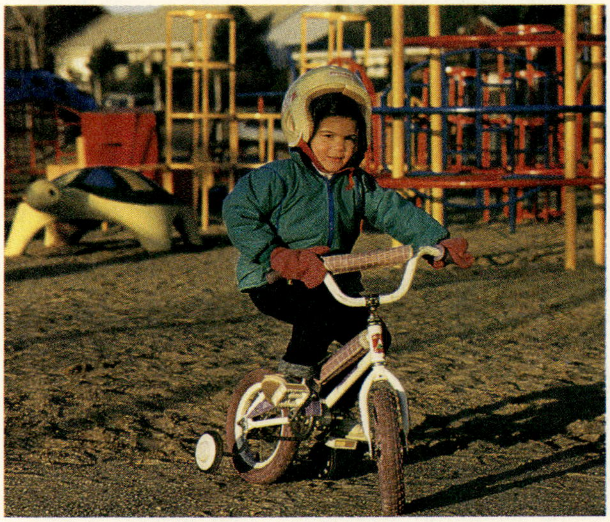

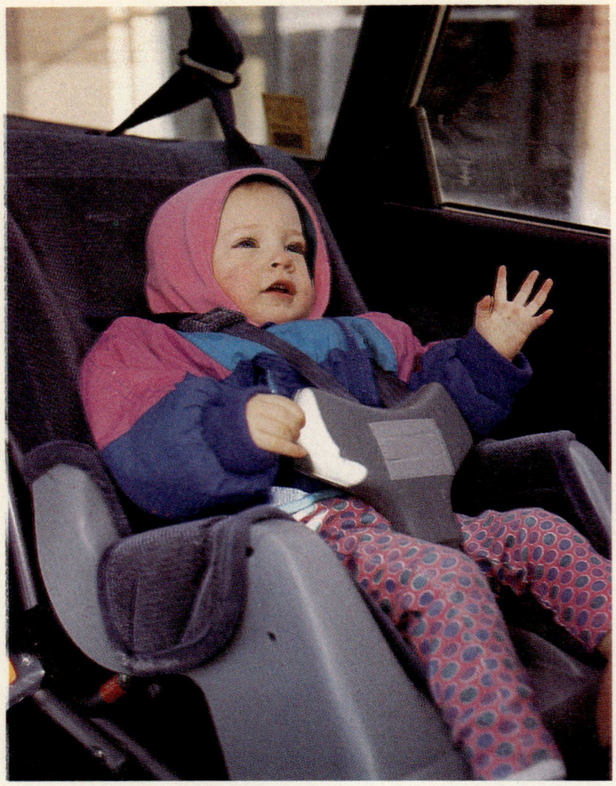

Injury prevention through an awareness of which dangers can, and frequently do, cause injuries, as well as knowledge about how we can make a child's environment safer, are all important components of first aid for children. Injury prevention can reduce the likelihood that first aid techniques will be needed.

Need for First Aid Training

Injuries can occur, however, no matter how caring and watchful adults are and despite the best safety plans. Because of the frequency of injury to children, it is likely that a child care provider will, at some time, be present when an injury or sudden illness strikes. The types of injuries that happen to children often directly relate to the child's age and developmental level. (Refer to the table in Chapter 13 which identifies typical injuries related to the child's developmental level.) Planning to prevent these injuries is essential. It is equally essential to master the first aid techniques presented in this text to be prepared if an injury or sudden illness occurs in the child care setting or home.

First aid is the immediate care given to the injured or suddenly ill child. First aid does not take the place of proper medical treatment. It consists only of furnishing temporary assistance until more complete medical care, if needed, is obtained, or until the chance for recovery without medical care is assured. Most injuries and illnesses require only first aid care.

Properly applied, first aid can mean the difference between life and death, rapid recovery and long hospitalization, or temporary disability and permanent disability.

Legal Aspects of First Aid

Duty to Act

No one is required to provide first aid unless a legal duty to do so exists. For example, even a physician can ignore a stranger experiencing a seizure or suffering from a fractured bone. Moral obligations exist, but they are not the same as legal obligations to give aid.

First aiders have a legal duty to act in the following situations:

1. ***When there is a contractual duty.*** If a preexisting relationship exists between two people such as a child care provider and a child, a teacher and a student, a lifeguard and a swimmer, or a driver and a passenger, a duty to give first aid exists.

2. ***After first aid has been started.*** Once first aiders begin treating an injury, they may not stop unless emergency medical help arrives to care for the child, they are relieved by another competent adult who can seek further appropriate treatment, or they become physically exhausted.

Standards of Care for First Aid

Standards of care ensure quality care and protection for the injured or suddenly ill child. They include:

1. ***A qualified training program.*** First aid and CPR programs must meet the requirements of state regulations and follow current first aid procedures and practices as established by national emergency care and safety-related organizations.

2. ***A qualified first aider.*** First aiders should be expected to provide appropriate care within the scope of their training. First aid treatment given should be similar to that given by an equally trained, responsible rescuer in a similar circumstance and should not endanger the child.

Obtaining Permission to Give First Aid

First aiders should always obtain permission before performing first aid. Most centers require parents to complete forms that provide the child care provider with a medical history and permission to have the child treated in an emergency situation.

In the event that the injured child is unknown to you, you must first obtain parental permission.

- Permission should be obtained from the parent or guardian of an injured child. Oral consent is valid. Tell the parent that you are a trained first aider and explain what you plan to do.
- If a parent or guardian is not available, emergency life-saving first aid may be given without consent.
- Combative older children who threaten to harm themselves or others can present a difficult management problem. Remember that, although infrequently needed, police officers have the authority to restrain and transport a person against the person's will.

Parent Refusing Permission to Help a Child

Rarely will a first aider encounter parents who refuse permission—usually on moral, ethical, or religious grounds—to care for a seriously injured or ill child. If parents refuse permission, make every effort to convince them of the seriousness of the problem and the need for first aid. If the parents remain unconvinced, call the police and document the situation and your actions.

Good Samaritan Laws

Some states have a Good Samaritan law that protects first aiders who provide care to an injured or suddenly ill person. Even in the absence of a Good Samaritan law, a first aider who acts in good faith and without gross negligence or willful misconduct is very unlikely to encounter litigation.

2

Injury Assessment

■ Approaching an Accident ■ Primary Survey ■
■ Secondary Survey ■ Calling for Emergency Medical Help ■

During an emergency involving the health of a child, it is essential to remain calm and in control. A calm attitude and methodical approach will inspire the confidence of an injured child and set a standard that other adults will follow.

Do no harm. First aiders should avoid making a health-related emergency worse by their own actions. To that end, always handle an injured child gently and avoid any unnecessary movements that might aggravate an undetected fracture or spinal injury. NEVER MOVE AN UNCONSCIOUS CHILD EXCEPT TO SAVE A LIFE.

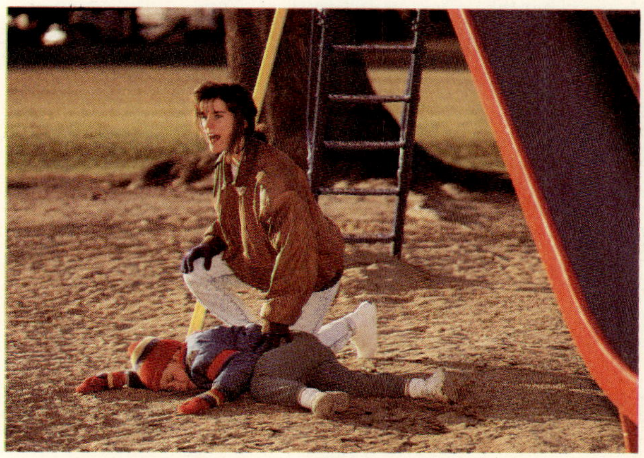

Shout for help.

Approaching an Injury

1. ***Survey the injury scene.*** Before approaching an injured child, scan the injury scene, making sure that it is safe to approach. Gather clues as to what happened. Look around to be certain that there is only one injured child. Be alert for unusual dangers facing rescuers, such as chemical fumes, live electrical wires, or deep water.

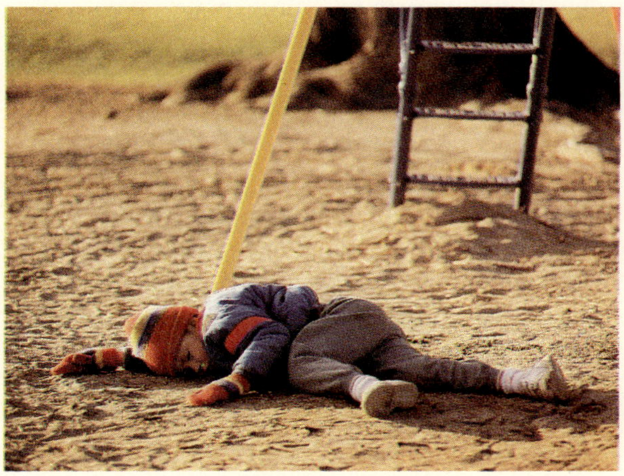

Survey the scene, gathering clues to what has happened.

2. ***Check for responsiveness.*** If the child does not respond when called by name or gently tapped on the shoulder, it is likely that the child is unconscious.

3. ***Shout for Help.*** This will alert others to the emergency. Direct a bystander to call for emergency medical help immediately.

The **primary** and **secondary surveys** provide a first aider with a methodical approach to help identify and prioritize a child's injuries or sudden illness. The primary survey should always be conducted first because it reveals immediate life-threatening problems. These problems must be corrected before going on to the secondary survey. The secondary survey helps to identify less serious injuries requiring care.

Primary Survey

The primary survey covers these areas:

A–Airway
B–Breathing
C–Circulation
H–Hemorrhage

The primary survey is the first step in assessing or evaluating the condition of an injured child. The purpose is to find, so that you can correct, conditions that threaten the most basic body functions of breathing and heartbeat.

Airway. Does the child have an open airway? If the child is talking, the airway is open.

Breathing. Is the child breathing? Conscious children are breathing. However, look for signs of breathing difficulties or unusual breathing sounds.

Circulation. Is the child's heart beating? It is beating if the child is conscious. If the child is unconscious check for the heartbeat by feeling for the pulse. The ABCs will be described in greater depth in Chapter 3.

Hemorrhage. Is the child bleeding severely? Severe bleeding is recognized by blood-soaked clothing or blood spurting from a deep cut or wound.

Sometimes the need for emergency medical help is apparent immediately, as in the event of heavy bleeding, unconsciousness, or the absence of breathing or of a heartbeat. At other times, it takes a few minutes of assessment before you can identify the injuries and know what additional help is necessary. The **secondary survey** provides a guideline for further assessment.

Secondary Survey

A first aider must not assume that the obvious injuries are the only injuries. Once you have completed the primary survey and attended to any life-threatening problems it reveals, take a closer look at the child. Use the secondary survey to locate and prioritize additional injuries that do not pose an immediate threat to life, but might become life threatening if untreated. The secondary survey has three parts:

- Interview
- Vital signs
- Head-to-toe exam

As you examine the child, look for important signs and symptoms of injury. A *sign* is something the first aider sees, hears, or feels, such as a pale face, difficulty breathing, and cool skin. A *symptom* is something the child describes to the first aider, such as nausea or back pain.

Interview

Identify yourself as a first aider and, if necessary, obtain the parent's permission before beginning first aid. See Chapter 1 for more information on obtaining permission and its legal implications.

Ongoing communication on the child's level is essential when providing first aid. Allow the child time

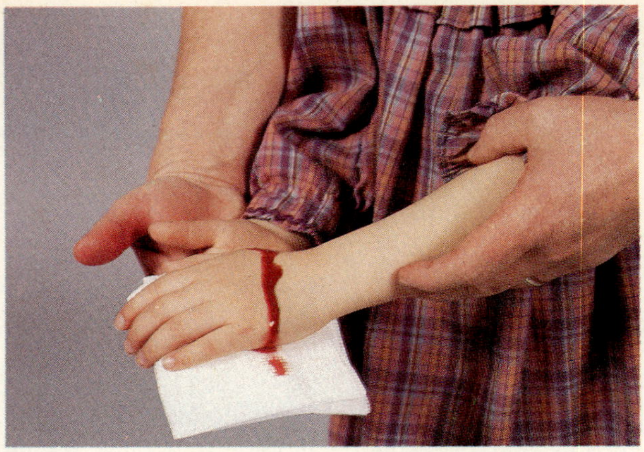

A sign

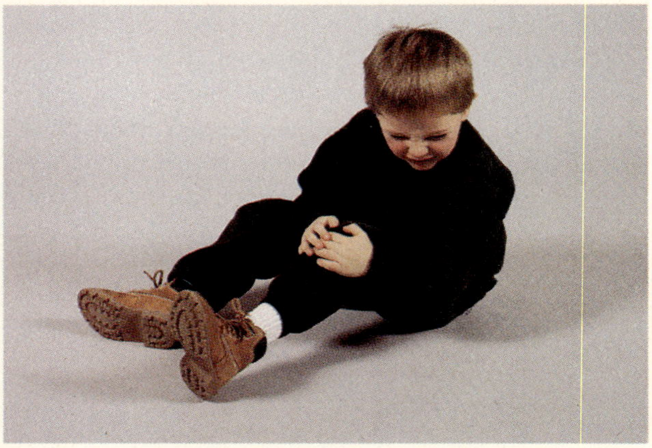

A symptom

to calm down. Ask other adults and children if they saw what happened.

Reassure the child by explaining that you will help. Ask simple, nonthreatening questions such as, "Tell me about what happened," and, "Point to where it hurts." Use short sentences and familiar words. Try to be as honest as possible. You might not know the extent of the injuries but you can say, "You are safe now," and "I am taking good care of you."

Ask the child about the major complaint. Sometimes it is obvious, such as with bleeding. Most injuries are accompanied by pain or abnormal function. The word S-A-M-P-L-E can help you to remember other important information that might be needed at a later time by emergency medical personnel.

Symptoms (the child's major complaint)
Allergies (might give a clue as to the problem)
Medications (might give a clue as to the problem)
Preexisting illnesses (a known health condition relating to the problem)
Last food (in case surgery is needed or food poisoning is suspected)
Events before the injury (such as a child on playground equipment or eating)

Medical Alert Tag

Always check for a medical alert tag worn as a necklace or a bracelet. These tags provide important information about allergies, medications, and preexisting illnesses and a 24-hour telephone number to call in case of an emergency. *Never* remove a child's medical alert tag.

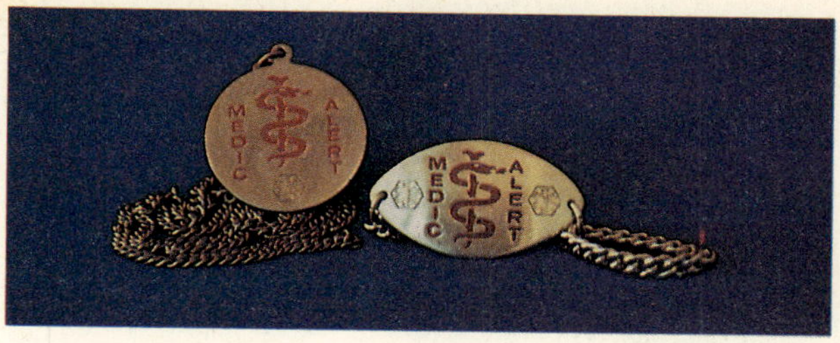

Medical alert tag

Vital Signs

Vital signs provide important information about basic heart and lung function and can provide clues to other injuries. You should check the vital signs of pulse, respirations, and skin condition as soon as you reach a seriously injured child and every 5 minutes while waiting for emergency medical help to arrive.

Pulse. Locate the pulse in one of the following three ways:

1. Place two fingertips over the brachial pulse point located on the inside of the upper arm, as illustrated in the Vital Signs Skill Scan. An infant's pulse is most easily felt here.
2. Place two fingertips over the carotid pulse point located on the neck, in the groove beside the Adam's apple, as illustrated in the Vital Signs Skill Scan. The pulse of a child over age 1 is most easily felt here. Do not feel both carotid arteries at the same time. Do not massage or press hard on the carotid pulse points because either will disturb the heart's rhythm.
3. Place two fingertips over the radial pulse point located on the thumb side of the inside wrist, as illustrated in the Vital Signs Skill Scan. The pulse of a child over age 1 can also be felt here.

Do not use your thumb to feel for a pulse because it has its own pulse.

Respiration. During the primary survey, you are concerned about whether the child is breathing. The secondary survey, however, focuses on the rate and character of the breathing.

Count the number of breaths per minute by watching the chest rise and fall or by gently placing your hand on the child's chest. Do not say you are counting his respirations as this might change the child's natural breathing pattern. As you are counting the number of breaths, listen to how the breathing sounds. For example:

- A whistle, wheezing, or crowing noise can indicate that the airway is constricted or partially obstructed.
- A gurgling noise can indicate that there is fluid in the airway.

Skin. Examine the child's skin condition by checking the following:

- ***Temperature.*** The child's temperature is best measured with a thermometer. If one is not available, you can get an idea of the temperature by putting the back of one hand on the child's cheek and the other on your own or that of another healthy person. If the child has an elevated temperature, you should feel the difference. Do not use your fingertips or palms because they are less sensitive to slight temperature differences. See Fevers, Chapter 11, for information on taking a child's temperature.
- ***Color.*** Skin color is an indicator of blood oxygen content. A blue or gray discoloration around a child's lips and nose in a light-skinned child is easily noticed and indicates that the child is having a respiratory problem. In darkly pigmented children, however, color changes are not as easily seen. For any skin type, color changes and blood oxygen content can be assessed by examining the nailbeds or the mucous membranes inside the mouth and inside the lower eyelids. Healthy mucous membranes are moist and appear pink because of their abundant supply of blood vessels. Mucous membranes that lack adequate oxygen appear blue or gray.

Normal Resting Pulse Rates	
Infants (under 1 year)	100–130 beats per minute
Toddlers (1–2 years)	90–120 beats per minute
Children (3–10 years)	80–110 beats per minute

Normal Resting Respiratory Rates	
Infants (under age 1)	30–40 breaths per minute
Toddlers (ages 1–2)	20–30 breaths per minute
Children (ages 3–10)	16–24 breaths per minute

Dilated pupils

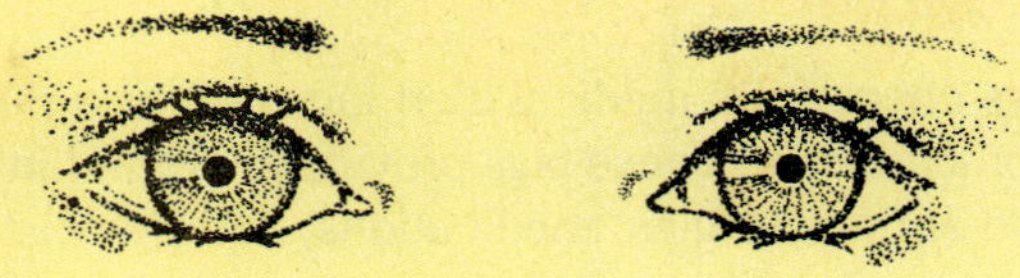

Constricted pupils

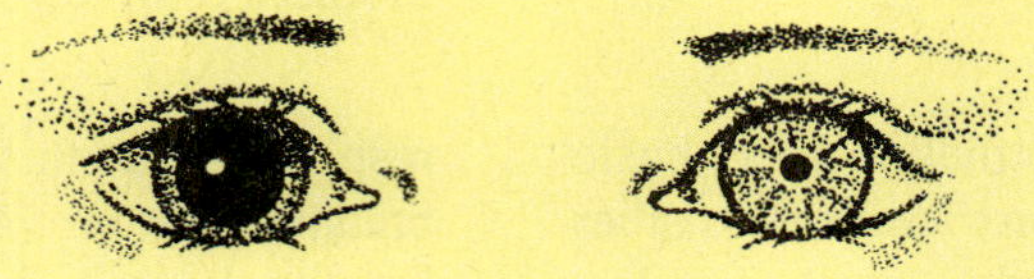

Unequal pupils

Head-to-Toe Exam

The final step in the injury assessment is a head-to-toe exam. A head-to-toe exam is necessary if the child has sustained an injury that was the result of a forceful impact, such as a fall from a climbing structure or a bicycle accident. A minor injury such as a scraped knee or sand in the eyes rarely requires a complete head-to-toe exam.

When performing a head-to-toe exam, explain what you are doing and why. Do not move the child if you suspect a spinal injury has occurred. Removing the clothing is usually unnecessary.

Head. Check the scalp for bleeding, swelling ("goose egg"), or depressions. Taking care not to move the head, check the ears and nose for clear fluid or bloody drainage. Look in the mouth for blood or foreign objects such as gum, candy, food, and small toy pieces.

Eyes. Gently separate the eyelids and look at the pupils, the small dark center of the eye. Normally, pupils become smaller when exposed to light. If pupils are unequal in size, the child might have experienced an internal head injury. Large or dilated pupils might indicate shock, internal bleeding, or cardiac arrest. Pupils that are constricted might indicate a drug overdose.

Spine. Tell the child not to move. If you suspect the child has suffered a spinal injury, ask if the child feels any pain or tingling in the arms or legs. Check the sensation, or feeling, and strength in the arms and legs by asking the child to press each foot against your hand and to squeeze your fingers with each hand.

Chest. Check for cuts, bruises, penetrations, tenderness or unusual position of the shoulders and ribs.

Abdomen. Gently feel the abdomen to check for bleeding, tenderness, and guarding (tightening of the abdominal muscles).

Arms and legs. Check the arms and legs for injury, deformity, and tenderness. Compare both sides of the body. (See the photo below.) Check to be sure that there is good circulation in an injured limb. To do this, use your thumb and index finger to squeeze the child's nailbed firmly. The nail should initially turn white and then immediately return to the normal pink color. (See the photo on the next page.) The child should be able to feel and move fingers or toes. The hands and feet should be warm to the touch.

Putting It All Together

The value of following the primary and secondary surveys will become apparent if you are faced with the responsibility of assessing and caring for an injured or suddenly ill child. This system helps a first aider

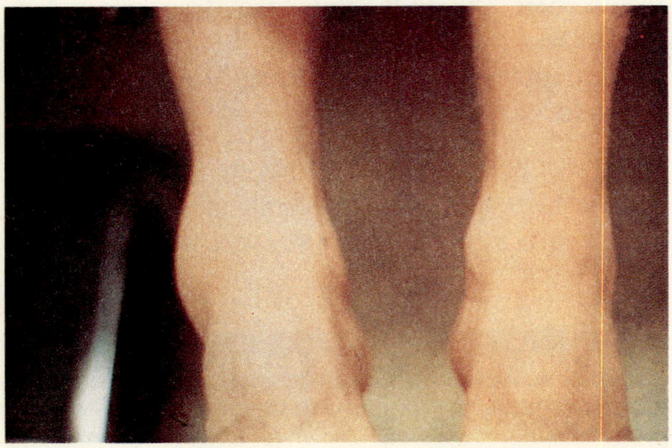

A sprained ankle

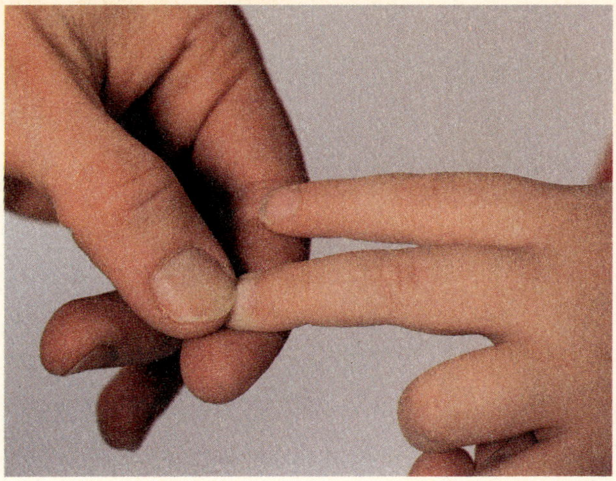

Check the circulation of hands and feet by pinching the fingernail and toenail (capillary refill).

react with confidence, prioritize problems, and initiate first aid in the order it is needed. Remember to conduct a primary survey first and correct any problems that it reveals before going on to the secondary survey.

Calling for Emergency Medical Help (EMS, Emergency Medical Services)

It is important to know that the 9-1-1 emergency number is not available in all communities. Know the emergency telephone numbers in your area and what services they provide. Make sure the following emergency numbers are posted next to each telephone in your child care center or home:

1. ***Fire.*** Many fire departments have a rescue squad with trained paramedics and are likely to respond quickly in an emergency situation.

2. ***Ambulance.*** The fastest way to transport an injured child to an emergency medical facility is by ambulance. Some ambulance services have trained paramedics; others do not.

3. ***Police.*** If necessary, they can transport an injured child to an emergency medical facility quickly. Many police officers are trained in basic life support.

4. ***The child's parent.*** Child care providers should have both the home and work telephone numbers of the child's parent. In addition, they should have the telephone number of a trusted neighbor or relative to contact if they are unable to reach the child's parent.

5. ***The child's health care provider.*** The child's health care provider might not be available but should be notified if an emergency occurs. This text uses the term, "health care provider" when referring to a medical professional who is responsible for the health of a child. A health care provider can be a doctor, nurse practitioner, physician's assistant, or a medical specialist such as an ophthalmologist or allergist.

6. ***Poison control center.*** Call your local operator for the number of the regional poison control center that serves your area. These centers are important sources of information and are available on a 24-hour basis.

When calling for emergency medical help, give the following information over the telephone:

1. ***The location of the injured child.*** Include the town, street name and number, and the nearest intersecting street. Be specific in describing the building. Send someone out to meet the ambulance. Ambulance drivers and paramedics too often waste precious minutes searching for an injured child because directions are not complete and street signs and numbers are not present or easily seen.

2. ***Nature of the emergency.*** Explain what happened, such as, the child has fallen and is unconscious, or the child has a cut that is bleeding heavily.

3. ***Treatment being given.*** Explain what first aid is being given to the injured child. The dispatcher sending emergency help can explain what other care should be given before emergency help arrives.

4. ***Your name and telephone number.*** If additional information is needed, the dispatcher can call you back.

It is important to speak slowly and clearly when giving the above information. Always be the last to hang up the telephone.

SKILL SCAN: Vital Signs

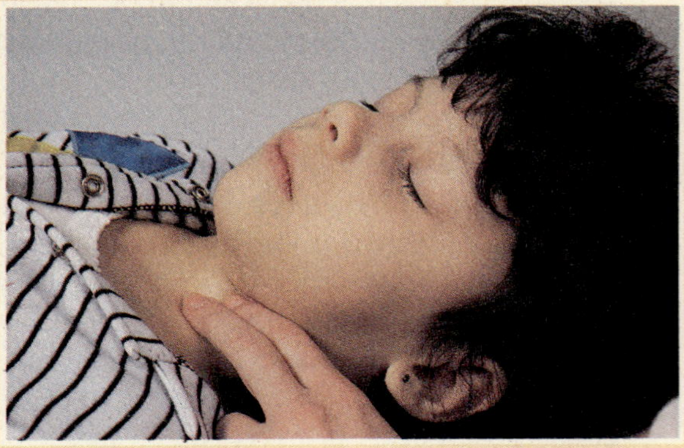

Location of carotid pulse.

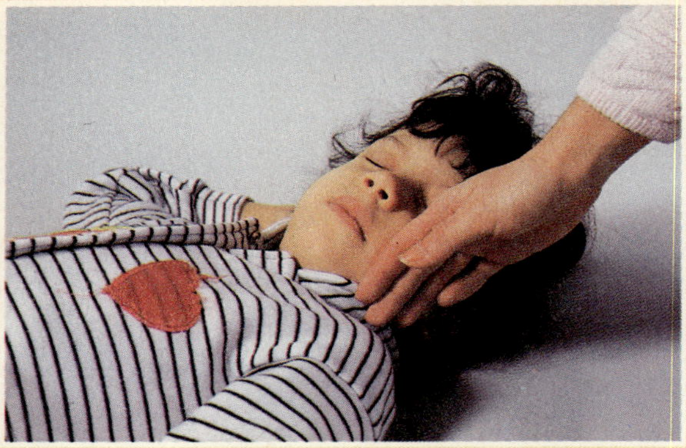

Checking child's skin temperature.

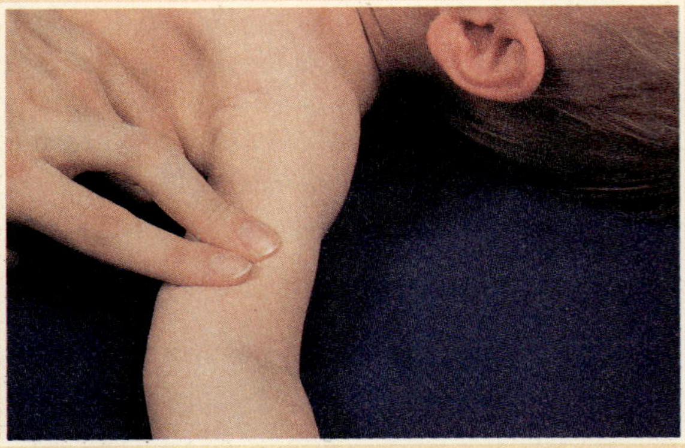

Location of brachial pulse.

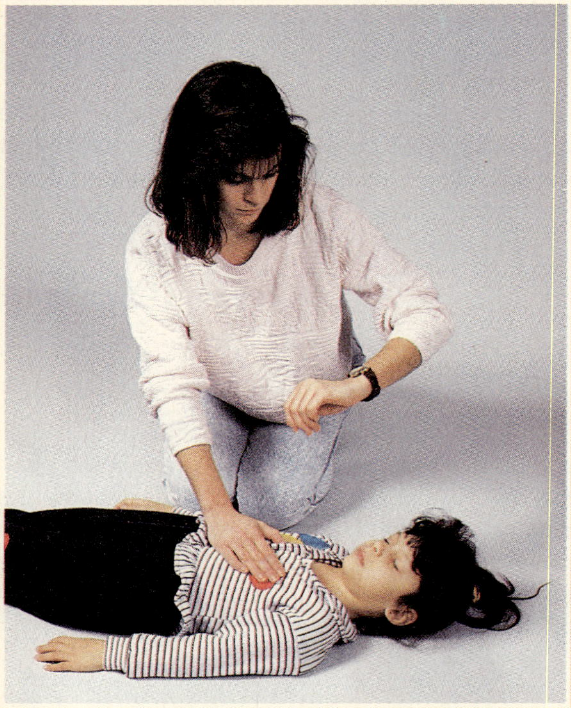

Checking child's respiration rate.

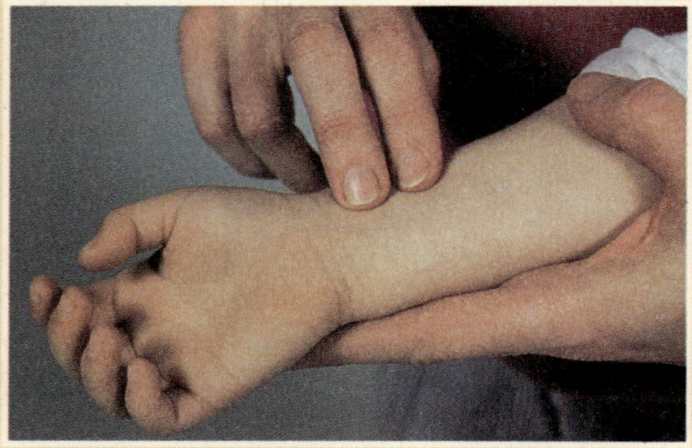

Location of radial pulse.

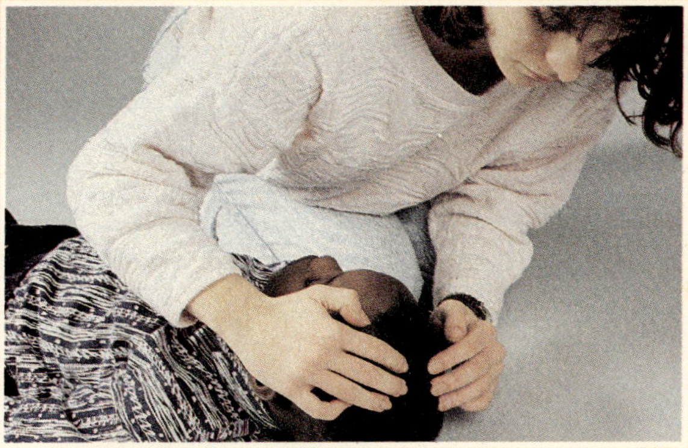

Check head for bleeding, bumps or indentations.

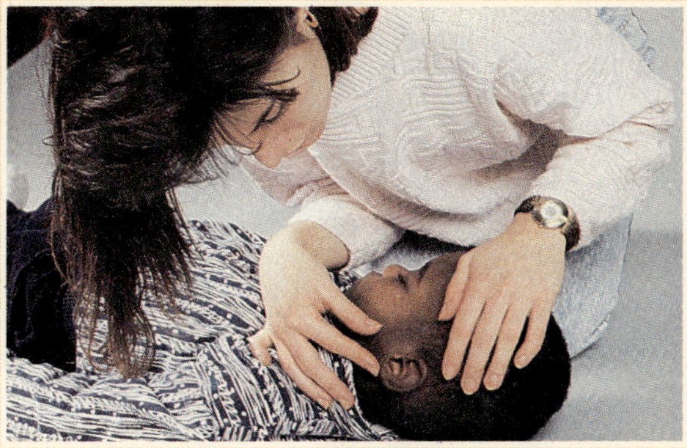

Check ears and nose for clear fluid or blood.

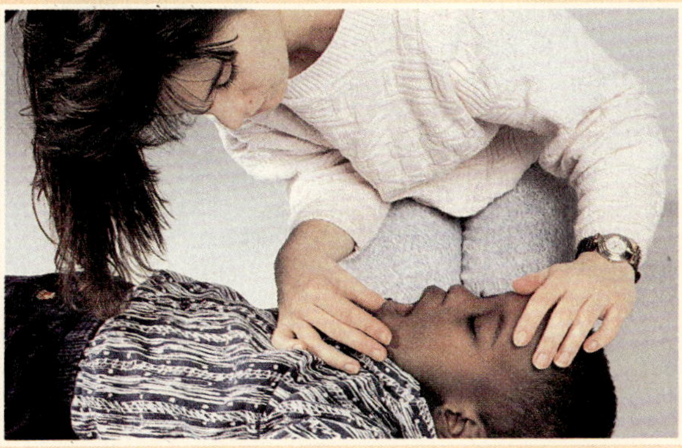

Check mouth for cuts or foreign objects.

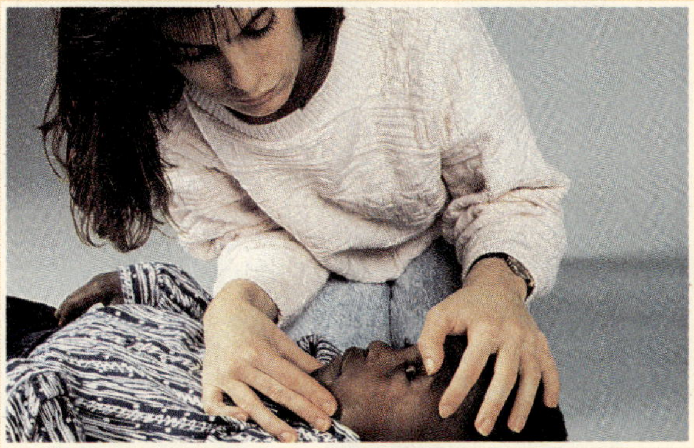

Check size of pupils.

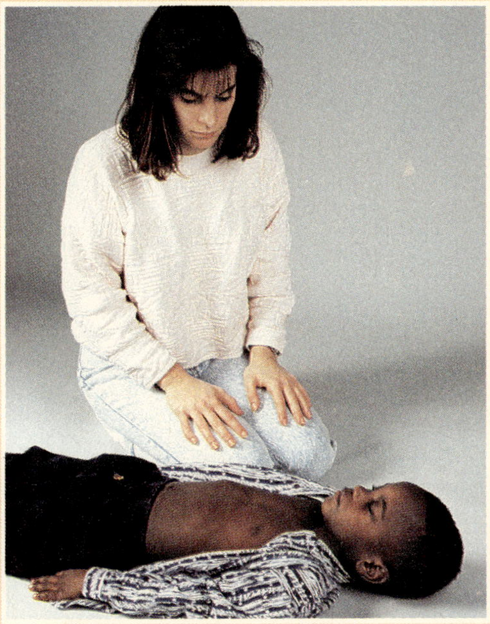

Check chest and abdomen for wounds.

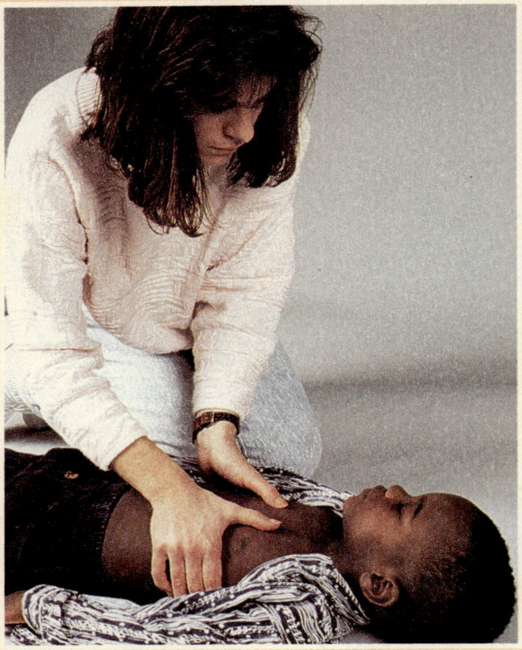

Check chest for wounds and tenderness.

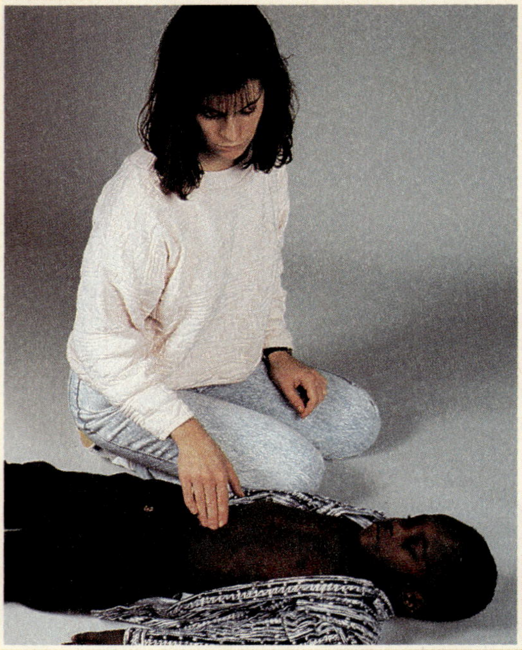

Check abdomen for tenderness and guarding.

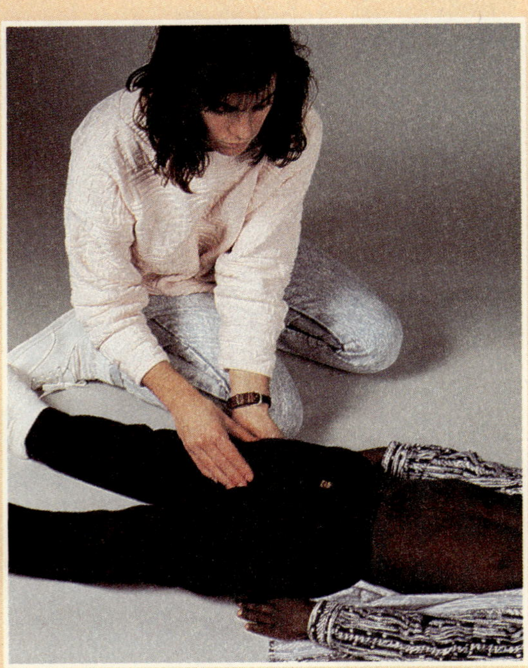

Check arms and legs for deformity and tenderness. Compare each side with the other.

Injury Assessment

Mark each statement true (T) or false (F).

1. ____ If you find an unconscious child and notice swelling and deformity of the right arm during your primary survey, continue your examination and come back to the injury later.
2. ____ Use your thumb to feel for an injured child's pulse.
3. ____ A child's pulse can be felt at either the wrist's radial point or the neck's carotid point.
4. ____ An infant's pulse can be felt most easily at the neck's carotid point.
5. ____ Feel for both carotid pulses at the same time.
6. ____ The normal pulse rate for a four-year-old child is 80 to 110 beats per minute.
7. ____ The normal respiration rate for infants is between 16 and 24 breaths per minute.
8. ____ The capillary refill technique can help a first aider determine if there is a problem with the blood circulation in an arm or leg.
9. ____ Clear fluid draining from the nose or ears might be spinal fluid.

Mark the following as either a sign (A) or a symptom (B).

1. ____ Lorraine says she feels like throwing up.
2. ____ Paul's skin is red and blistered.
3. ____ Dan begins to vomit.
4. ____ After falling, Angela's ankle becomes swollen.
5. ____ Carlos says he has a headache.

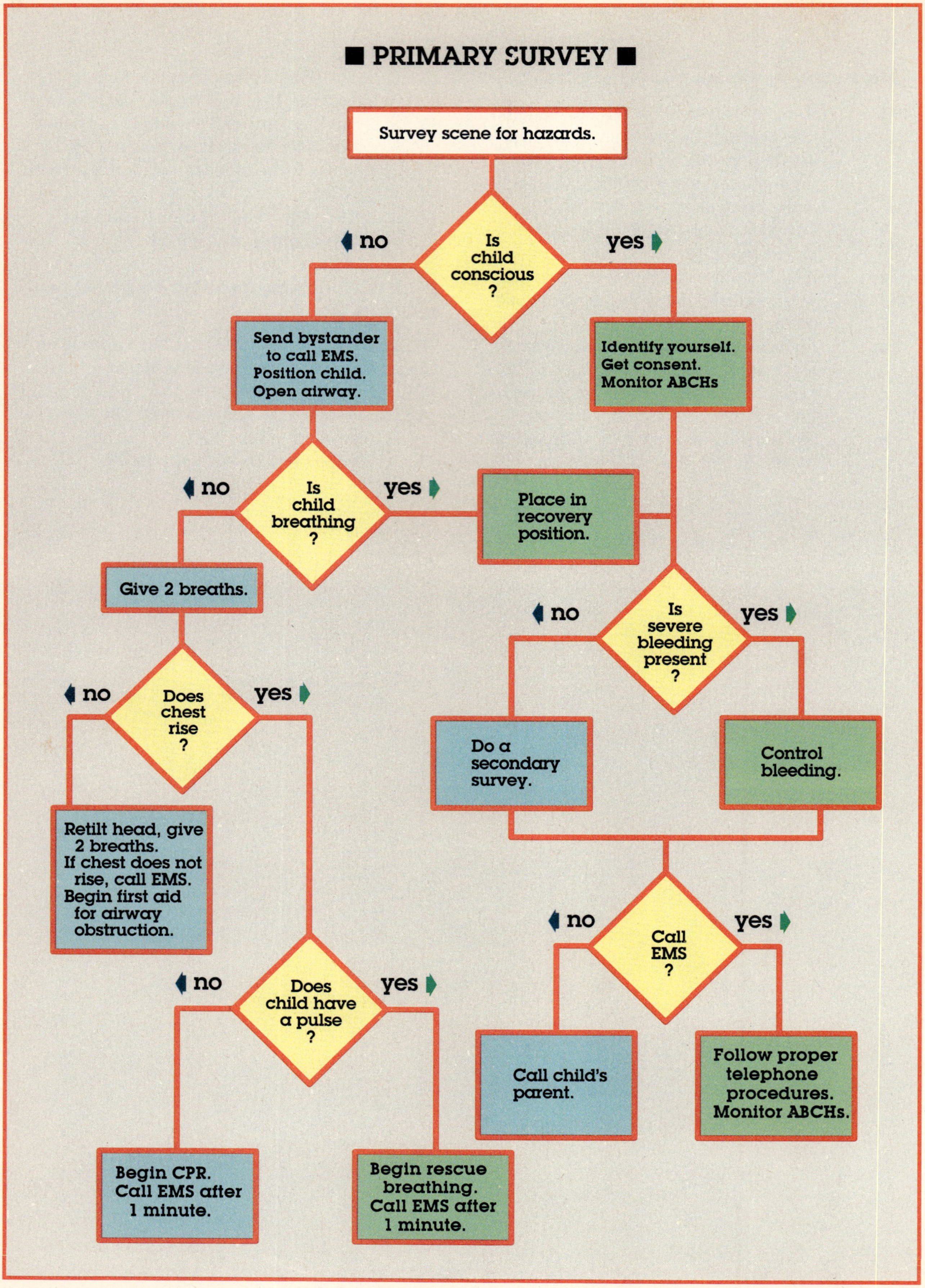
■ PRIMARY SURVEY ■
Survey scene for hazards.
Is child conscious ?
no
yes
Send bystander to call EMS. Position child. Open airway.
Identify yourself. Get consent. Monitor ABCHs
Is child breathing ?
no
yes
Place in recovery position.
Give 2 breaths.
Is severe bleeding present ?
no
yes
Does chest rise ?
no
yes
Do a secondary survey.
Control bleeding.
Retilt head, give 2 breaths. If chest does not rise, call EMS. Begin first aid for airway obstruction.
Call EMS ?
no
yes
Does child have a pulse ?
no
yes
Call child's parent.
Follow proper telephone procedures. Monitor ABCHs.
Begin CPR. Call EMS after 1 minute.
Begin rescue breathing. Call EMS after 1 minute.

3

Basic Life Support

■ Child Rescue Breathing ■ Child CPR ■ Conscious Choking Child ■ Unconscious Choking Child ■ Infant Rescue Breathing ■ Infant CPR ■ Conscious Choking Infant ■ Unconscious Choking Infant ■

Providing basic life support means providing the most essential emergency first aid to a person in need until more skilled emergency medical care arrives to relieve you. Rhythmic and uninterrupted breathing and heartbeat are essential for sustaining life. First aid for an interruption of these two vital functions is known as **cardiopulmonary resuscitation (CPR).**

Cardiopulmonary resuscitation is a series of skills that combines breathing into another person's lungs—rescue breaths—*with repeated chest compressions* on the sternum (breastbone). *Cardio* refers to the heart, and *pulmonary* refers to the lungs. Together they represent the intimate connection between the work of the heart and lungs in sustaining life. CPR can keep a person alive by circulating blood and oxygen to the most vital organs of the body—the heart, lungs, and brain—while waiting for emergency medical help to arrive.

The health problems that first come to mind when we think about basic life support and CPR are heart attacks and strokes. Middle-aged and elderly American adults who experience sudden death due to some form of heart or artery disease are clearly the largest group for whom CPR techniques are intended.

But what about children? For most children, the heart is a healthy, strong muscle, pumping blood through open, unobstructed blood vessels. When a healthy child's heart stops beating, the most likely cause is an injury that causes the child to stop breathing. If breathing stops (respiratory arrest), the supply of oxygen to the heart muscle is cut off. Without oxygen, the heart slows and, within minutes, it too stops (cardiac arrest). Incidents that cause a child to stop breathing might include electrocution, drowning, poisoning, smoke inhalation, severe head injury, or choking. If the heart stops beating, breathing stops immediately.

The Heart, Lung, and Brain Connection

The heart is about the size of one's clenched fist and is located in the center of the chest behind the sternum. The lungs lie on either side of the heart. Both heart and lungs are protected by the rib cage.

The heart is a muscle that pumps oxygen-containing blood throughout the body. All body tissues need oxygen to live. Oxygen enters the body through the lungs where it passes into the blood and is then pumped by the heart throughout the body to every cell including those in the heart. While passing through the lungs, blood picks up oxygen and expels its waste—primarily carbon dioxide—into the lungs to be exhaled.

The air we breathe contains 21 percent oxygen. The body uses what it needs and then exhales air that contains 16 percent oxygen. Therefore, **when per-**

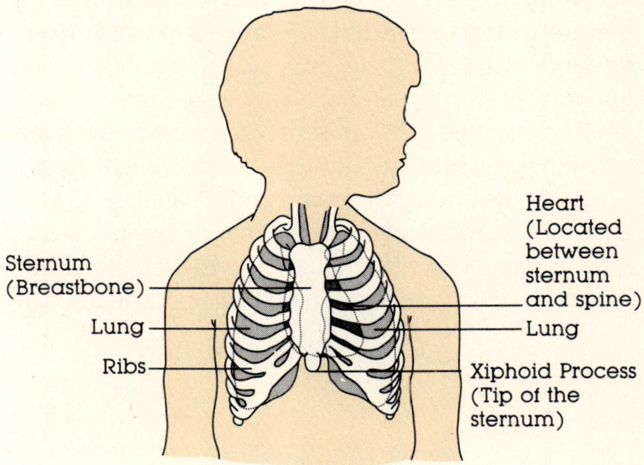

Location of heart and lungs

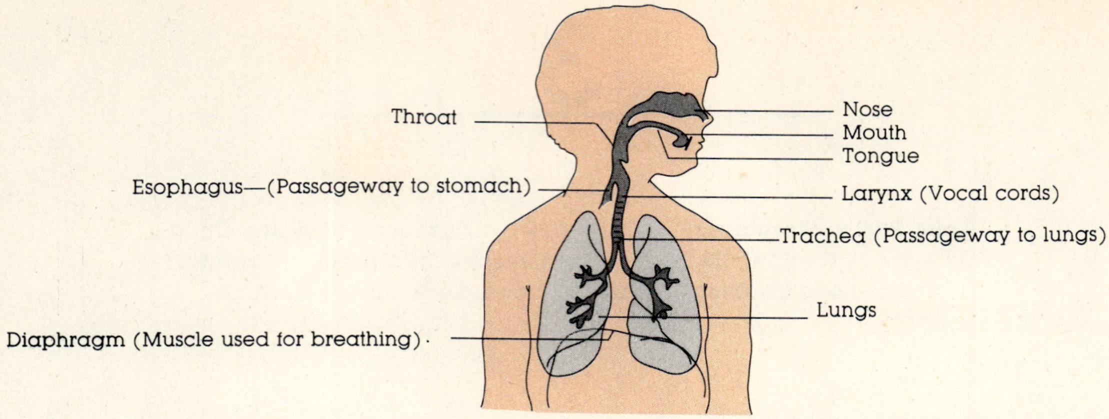

Parts of the body used for breathing

forming CPR, the exhaled air breathed into another person contains more than enough oxygen to keep that person alive.** The chest compressions produce only 20 to 30 percent of the normal output of the heart. The body uses this circulation effectively, however, and sends the blood primarily to the heart muscle, lungs, and brain.

The biggest user of oxygen is the brain, the master control center of the body. A network of blood vessels supplies the brain with the large amount of oxygen it requires. This single organ needs about 20 percent of the total amount of oxygen used by the entire body. Consequently, **the brain can survive without oxygen for only 4 to 6 minutes before risking serious damage.** This is why beginning CPR immediately on finding a person in cardiac arrest is so crucial.

The condition that exists at the moment the heart and lungs stop functioning is called *clinical death.* However, the brain can remain undamaged for as long as 4 to 6 minutes after the supply of oxygen stops. After 6 minutes without oxygen, irreversible brain damage is likely and can result in brain death. The condition that exists when the brain can no longer function is called *biological death.*

The condition of the brain determines the quality of life for the injured person after recovery. Promptly starting CPR helps ensure that the brain will not be damaged during the emergency and gives the brain and the heart muscle the best chance for surviving unharmed.

Your assessment of an injured child should always begin with the ABCs. These letters stand for *airway, breathing,* and *circulation* and will help you to identify life-threatening problems in their correct sequence. Although many injuries can wait until emergency medical help arrives, first aid for the ABCs cannot. The importance of the ABCs will become obvious in the emergencies described in this book.

CPR is a skill that must be practiced repeatedly on a manikin to be mastered. It is NEVER practiced on another person. Reading the material alone does not make a skilled rescuer.

The CPR techniques in this chapter are based on the Standards and Guidelines established by the 1992 National Conference on Cardiopulmonary Resuscitation and Emergency Cardiac Care.

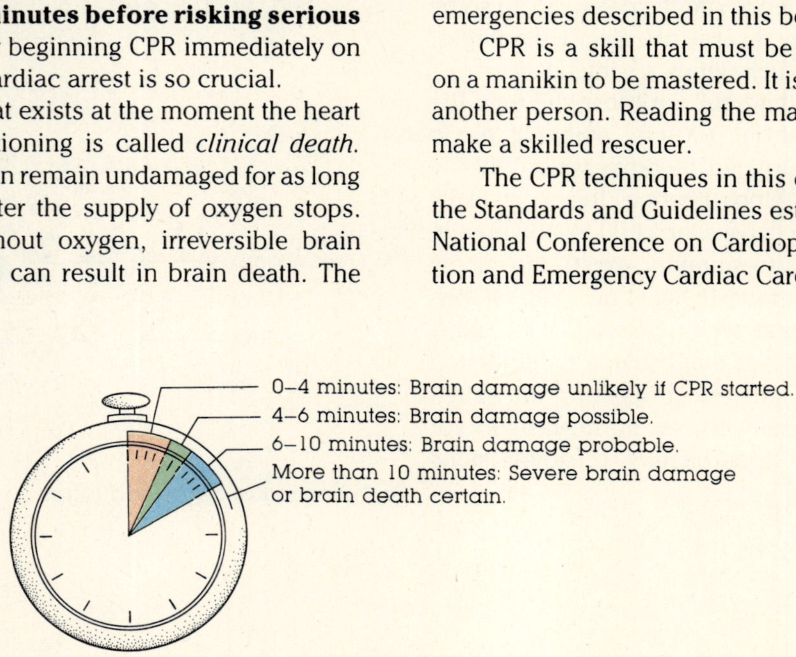

CHILD RESCUE BREATHING | CHILD CPR
(approximately 1 to 8 years)

Child Rescue Breathing

- Necessary when breathing has stopped.
- If started immediately after breathing stops, there is a good chance of preventing heart from stopping.

Child CPR

- Necessary when both heartbeat and breathing have stopped.

If you find a motionless child, THEN check the scene for hazards and clues to what happened.

□ **1.** CHECK RESPONSIVENESS:

- Gently tap child's shoulder or back.
- Shout child's name and ask, "Are you O.K.?"

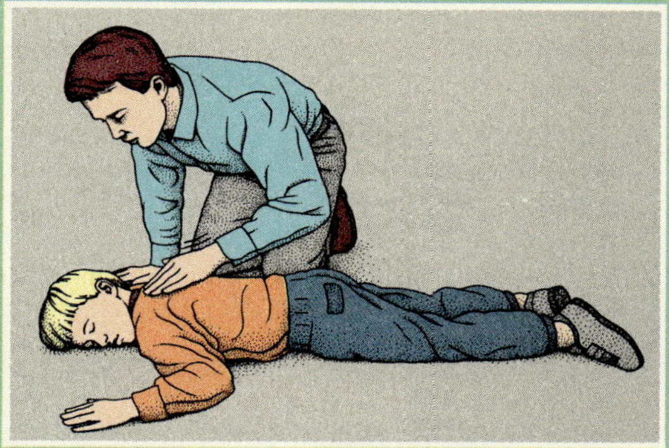

IF child responds, THEN STOP numbered rescue steps. Do a secondary survey by checking child from head to toe for injuries.

IF child does not respond, THEN CONTINUE numbered rescue steps.

2. SEND SOMEONE TO ACTIVATE EMS SYSTEM. Check for breathing without changing child's position.

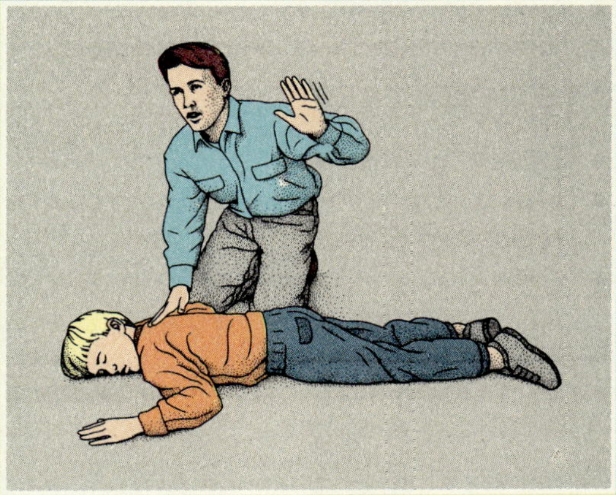

□ **3.** POSITION CHILD ON BACK if breathing cannot be detected . If neck or spinal injury is suspected, avoid any twisting motion by taking the following steps.

- Straighten child's legs, if necessary.
- Move child's arm closest to you above child's head.
- Place one hand on child's shoulder and other hand on child's hip.

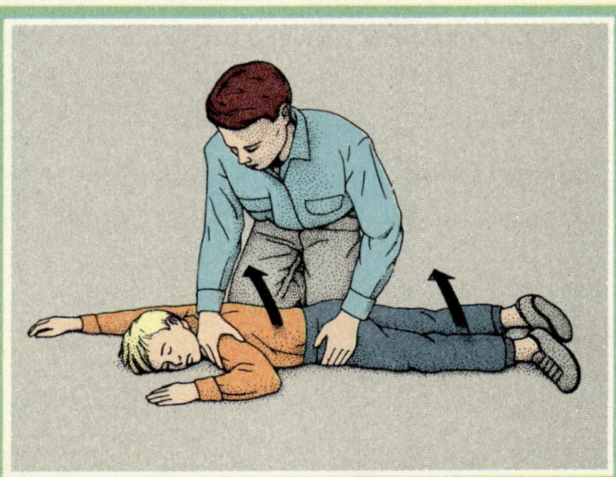

- Roll child toward you as a unit. Move your hand from child's shoulder to support back of head and neck.
- Place child's arms alongside body.

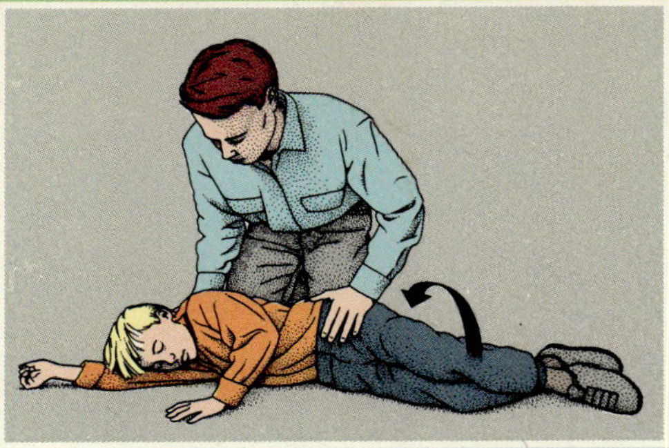

□ **4.** OPEN AIRWAY using head-tilt/chin-lift method:

- Place hand nearest child's head on child's forehead and apply pressure to tilt head back to an above-neutral position. (Dotted line in diagram indicates above-neutral position.)
- Place index and middle fingers of other hand under bony part of jaw near chin, and lift. Avoid pressing on soft tissue under jaw.
- Do not close child's mouth when tilting head.

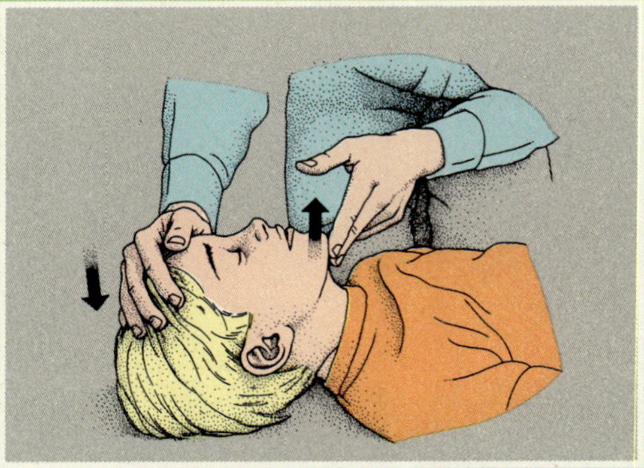

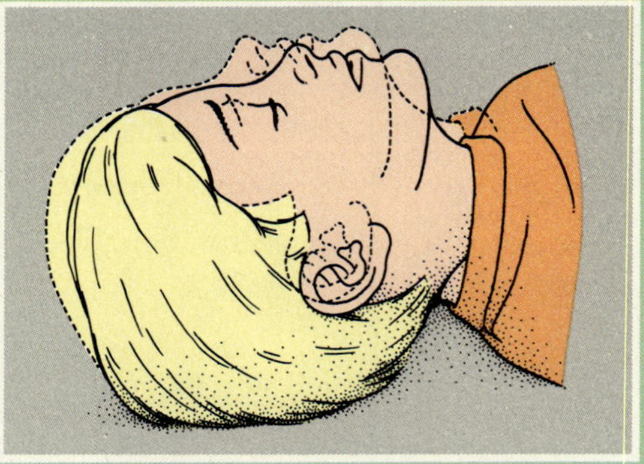

Above-neutral position

IF you see vomitus, THEN wipe it out with fingers covered by a cloth, if available, and CONTINUE numbered rescue steps.

IF you see a solid object, THEN remove it by hooking it with your little finger and CONTINUE numbered rescue steps.

□ **5.** CHECK FOR BREATHING (allow 5 seconds).

- Place your ear over child's mouth and nose while keeping airway open.
- LOOK for child's chest to rise and fall.
- LISTEN for breathing.
- FEEL for breath against your cheek.

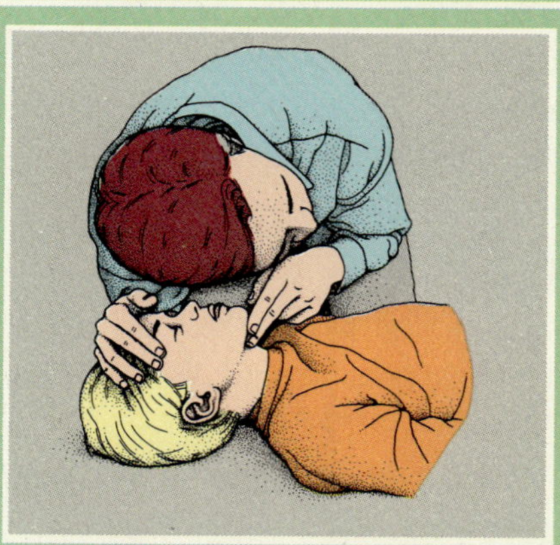

IF child is breathing, (anyone breathing also has a pulse) THEN STOP numbered rescue steps and:

- Keep airway open.
- Monitor breathing until EMS arrives.

□ **6.** GIVE TWO SLOW BREATHS.

- Use head-tilt/chin-lift to keep airway open in an above-neutral position.
- Pinch child's nose shut.
- Make a seal around child's mouth with your mouth.
- Give two slow breaths, each lasting 1 to 1½ seconds.
- Give breaths with just enough force to see child's chest rise.
- Remove your mouth from child's after each breath to allow for chest deflation.

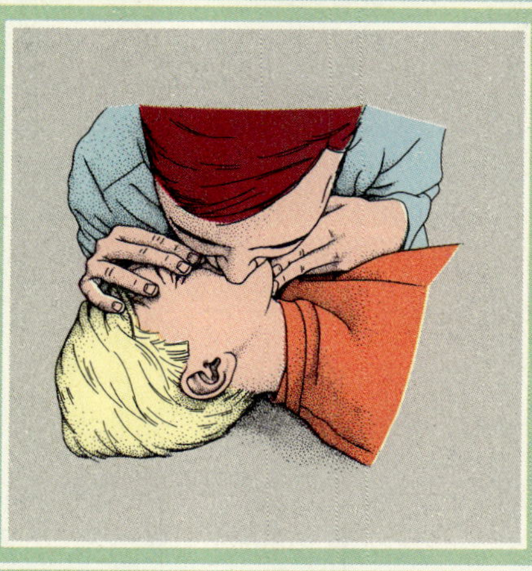

IF first two breaths will not go in and resistance is felt, THEN retilt child's head further back and try another two breaths.

IF second two breaths will not go in and resistance is felt, THEN STOP numbered rescue steps and:

- Assume foreign body airway obstruction.
- Proceed to Step 7 of Unsconscious Choking Child to remove airway obstruction.

□ **7.** CHECK FOR PULSE.

- Keep hand on child's forehead to maintain head tilt in an above-neutral position.
- Use index and middle fingers to locate Adam's apple with hand nearest child's feet.
- Slide your fingers down into groove of neck on side closest to you.
- Feel for carotid pulse (allow 10 seconds).
- Do not use thumb to feel for pulse because it has a pulse of its own.

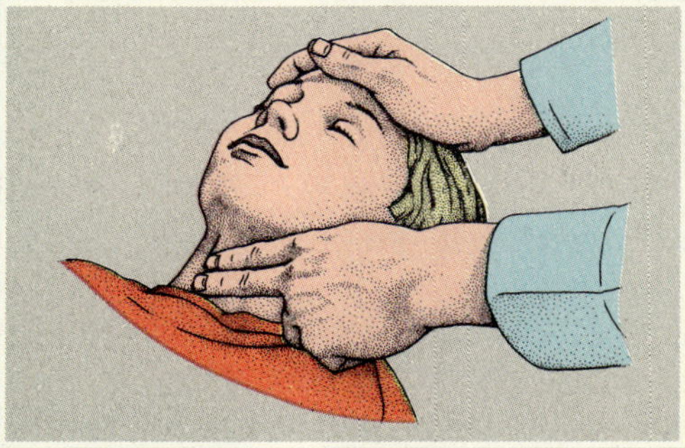

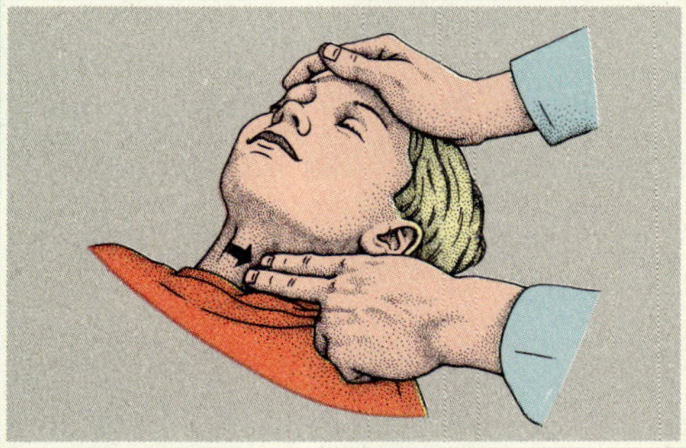

CHILD RESCUE BREATHING	CHILD CPR

IF child has no pulse and is not breathing, THEN **CPR** is necessary.
IF child has a pulse but is not breathing, THEN **rescue breathing** is necessary.

If no one activated EMS system, THEN:

Child Rescue Breathing

- Perform **rescue breathing** for about 1 minute (20 breaths).
- Quickly locate a nearby telephone and phone EMS system.
- Return to child and continue rescue breathing until EMS arrives.

8. BEGIN RESCUE BREATHING.

- Maintain open airway with head-tilt/chin-lift.
- Pinch child's nose shut.
- Make a seal around child's mouth with your mouth.
- Give one breath every 3 seconds. To do this, count: one one-thousand, take a breath on two one-thousand, and breathe into child on three one-thousand.

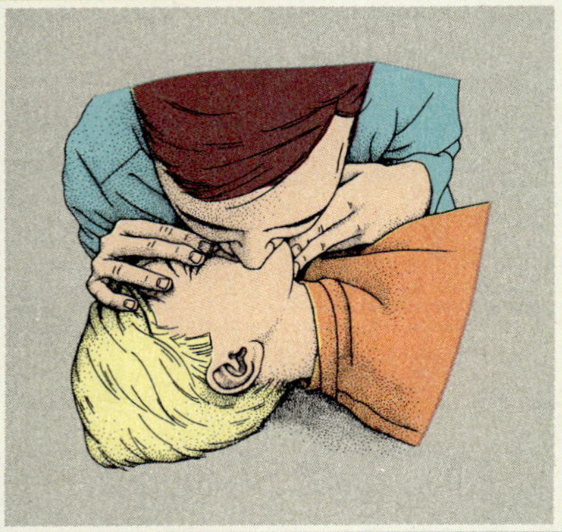

- Watch for chest to rise to see if your breaths go in.
- Remove your mouth from child's after each breath to allow for chest deflation.
- Continue for about 1 minute (20 breaths).

Child CPR

- Perform **CPR** for about 1 minute (12 cycles).
- Quickly locate a nearby telephone and phone EMS system.
- Return to child and continue CPR until EMS arrives.

8. BEGIN CPR.

- FIND COMPRESSION LOCATION.
  - Keep one hand on child's forehead to maintain head tilt.
  - Slide fingers of other hand along edge of rib cage to notch at end of sternum.

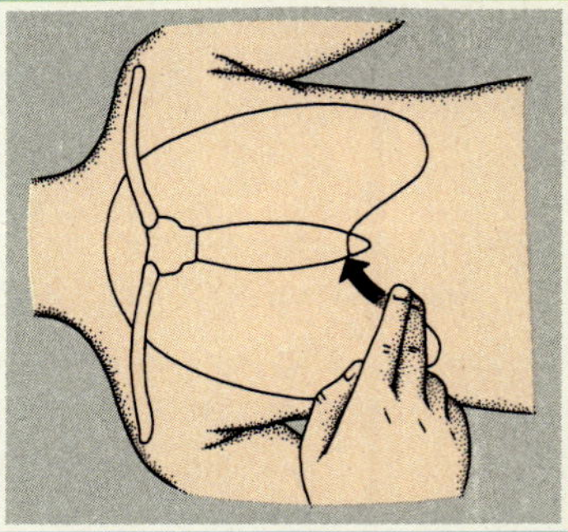

  - Cover notch with your middle finger and place your index finger beside it.

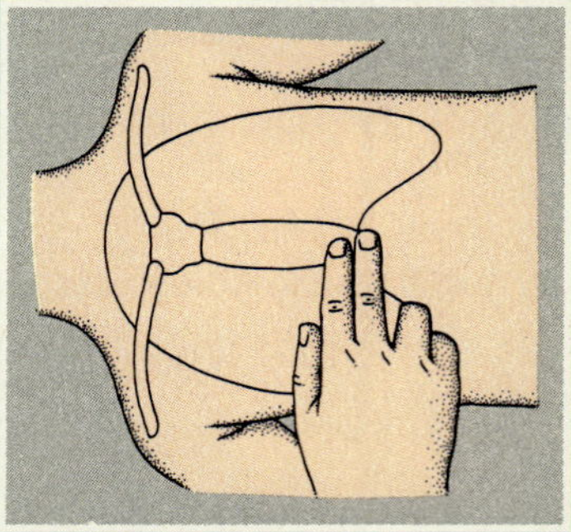

- Remember location of index finger while you remove hand and place heel on sternum next to index finger's prior location.

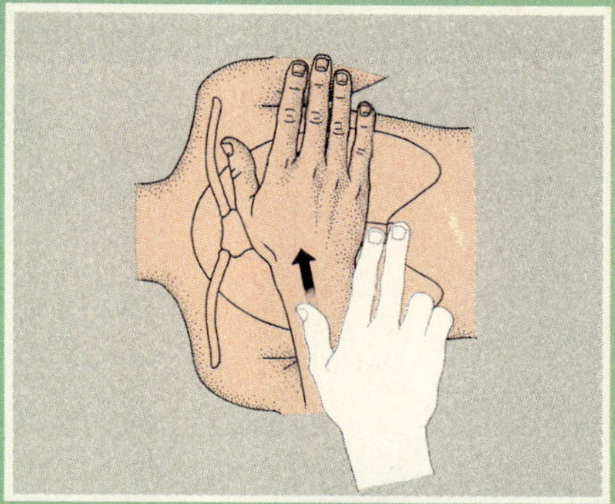

- Keep fingers off child's chest and deliver one compression with heel only of one hand.

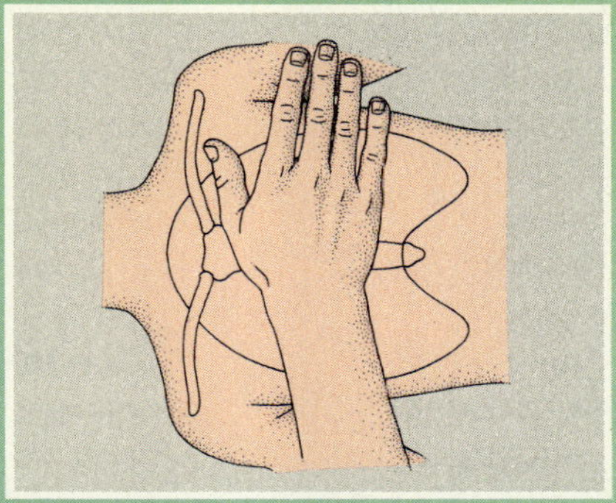

- GIVE FIVE CHEST COMPRESSIONS.
  - Do five compressions at a rate of 100 per minute or 5 compressions in about 3 seconds. Count as you push down: "One, two, three, four, five."
  - Compress sternum 1 to 1½ inches.
  - Deliver compressions smoothly and rhythmically. Compression time should equal relaxation time. Blood is forced out of heart during compressions and it flows into heart during relaxation or when pressure is released.
  - Keep heel of hand in contact with child's chest. Fingers should point across child's chest and away from you.

CHILD RESCUE BREATHING	CHILD CPR
	• Keep one hand on child's forehead to maintain head tilt. 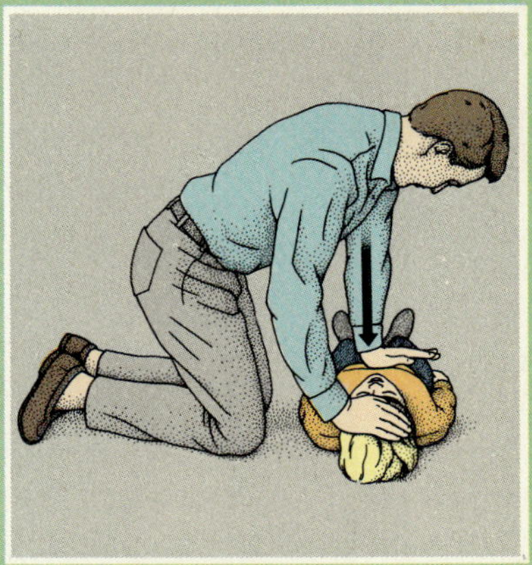 ■ GIVE ONE BREATH. • Use head-tilt/chin-lift to keep airway open in an above-neutral position. • Pinch child's nose shut. • Make a seal around child's mouth with your mouth. • Give one slow breath with just enough force to see child's chest rise. 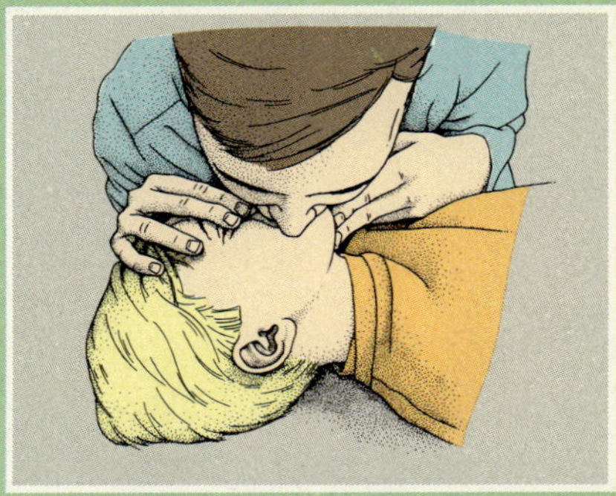 • Allow for chest deflation after each breath. ■ Give compressions and breaths in cycles of 5 compressions to 1 breath. Repeat for about 1 minute (12 cycles).
□ **9.** RECHECK PULSE AND BREATHING once every minute (20 breaths). ■ Check for carotid pulse as in Step 7. ■ Check for breathing using LOOK, LISTEN, and FEEL as in Step 5.	□ **9.** RECHECK PULSE after 1 minute and every few minutes thereafter. ■ Keep hand on child's forehead to maintain open airway. ■ Feel for carotid pulse (allow 5 seconds).

IF child has a pulse and is breathing, THEN:

- Keep airway open.
- Monitor pulse and breathing.
- Wait for EMS to arrive.

CHILD RESCUE BREATHING	CHILD CPR
IF child has a pulse but is not breathing, THEN: ■ Begin or continue rescue breathing. ■ Wait for EMS to arrive.	
IF child has no pulse and is not breathing, THEN: ■ Begin or continue CPR. ■ Wait for EMS to arrive.	
10. CONTINUE RESCUE BREATHING until: ■ Child begins to breathe. ■ A second trained rescuer arrives to relieve you. ■ EMS arrives to relieve you. ■ You are too exhausted to continue rescue breathing.	**10.** CONTINUE CPR until: ■ Child has pulse and is breathing. ■ A second trained rescuer arrives to relieve you. ■ EMS arrives to relieve you. ■ You are too exhausted to continue CPR.
	IF second CPR-trained rescuer arrives, THEN: ■ Ask second rescuer to determine if EMS system has been called. ■ Ask if second rescuer knows CPR. ■ Finish your compression/breathing cycle with breath. ■ Tell second rescuer to take over CPR. ■ Second rescuer begins CPR by checking pulse for 5 seconds. If no pulse, second rescuer restarts CPR by giving chest compressions. ■ Second rescuer continues cycles of five chest compressions and one breath until tired and asks first rescuer to take over again. ■ Rescuer who is not performing CPR can check the effectiveness of the chest compressions by feeling for the carotid pulse during compressions.
	IF you arrive on scene where a first rescuer is performing CPR, THEN: ■ Phone EMS system, if it has not already been done. ■ Tell first rescuer that EMS system has been called and that you know CPR and are able to help.
	IF a rescuer performing CPR asks you to take over, THEN: ■ Wait until rescuer finishes cycle of five chest compressions and 1 breath. ■ Check pulse for 5 seconds. ■ If no pulse, restart CPR by giving chest compressions.

CONSCIOUS CHOKING CHILD
(approximately 1 to 8 years)

- Necessary when airway is obstructed.

IF child is coughing forcefully (wheezing might be present between coughs), but child has good air exchange, THEN suspect airway is partially obstructed and:

- Encourage child to continue coughing.
- Do not interfere with child's attempts to cough up object.
- Do not slap child on back.
- Do not attempt choking rescue techniques.

IF child:

- Is coughing weakly or cannot speak, cough, or cry
- Is making high-pitched noises
- Has a panicked expression
- Clutches throat, known as universal distress signal for choking
- Has blue lips and nails

THEN ask child, "Are you choking?" Assume that either the partially obstructed airway now has poor air exchange or that airway is completely obstructed. Begin choking rescue techniques.

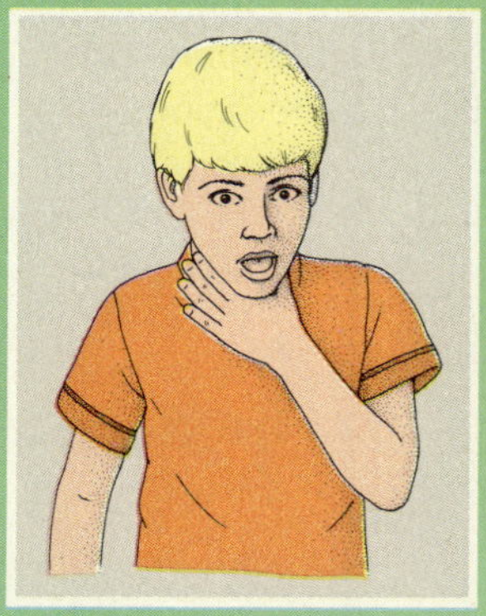

□ **1.** SHOUT FOR HELP to alert others of the emergency.

□ **2.** GIVE FIVE ABDOMINAL THRUSTS (Heimlich Maneuver):

- Stand or kneel behind child (who is standing) with your shoulders at about same level as child's. You will need to be on your knees for a small child.
- Wrap your arms around child's waist.
- Make a fist with one hand and place thumb side just above child's navel and well below tip of sternum (a).
- Grasp fist with your other hand (b).
- Press fist into child's abdomen with quick upward thrust (c).
- Each thrust should be a separate and distinct effort to dislodge object.
- Pause after every series of 5 abdominal thrusts to check the child and your hand placement.

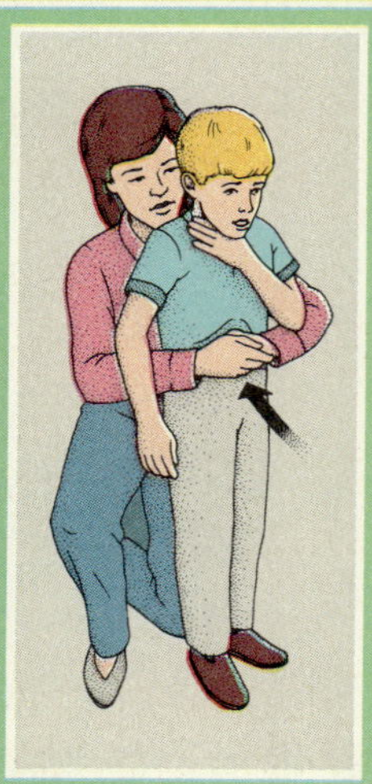

c

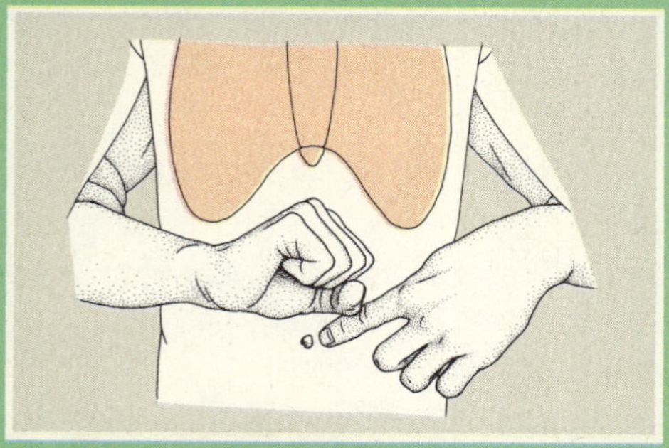

a

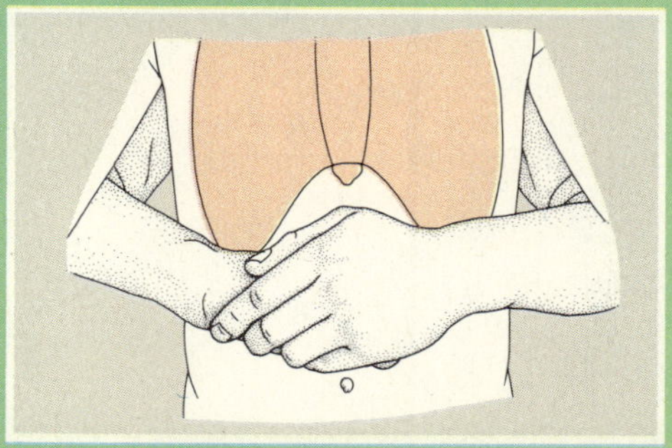

b

CONSCIOUS CHOKING CHILD

□ **3.** REPEAT SERIES OF FIVE ABDOMINAL THRUSTS until:

- Child coughs up object, or
- Child starts to breathe, or
- Child becomes unconscious.

IF object is dislodged or expelled, THEN have child examined by health care provider.

IF child becomes unconscious and object is not dislodged or expelled, THEN:

- Tell someone to phone EMS system for help.
- Lay child on floor, face up.
- Proceed to Step 8 of Unconscious Choking Child for how to continue rescue steps when child becomes unconscious before obstruction is relieved.

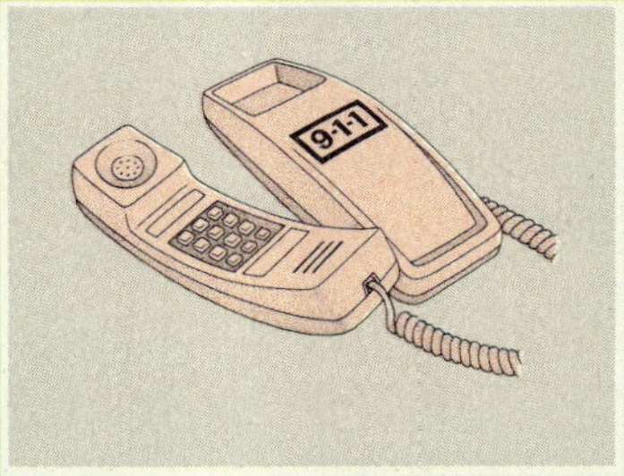

UNCONSCIOUS CHOKING CHILD

(approximately 1 to 8 years)

- Necessary when airway is obstructed.

IF you find a motionless child, THEN check the scene for hazards and clues to what happened.

□ **1.** CHECK RESPONSIVENESS:

- Gently tap child's shoulder or back.
- Shout child's name and ask, "Are you O.K.?"

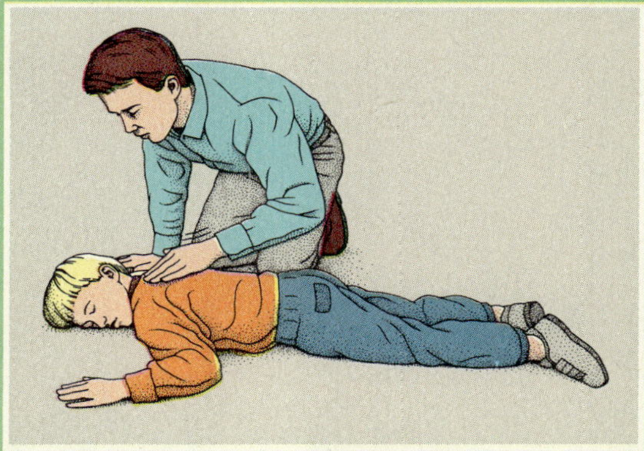

□ **2.** SEND SOMEONE TO ACTIVATE EMS SYSTEM. Check for breathing without changing child's position.

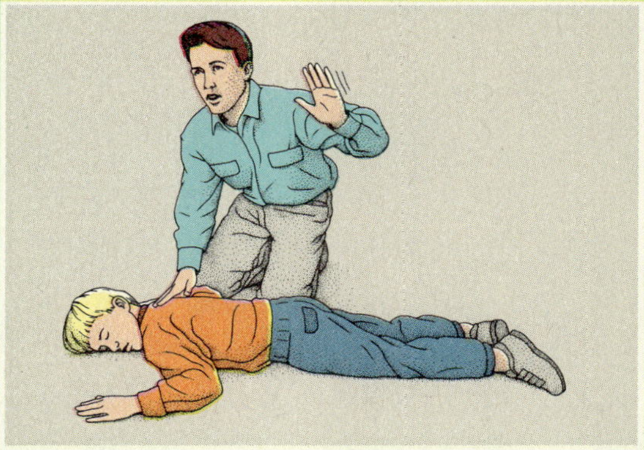

□ **3.** POSITION CHILD ON BACK if breathing cannot be detected. If neck or spinal injury is suspected, move child as a unit to avoid any twisting motion by taking the following steps:

- Straighten child's legs, if necessary.
- Move child's arm closest to you above child's head.
- Place one hand on child's shoulder and other hand on child's hip.
- Roll child toward you as a unit. Move your hand from child's shoulder to support back of head and neck.
- Place child's arms alongside body.

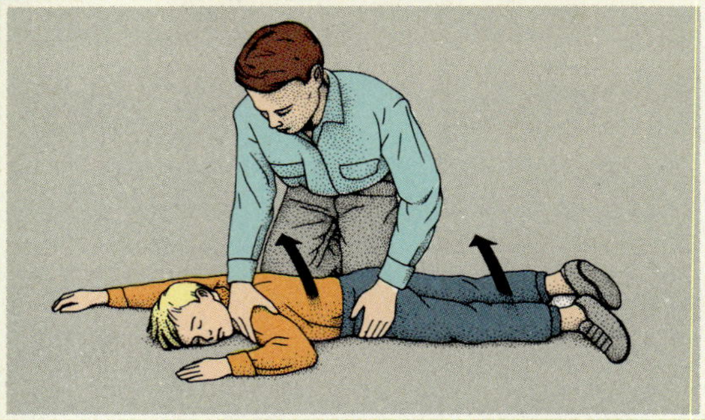

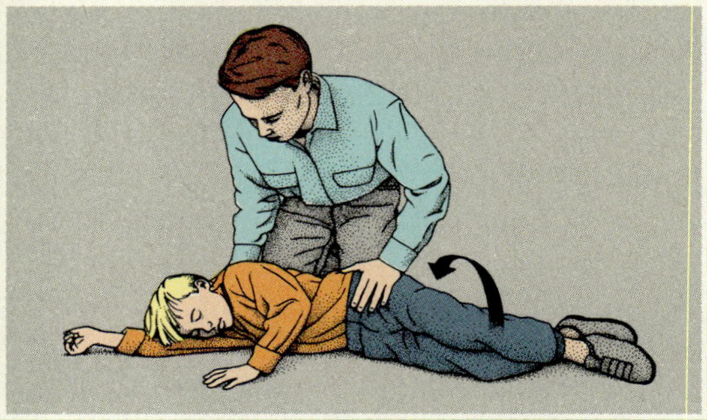

□ **4.** OPEN AIRWAY using head-tilt/chin-lift method:

- Place hand nearest child's head on child's forehead and apply pressure to tilt head back to an above-neutral position.
- Place index and middle fingers of other hand under bony part of jaw near chin, and lift. Avoid pressing on soft tissue under jaw.
- Do not close child's mouth when tilting head.

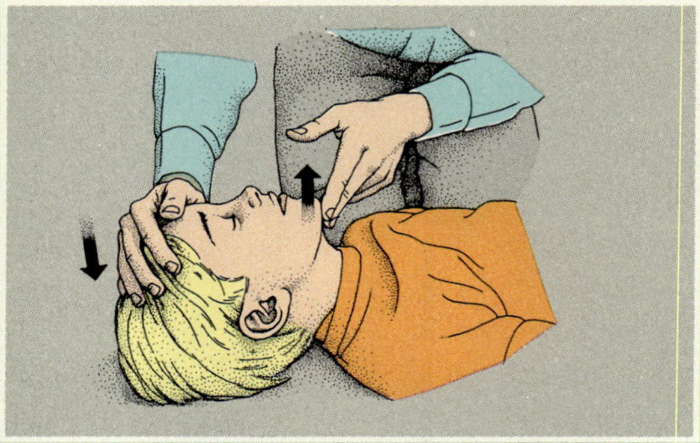

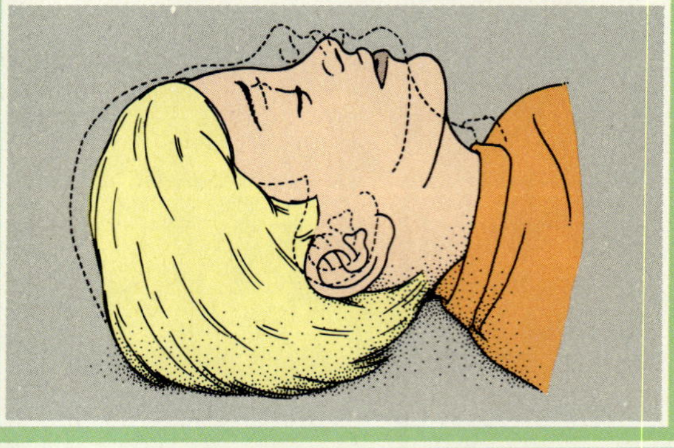

Above-neutral position

IF you see vomitus, THEN wipe it out with fingers covered by a cloth, if available, and CONTINUE numbered rescue steps.

IF you see a solid object, THEN remove it by hooking it with your little finger and CONTINUE numbered rescue steps.

□ **5.** CHECK FOR BREATHING (allow 5 seconds).

- Place your ear over child's mouth and nose while keeping airway open.
- LOOK for child's chest to rise and fall.
- LISTEN for breathing.
- FEEL for breath against your cheek

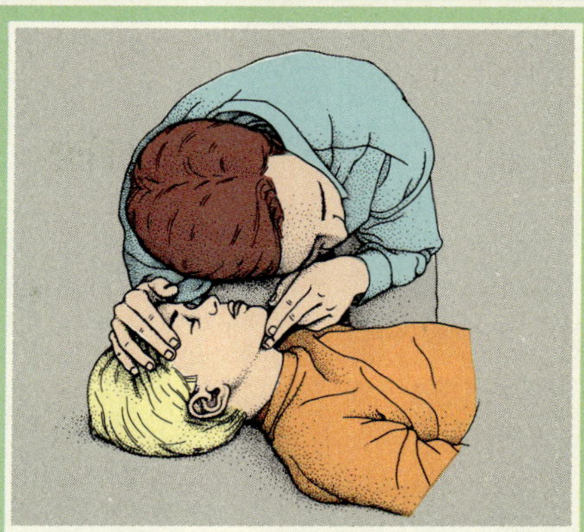

□ **6.** GIVE TWO SLOW BREATHS.

- Use head-tilt/chin-lift to keep airway open in an above-neutral position.
- Pinch child's nose shut.
- Make a seal around child's mouth with your mouth.
- Give two slow breaths, each lasting 1 to 1½ seconds.
- Give breaths with just enough force to see child's chest rise.

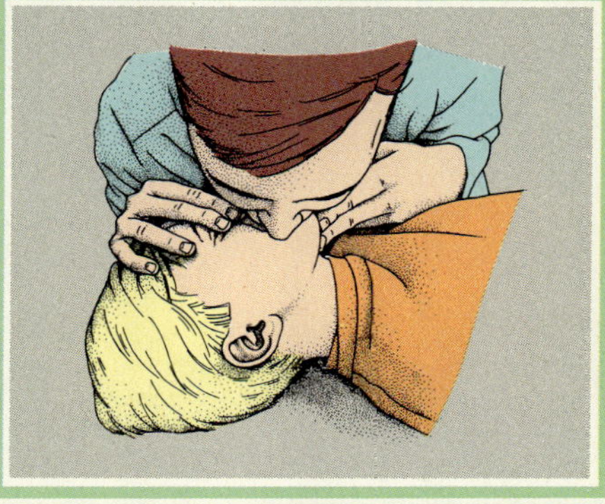

IF first two breaths will not go in and resistance is felt, THEN retilt child's head further back and try another two breaths.

IF second two breaths will not go in and resistance is felt, THEN assume airway is obstructed and CONTINUE with numbered rescue steps.

□ **7.** GIVE FIVE ABDOMINAL THRUSTS.

- Kneel at child's feet or straddle child's thighs.
- Put heel of one hand against middle of child's abdomen, slightly above navel and well below notch at end of sternum.
- Place your other hand directly on top of first hand. Fingers should point toward child's head.

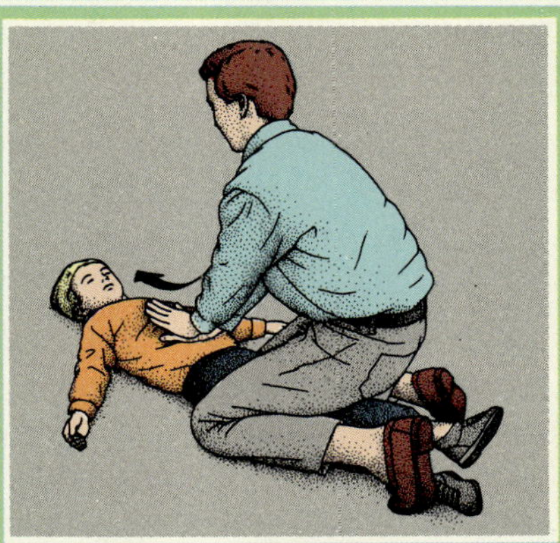

- Press inward and upward using both hands as a single unit, but allowing heel only of lower hand to touch abdomen. Keep heel of hand in contact with abdomen between abdominal thrusts.
- Give five abdominal thrusts. Deliver each thrust firmly and separately, as if each one will expel object.

□ **8.** CHECK FOR FOREIGN OBJECT.

- Position yourself at the child's head.
- Grasp both tongue and jaw between your thumb and fingers and lift jaw upward.

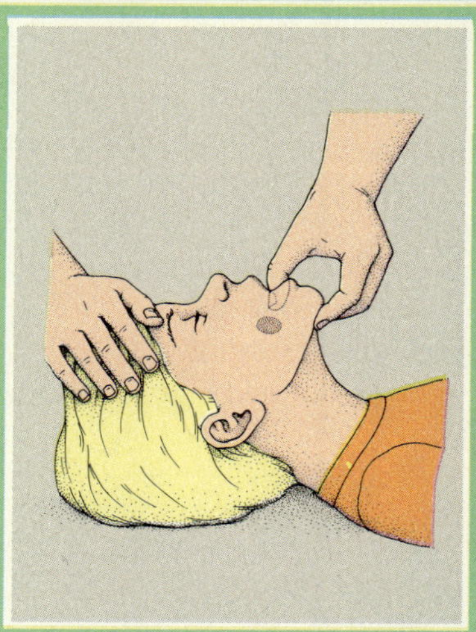

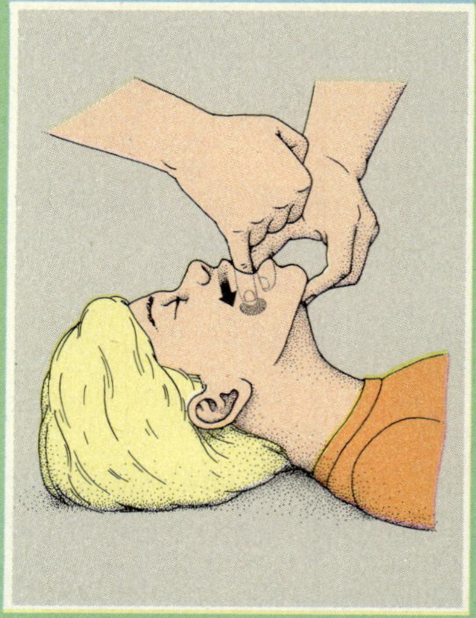

- If object is seen, then remove it with a finger sweep by sliding little finger of your free hand along inside of cheek to base of tongue, using a hooking action.
- Do not try to remove object if you cannot see it because the attempt could push object deeper into airway.

□ **9.** GIVE TWO BREATHS.

- Open airway with head-tilt/chin-lift.
- Pinch child's nose shut.
- Seal your mouth around child's mouth.
- Attempt to give two breaths.

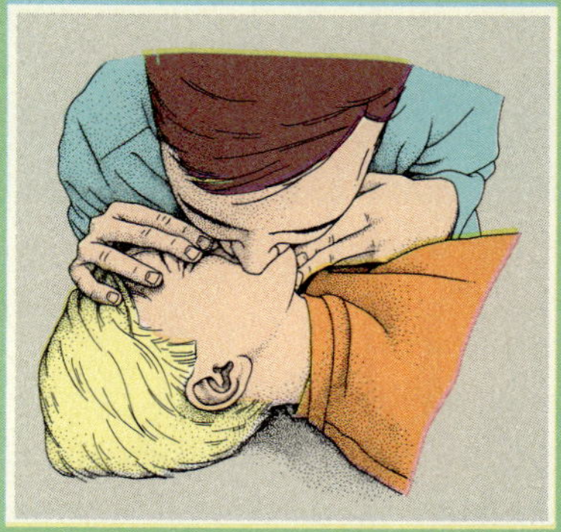

UNCONSCIOUS CHOKING CHILD

□ **10.** REPEAT STEPS 7, 8, and 9 until object is dislodged or expelled:

- Give five abdominal thrusts.
- Check for foreign object.
- Give two breaths.

□ **11.** CHECK FOR PULSE AND BREATHING once object has been dislodged or expelled and airway is open.

IF child has a pulse and is breathing, THEN:

- Keep airway open.
- Monitor pulse and breathing.
- Wait for EMS to arrive.

IF child has a pulse but is not breathing, THEN:

- Begin rescue breathing.
- Wait for EMS to arrive.

IF child has no pulse and is not breathing, THEN:

- Begin CPR.
- Wait for EMS to arrive.

INFANT RESCUE BREATHING / INFANT CPR

(up to approximately 1 year)

INFANT RESCUE BREATHING	INFANT CPR
■ Necessary when breathing has stopped. ■ If started immediately after breathing stops, there is a good chance of preventing heart from stopping.	■ Necessary when both heartbeat and breathing have stopped.

IF you find a motionless infant, THEN check the scene for hazards and clues to what happened.

□ **1.** CHECK RESPONSIVENESS.

- Gently tap infant's shoulder or back.
- Call infant's name.

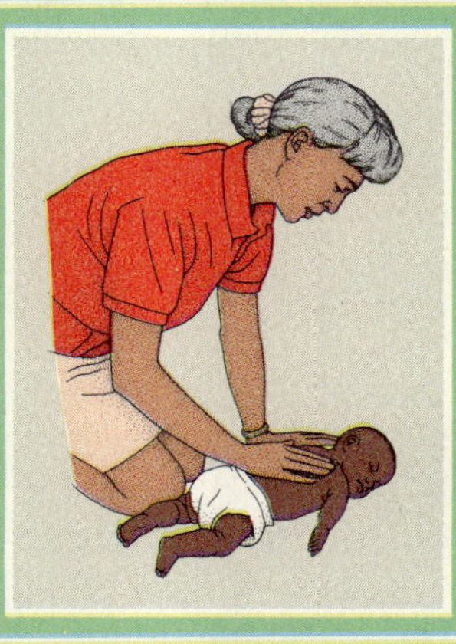

IF infant responds, THEN STOP numbered rescue steps. Do a secondary survey by checking infant from head to toe for injuries.

IF infant does not respond, THEN CONTINUE numbered rescue steps.

□ **2.** SEND SOMEONE TO ACTIVATE EMS SYSTEM. Check for breathing without changing infant's position.

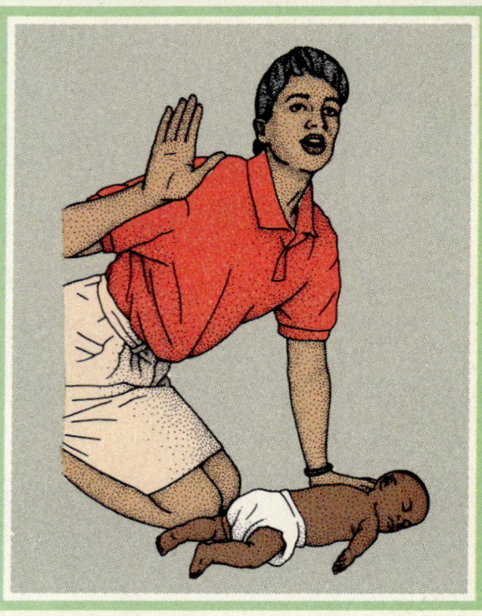

□ **3.** POSITION INFANT ON BACK if breathing cannot be detected. If neck or spinal injury is suspected, move infant as a unit to avoid any twisting motion by taking the following steps:

- Move infant's arm closest to you above infant's head.
- Place one hand on infant's shoulder and other hand on infant's hip (a).
- Roll infant toward you as a unit. Move your hand from infant's shoulder to support back of head and neck (b).
- Place infant's arms alongside body.

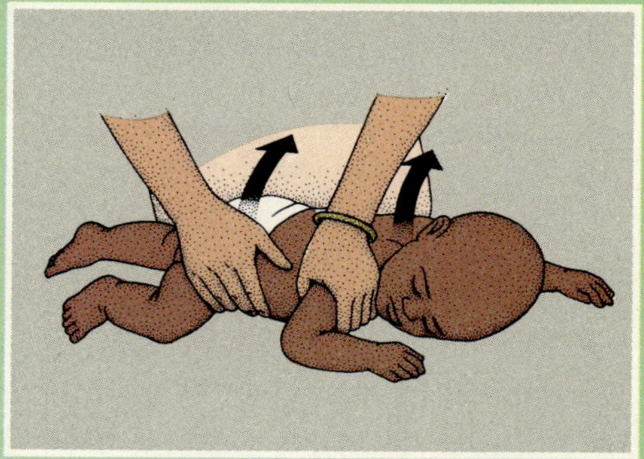

a

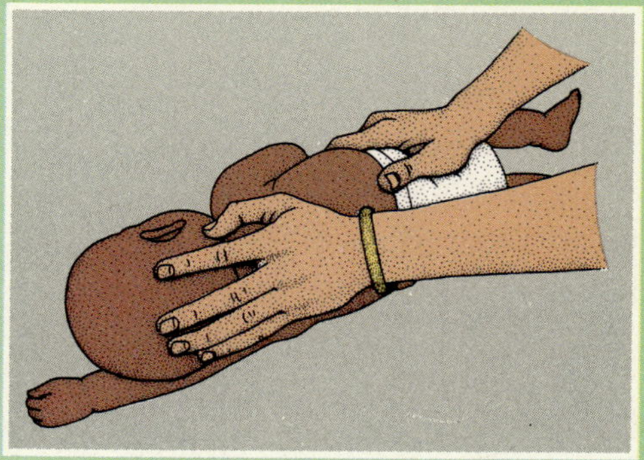

b

□ **4.** OPEN AIRWAY using head-tilt/chin-lift method:

- Place hand nearest infant's head on infant's forehead and apply pressure to tilt head back slightly into a neutral position.
- Place index finger of other hand under bony part of jaw near chin, and lift. Avoid pressing on soft tissue under jaw.
- Do not close infant's mouth when tilting head.

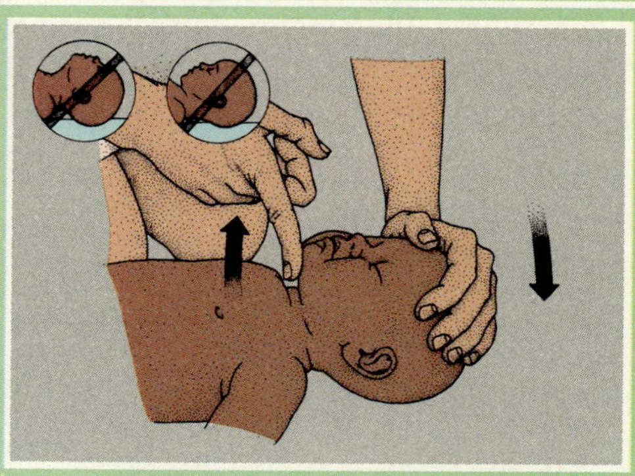

IF you see vomitus, THEN wipe it out with fingers covered by a cloth, if available, and CONTINUE numbered rescue steps.

IF you see a solid object, THEN remove it by hooking it with your little finger and CONTINUE numbered rescue steps.

□ **5.** CHECK FOR BREATHING (allow 5 seconds).

- Place your ear over infant's mouth and nose while keeping airway open.
- LOOK for infant's chest to rise and fall.
- LISTEN for breathing.
- FEEL for breath against your cheek.

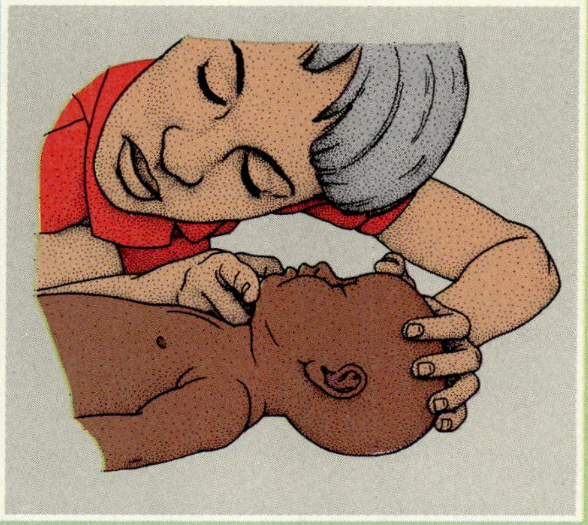

IF infant is breathing (anyone breathing also has a pulse), THEN STOP numbered rescue steps and:

- Keep airway open.
- Monitor breathing until EMS arrives.

□ **6.** GIVE TWO SLOW BREATHS.

- Use head-tilt/chin-lift to keep airway open in a neutral position.
- Make a seal around infant's mouth and nose with your mouth.
- Give two slow breaths, each lasting 1 to 1½ seconds.
- Give breaths with just enough force to see infant's chest rise.
- Remove your mouth from infant's after each breath to allow for chest deflation.

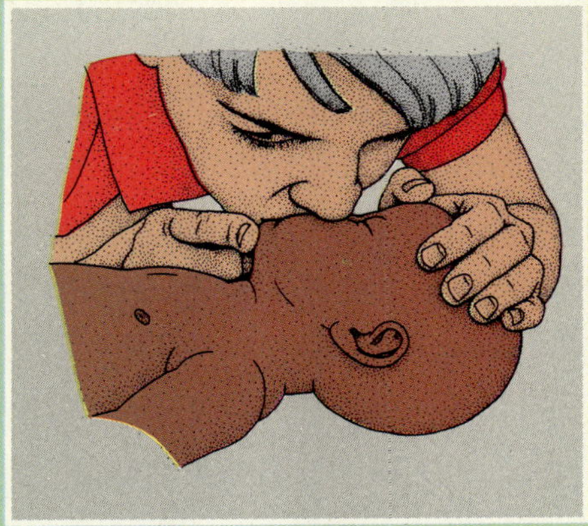

IF first two breaths will not go in and resistance is felt, THEN retilt infant's head and try another two breaths.

IF second two breaths will not go in and resistance is felt, THEN STOP numbered rescue steps and:

- Assume foreign body airway obstruction.
- Proceed to Step 7 of Unconscious Choking Infant to remove airway obstruction.

□ **7.** CHECK FOR PULSE.

- Keep hand on infant's forehead to maintain head-tilt in neutral position.
- Feel for brachial pulse on inside of upper arm between elbow and shoulder using flats of fingers. Allow 10 seconds.
- Do not use thumb to feel for pulse because it has a pulse of its own.

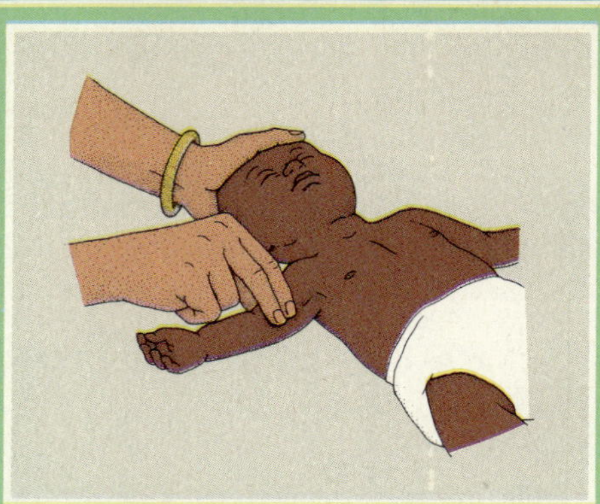

IF infant has no pulse and is not breathing, THEN **CPR** is necessary.
IF infant has a pulse but is not breathing, THEN **rescue breathing** is necessary.

IF no one responded to your initial shout for help, THEN:

Infant Rescue Breathing

- Perform **rescue breathing** for about 1 minute (20 breaths).
- Quickly locate a nearby telephone and phone EMS system.
- Return to infant and continue rescue breathing until EMS arrives.

Infant CPR

- Perform **CPR** for about 1 minute (12 cycles).
- Quickly locate a nearby telephone and phone EMS system.
- Return to infant and continue CPR until EMS arrives.

□ **8.** BEGIN RESCUE BREATHING.

- Maintain open airway with head-tilt/chin-lift.
- Make a seal around infant's mouth and nose with your mouth.

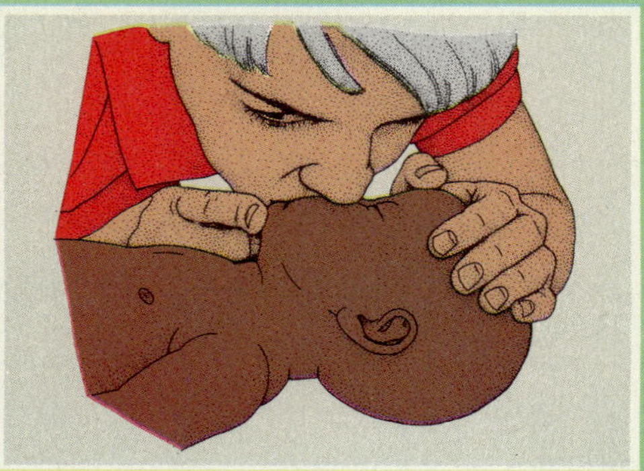

□ **8.** BEGIN CPR.

- FIND COMPRESSION LOCATION.
  - Keep one hand on infant's forehead to maintain head-tilt.
  - Imagine a line connecting the nipples.
  - Place three fingers on sternum with index finger touching, but below, imaginary nipple line.

INFANT RESCUE BREATHING

- Give one breath every 3 seconds. To do this, count: one one-thousand, take a breath on two one-thousand, and breathe into infant on three one-thousand.
- Watch for chest to rise to see if your breaths go in.
- Remove your mouth from infant's mouth and nose after each breath to allow for chest deflation.
- Continue for about 1 minute (20 breaths).

INFANT CPR

- Raise your index finger and use middle and ring fingers for compression. If you feel notch at end of sternum (xiphoid process), move your fingers up a little.

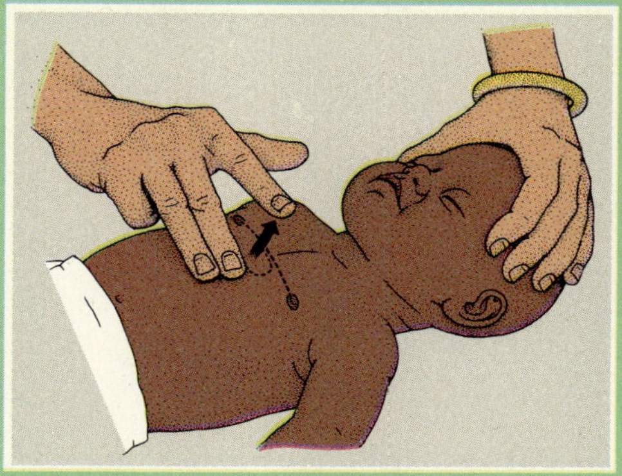

- GIVE FIVE CHEST COMPRESSIONS.
  - Do five compressions at a rate of at least 100 per minute, or five compressions in about 3 seconds. Count as you push down: "One, two, three, four, five."
  - Compress sternum ½ to 1 inch.
  - Deliver compressions smoothly and rhythmically. Compression time should equal relaxation time. Blood is forced out of heart during compressions and it flows into heart during relaxation or when pressure is released.
  - Keep tips of fingers in contact with infant's chest. Knuckles should point across infant's chest and away from you.
  - Keep one hand on infant's forehead to maintain head-tilt.

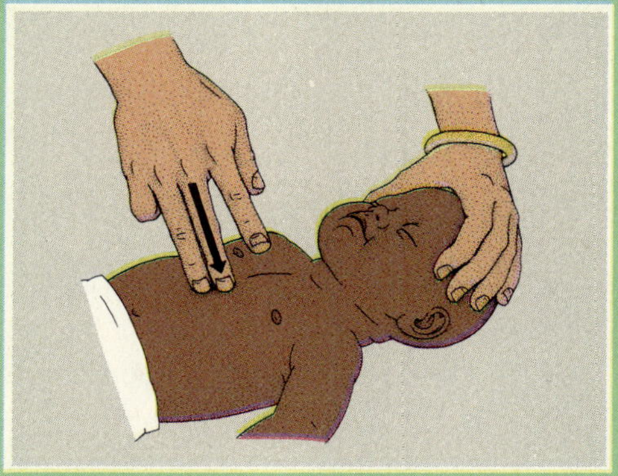

- GIVE ONE BREATH.
  - Use head-tilt to keep airway open in a neutral position.
  - Make a seal around infant's mouth and nose with your mouth.

INFANT RESCUE BREATHING	INFANT CPR

INFANT CPR

- Give one slow breath from cheeks of your mouth, with just enough force to see infant's chest rise.

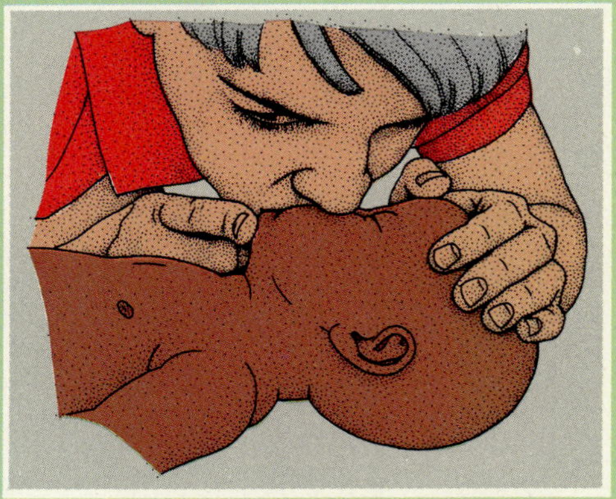

- Allow for chest deflation after each breath.
- Give compressions and breaths in cycles of 5 compressions to 1 breath. Repeat for about 1 minute (12 cycles).

INFANT RESCUE BREATHING

□ **9.** RECHECK PULSE AND BREATHING once every minute.

- Check for brachial pulse as in Step 7.
- Check for breathing using LOOK, LISTEN, and FEEL as in Step 5.

INFANT CPR

□ **9.** RECHECK PULSE after one minute and every few minutes thereafter.

- Keep hand on infant's forehead to maintain open airway.
- Feel for brachial pulse (allow 5 seconds).

IF infant has a pulse and is breathing, THEN:

- Keep airway open.
- Monitor pulse and breathing.
- Wait for EMS to arrive.

IF infant has a pulse but is not breathing, THEN:

- Begin or continue rescue breathing.
- Wait for EMS to arrive.

IF infant has no pulse and is not breathing, THEN:

- Begin or continue CPR.
- Wait for EMS to arrive.

INFANT RESCUE BREATHING

□ **10.** CONTINUE RESCUE BREATHING until:

- Infant begins to breathe.
- A second trained rescuer arrives to relieve you.
- EMS arrives to relieve you.
- You are too exhausted to continue rescue breathing.

INFANT CPR

□ **10.** CONTINUE CPR until:

- Infant has pulse and is breathing.
- A second trained rescuer arrives to relieve you.
- EMS arrives to relieve you.
- You are too exhausted to continue CPR.

IF second CPR-trained rescuer arrives, THEN:

- Ask second rescuer to determine if EMS system has been called.
- Ask if second rescuer knows CPR.
- Finish your compression/breathing cycle with breath.

INFANT RESCUE BREATHING	INFANT CPR
	■ Tell second rescuer to take over CPR. ■ Second rescuer begins CPR by checking pulse for 5 seconds. If no pulse, second rescuer restarts CPR by giving one breath and five chest compressions. ■ Second rescuer continues cycles of one breath and five chest compressions until tired and asks first rescuer to take over again. ■ Rescuer who is not performing CPR can check the effectiveness of the chest compressions by feeling for the brachial pulse during compressions.
	IF you arrive on scene where a first rescuer is performing CPR, THEN: ■ Phone EMS system, if it has not already been done. ■ Tell first rescuer that EMS system has been phoned and that you know CPR and are able to help.
	IF a rescuer performing CPR asks you to take over, THEN: ■ Wait until rescuer finishes cycle of five chest compressions and 1 breath. ■ Check pulse for 5 seconds. ■ If no pulse, restart CPR by giving one breath and five chest compressions.

CONSCIOUS CHOKING INFANT
(up to approximately 1 year)

- Necessary when airway is obstructed.

IF infant is coughing forcefully but has good air exchange, THEN suspect airway is partially obstructed, and:

- Encourage infant to continue coughing.
- If necessary, position infant sitting upright.
- Stay with infant.
- Do not interfere with infant's attempts to cough up object.
- Do not slap infant on back.
- Do not attempt choking rescue techniques.

IF infant:

- Is coughing weakly or cannot cough or cry
- Is making high-pitched noises
- Has a panicked expression
- Has blue lips and nails

THEN assume that either the partially obstructed airway now has poor air exchange or that airway is completely obstructed. Begin choking rescue techniques.

CONSCIOUS CHOKING INFANT

□ **1.** SHOUT FOR HELP to alert others of the emergency.

□ **2.** GIVE FIVE BACK BLOWS.

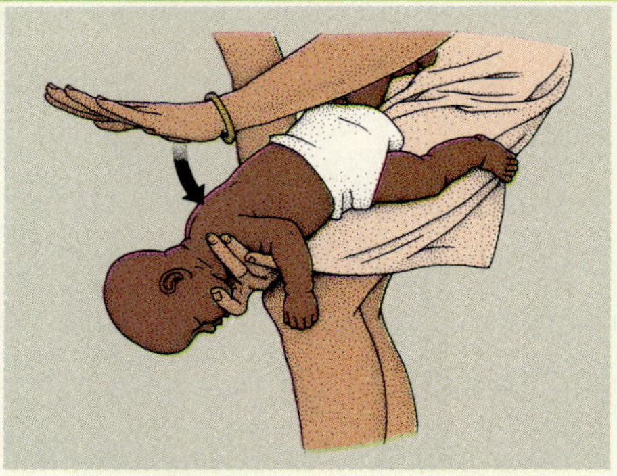

- Lay infant face down along your forearm. Support infant's head and neck by holding jaw between your thumb and fingers.
- Support your forearm against your thigh. Infant's head will be lower than chest.
- Give five back blows between shoulder blades with heel of one hand.
- Deliver each blow firmly and separately as if each one will expel obstruction.

□ **3.** GIVE FIVE CHEST THRUSTS.

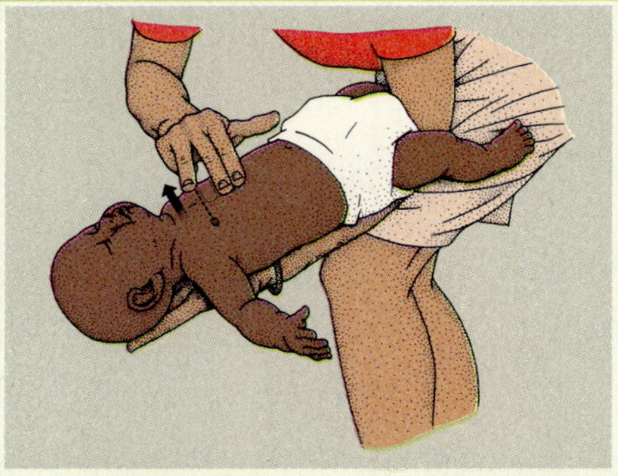

- Sandwich infant between your hands and forearms, and turn infant onto back with head lower than chest.
- Support back of infant's head with your hand.
- Imagine a line connecting infant's nipples.
- Place three fingers on sternum, or breast bone, with ring finger just below imaginary nipple line.
- Lift your ring finger off chest. If you feel notch at end of sternum (xiphoid process), move your fingers up slightly.
- Give five chest thrusts by compressing sternum approximately ½ to 1 inch with index and middle fingers.
- Keep fingers in contact with chest between chest thrusts.

□ **4.** REPEAT cycles of five back blows alternating with five chest thrusts until:

- Infant coughs up object.
- Infant starts to breathe.
- Infant becomes unconscious.

IF object is dislodged or expelled, THEN have infant examined by health care provider.

IF infant becomes unconscious and object is not dislodged or expelled, THEN:

- Tell someone to phone EMS system for help.
- Lay infant on floor face up.
- Proceed to Step 9 of Unconscious Choking Infant for how to continue when a conscious infant becomes unconscious before obstruction is relieved.

UNCONSCIOUS CHOKING INFANT
(up to approximately 1 year)

- Necessary when airway is obstructed.

IF you find a motionless infant, THEN check the scene for hazards and clues to what happened.

□ **1.** CHECK RESPONSIVENESS.

- Gently tap infant's shoulder or back.
- Call infant's name.

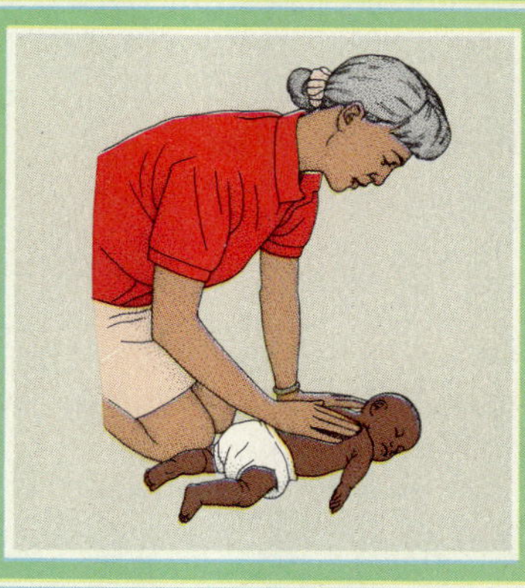

□ **2.** SEND SOMEONE TO ACTIVATE EMS SYSTEM. Check for breathing without changing infant's position.

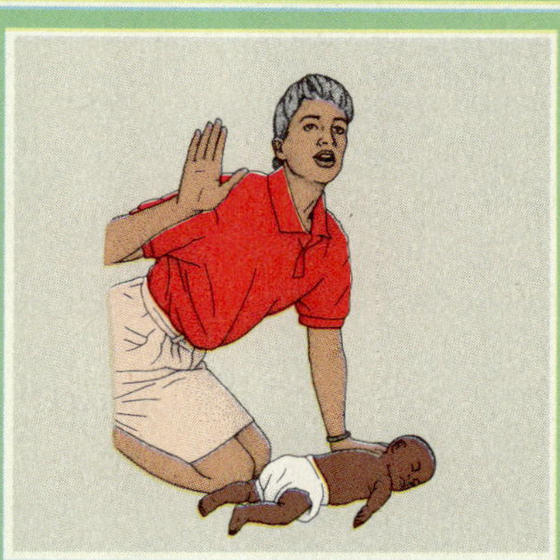

□ **3.** POSITION INFANT ON BACK if breathing cannot be detected. If neck or spinal injury is suspected, move infant as a unit to avoid any twisting motion by taking the following steps:

- Move infant's arm closest to you above infant's head.
- Place one hand on infant's shoulder and other hand on infant's hip (a).
- Roll infant toward you as a unit. Move your hand from infant's shoulder to support back of head and neck (b).
- Place infant's arms alongside body.

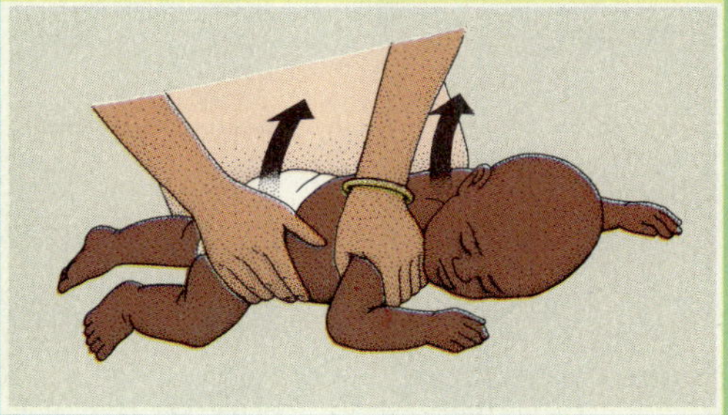

a

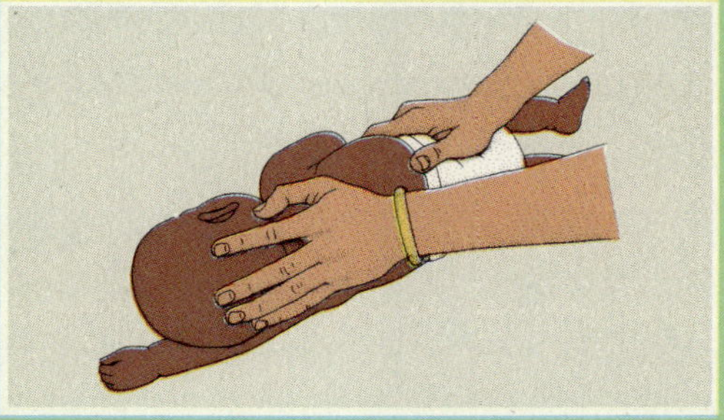

b

- ☐ **4.** OPEN AIRWAY using head-tilt/chin-lift method:
  - Place hand nearest infant's head on infant's forehead and apply pressure to tilt head back slightly into a neutral position.
  - Place index finger of other hand under bony part of jaw near chin, and lift. Avoid pressing on soft tissue under jaw.
  - Do not close infant's mouth when tilting head.

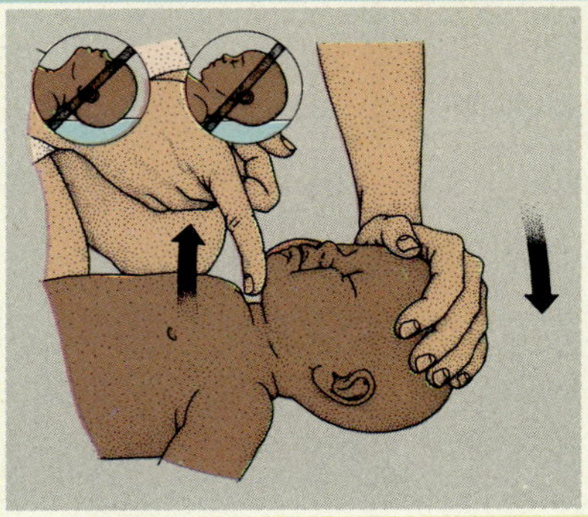

IF you see vomitus, THEN wipe it out with fingers covered by a cloth, if available, and CONTINUE numbered rescue steps.

IF you see a solid object, THEN remove it by hooking it with your little finger and CONTINUE numbered rescue steps.

- ☐ **5.** CHECK FOR BREATHING (allow 5 seconds).
  - Place your ear over infant's mouth and nose while keeping airway open.
  - LOOK for infant's chest to rise and fall.
  - LISTEN for breathing.
  - FEEL for breath against your cheek.

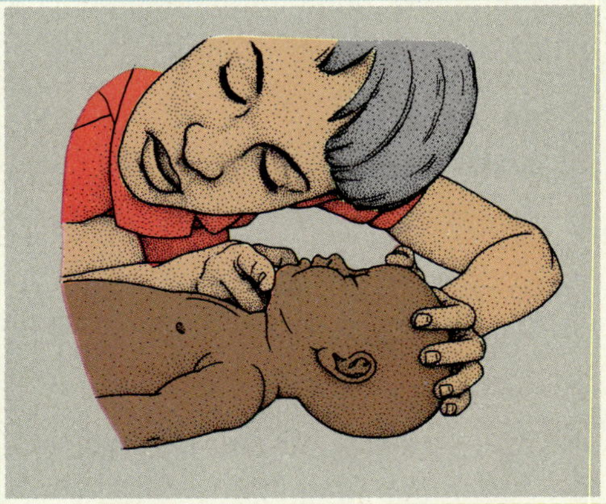

- ☐ **6.** GIVE TWO SLOW BREATHS.
  - Use head-tilt/chin-lift to keep airway open in a neutral position.
  - Make a seal around infant's mouth and nose with your mouth.
  - Give two slow breaths, each lasting 1 to 1½ seconds.
  - Give breaths with just enough force to see infant's chest rise.

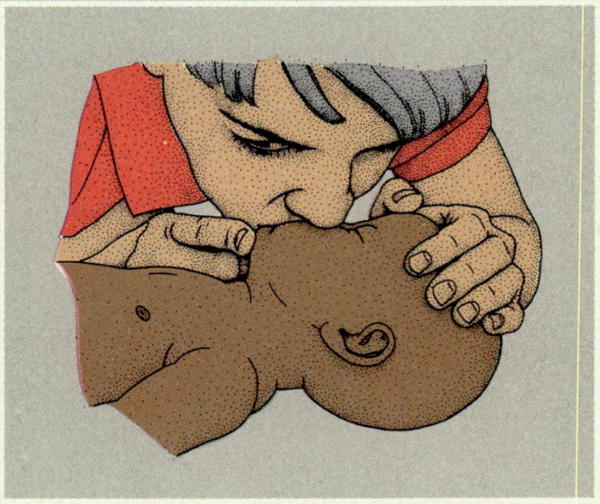

IF first two breaths will not go in and resistance is felt, THEN retilt infant's head and try another two breaths.

IF second two breaths will not go in and resistance is felt, THEN assume airway is obstructed and CONTINUE with numbered rescue steps.

□ **7.** GIVE FIVE BACK BLOWS.

- Lay infant face down along your forearm. Support infant's head and neck by holding jaw between your thumb and fingers.
- Support your forearm against your thigh. Infant's head will be lower than chest.
- Give five back blows between shoulder blades with heel of one hand.
- Deliver each blow firmly and separately, as if each one will expel obstruction.

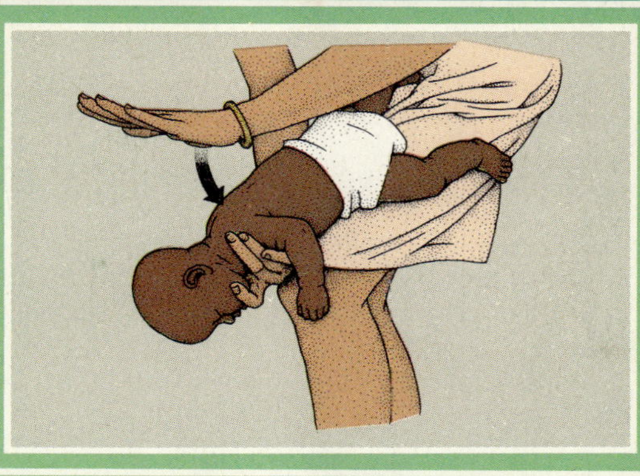

□ **8.** GIVE FIVE CHEST THRUSTS.

- Sandwich infant between your hands and forearms, and turn infant onto back with head lower than chest.
- Support back of infant's head with your hand.
- Imagine a line connecting infant's nipples.
- Place three fingers on sternum, or breast bone, with ring finger just below imaginary nipple line.
- Lift your ring finger off chest. If you feel notch at end of sternum (xiphoid process), move your fingers up slightly.
- Give five chest thrusts by compressing sternum approximately ½ to 1 inch with index and middle fingers.
- Keep fingers in contact with chest between chest thrusts.

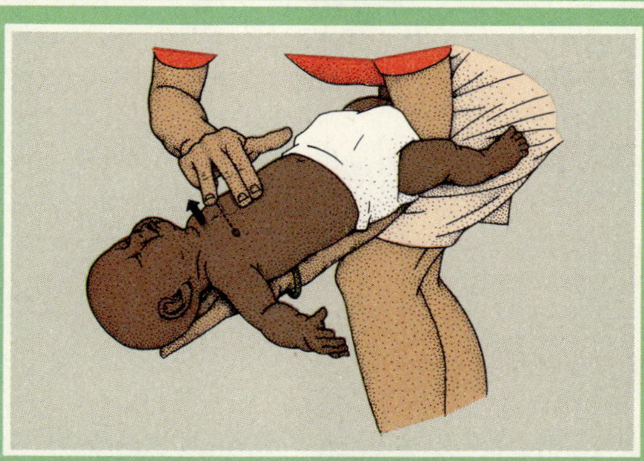

□ **9.** CHECK FOR FOREIGN OBJECT.

- Lay infant on floor or table, face up.
- Grasp both tongue and jaw between your thumb and fingers and lift jaw upward.
- If object is seen, remove it with a finger sweep by sliding little finger of your free hand along inside of cheek to base of tongue, using a hooking action.

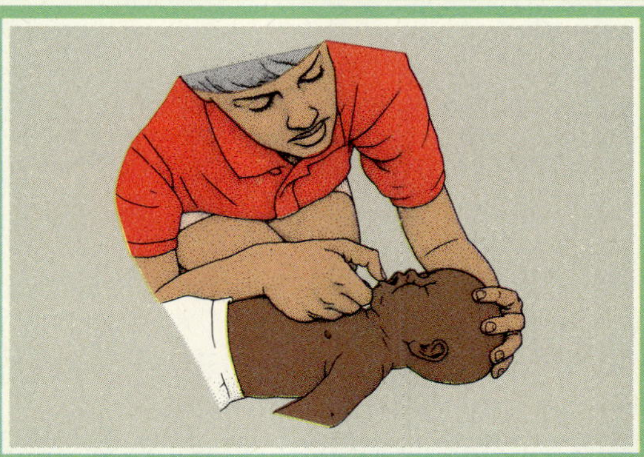

- Do not try to remove object if you cannot see it because the attempt could push object deeper into airway.

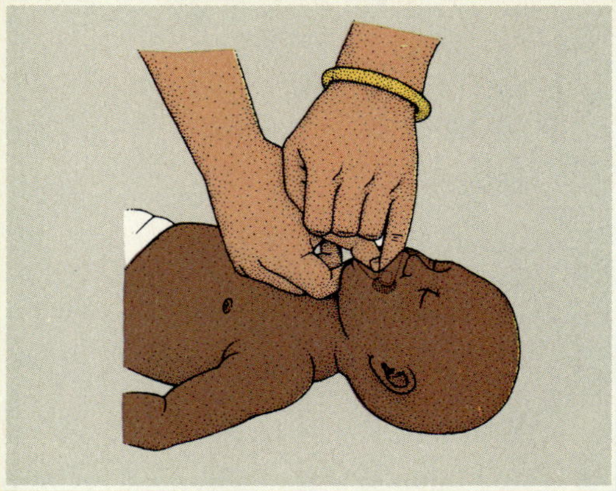

□ **10.** GIVE TWO BREATHS

- Open airway using head-tilt/chin-lift.
- Seal your mouth around infant's mouth and nose.
- Attempt to give two breaths.

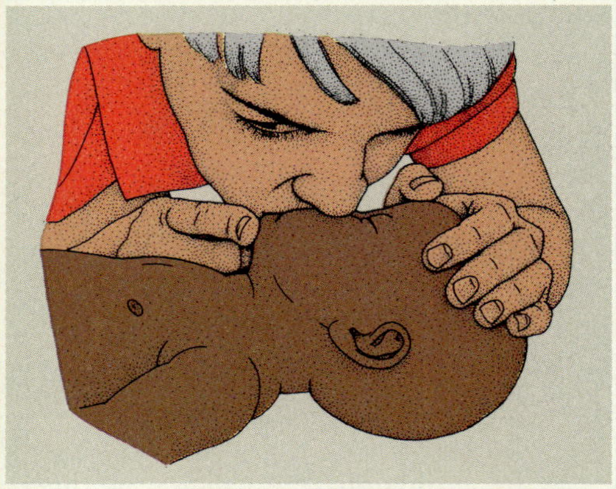

□ **11.** REPEAT STEPS 7, 8, 9, and 10 until object is dislodged or expelled.

- Give five back blows.
- Give five chest thrusts.
- Check for foreign object.
- Give two breaths.

□ **12.** CHECK FOR PULSE AND BREATHING once object has been dislodged or expelled and airway is open.

IF infant has a pulse and is breathing, THEN:

- Keep airway open.
- Monitor pulse and breathing.
- Wait for EMS to arrive.

IF infant has a pulse but is not breathing, THEN

- Begin rescue breathing.
- Wait for EMS to arrive.

IF infant has no pulse and is not breathing, THEN:

- Begin CPR.
- Wait for EMS to arrive.

Recovery Position

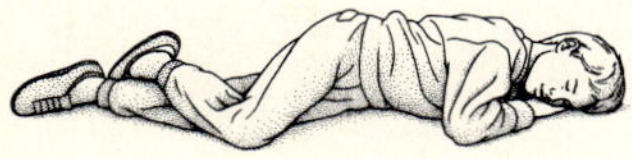

If a child is unconscious and breathing and you do not suspect a neck or spinal injury, place him or her in the **recovery position**. This position keeps the airway open and is the safest position if the child begins to vomit.

To Provide the Most Effective Chest Compressions:

- Perform CPR only on a flat, hard surface such as the floor or a table. It cannot be performed efficiently on a soft surface such as a bed or sofa.
- Compress straight up and down in a smooth motion. Jerking and rocking back and forth reduce the force of the compression and can cause damage.
- Use the hips, not the knees, as the pivot point when compressing the child's chest.
- Keep the elbows locked and your shoulders positioned over the child's sternum.
- Always use correct hand placement because this will avoid accidentally compressing the tip of the sternum. This soft cartilage notch (xiphoid process) can be injured and pushed into nearby tissues and organs.
- Keep the hand in contact with the chest between compressions. This will help to maintain correct hand position.
- When performing CPR on a child, allow only the heel of the hand, not the fingers, to come in contact with the chest at the compression site.

Important Points in CPR Emergencies

- If a spinal injury is suspected, first attempt to determine if child is breathing by performing the look, listen, and feel step with the child in the position in which you found him or her.
- Because there is a risk of damage when performing CPR, no part of CPR should be performed on a child who does not need it. Be absolutely certain that the infant or child victim is unconscious and not just sleeping. Also, never practice CPR on a child.
- If you are alone and cannot summon help by shouting, perform 1 full minute of rescue breathing or CPR, whichever is necessary, before calling for emergency medical help.
- An infant's airway is opened by tipping the head backward slightly into a neutral position. Over-extending the backward tip of the head can reduce or close the airway. A child's airway is opened by tipping the head back into an above-neutral position. The larger the child, the farther back the head must be tipped to open the airway.
- Touch only the bony part of the jaw near the chin when opening the airway. Do not touch the soft tissue of the throat.
- When breathing into the lungs of an infant or child, use only enough force to see the chest rise. Never use the full volume of air from your lungs when breathing into an infant or child.
- Do not use your thumb to locate a pulse because the thumb has a pulse of its own.
- Post the emergency medical telephone numbers by each telephone.
- Any child who requires any basic life support technique must be examined in an emergency medical facility even if the child appears to have recovered.
- If the child who requires CPR is not revived within 1 minute, it is unlikely that CPR alone will revive the child. CPR, however, can keep the child alive until further emergency medical treatment can be started.
- If you are able and if you do not suspect a head or spinal injury, carry the child to the telephone. This allows you to perform rescue breathing or CPR while calling for emergency medical help.
- If injuries around the mouth prevent you from being able to make a tight seal, close the mouth by pushing the chin and deliver breaths through the nose.
- Opening the airway by tilting the head back moves the tongue out of the airway. In an unconscious person the tongue is the most common airway obstruction.

Complications of Performing CPR

Air in the stomach. Sometimes air can be forced into a child's stomach when the rescuer is delivering breaths. This can lead to vomiting, which is especially dangerous if the vomitus enters the lungs.

Air can be forced into the child's stomach by:

- Giving breaths too quickly.
- Giving breaths too forcefully.
- Not tilting the child's head back far enough.

To keep air from being forced into the stomach while giving breaths:

- Allow enough time for the lungs to deflate between breaths.
- Give only enough breath to see the chest rise.
- Make certain that the child's head is tilted back far enough.

If you notice that the child's stomach is beginning to look bloated, do not attempt to remove the air by

Airway Obstruction Due to Illness

Occasionally in children, breathing difficulty leading to airway obstruction is caused by infection in the respiratory tract or by a severe allergic reaction. A child who is ill, with or without fever, and experiencing a barking cough and progressive difficulty breathing needs immediate care in an emergency medical facility.

The Heimlich maneuver and rescue breathing techniques will not help this child because the airway blockage is due to swollen throat tissue, not a foreign object. Attempting these techniques can be dangerous, and can postpone providing the care the child urgently needs. It is important to understand the difference between the sick child's emergency and the otherwise healthy child who suddenly begins to choke.

Choking Prevention

A small, solid object, such as a piece of food, small toy, or part of a toy, that suddenly becomes caught in the throat causes a child to choke by partially or completely blocking the airway. Choking is a life-threatening emergency that must be recognized and corrected immediately. Some safety rules regarding mealtime can help prevent choking emergencies.

- Teach children not to speak with their mouths full of food. A laugh or sudden gasp can direct food into the airway.
- Make sure children always sit while eating. Moving about or running while eating can lead to an accidental choking.
- Cut up or break food into small, manageable pieces.
- Avoid giving foods that are dangerous due to size, consistency, or have dangerous parts to children under 3. See Food Safety, Chapter 13.

CPR Mouth Barriers

Current practice now recommends that an infant-size and child-size CPR shield, mask, or other mouth barrier with a one-way valve be part of the first aid kit for use in a respiratory or cardiac emergency.

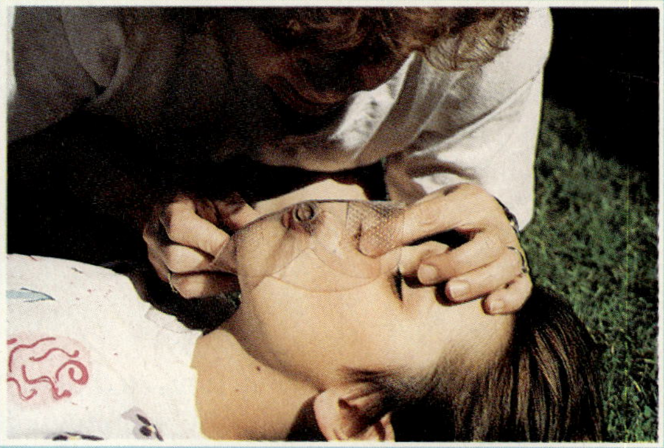

pressing on the stomach. Recheck your technique and continue breaths.

Vomiting. If a child or infant begins to vomit while you are performing CPR, immediately turn the head and body to one side to allow the vomitus to drain. Sweep the mouth clean and continue CPR.

Compression injuries. The actions necessary to perform CPR correctly require some degree of force. It is possible, although infrequent, that an injury to the ribs, lungs, or other organs can occur, despite correct CPR technique. Continue CPR, even if you think a compression injury might have occurred. Such an injury can receive medical treatment later, but basic life support must not be interrupted.

Keeping a Heart Healthy

The number one killer of Americans is heart disease. Although heart disease is usually seen in adults, routine blood cholesterol screening of grade school children shows that, for some, high blood cholesterol levels are already present. These high cholesterol levels are known to contribute to heart disease. For many, lifestyle changes such as diet and exercise can reduce these levels and reduce the chance of developing heart disease later in life.

Both parents and child care providers are in a position to influence the behaviors, attitudes, and habits of young children in a positive way. Be a good role model and teach these heart-healthy habits:

- ***Teach children not to smoke.*** If you smoke, avoid doing so in front of children or in an area that will cause children and other staff to breathe the smoke. Both smokers and nonsmokers should be aware of the dangers of smoking. Teach children that it is unhealthy to smoke cigarettes. Consider stopping smoking for yourself and for the people who love you.
- ***Teach children to eat healthy foods.*** A lifetime of poor dietary habits can contribute to heart disease, especially diets that are high in fat. Children need to eat a variety of foods including cereals, breads, and pastas, vegetables, fruits, low-fat dairy products, poultry, fish, and lean meats. Fats and sweets, although enjoyable, should be eaten sparingly. Talk about healthy foods at mealtimes and compliment the good choices that children make. If you eat with the children, be sure your meal has heart-healthy choices, as well.
- ***Teach children to exercise.*** Most young children enjoy physical activity. Those who remain physically active over the years will reap the benefits as adults. Teach children that activities like running, swimming, outdoor games, riding bicycles, and even jumping rope keep their heart muscles strong and healthy.

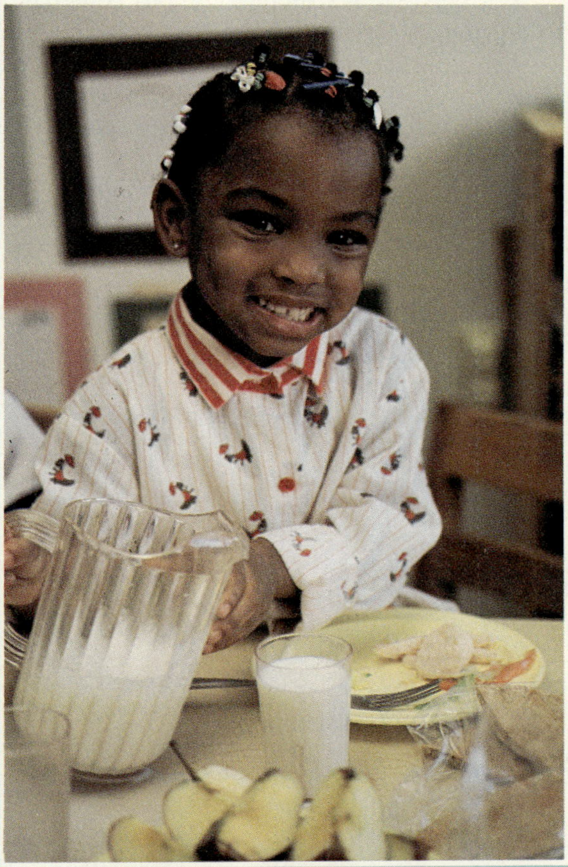

School-age children and adolescents need to learn about the additional factors of keeping both blood pressure and weight under control.

Call your local chapters of the American Heart Association and American Lung Association to learn about their educational materials for young children.

Rescue Breathing and CPR

Choose the best answer.

1. When giving rescue breaths to an infant, give one breath every_____seconds.
   A. ____ 6
   B. ____ 5
   C. ____ 4
   D. ____ 3

2. To determine if an unconscious child has stopped breathing, you should:
   A. ____ check for a pulse
   B. ____ look at the pupils
   C. ____ look, listen, and feel for breaths

3. When performing rescue breaths, give:
   A. ____ just enough breath to see the chest rise
   B. ____ enough air until you feel resistance

4. To open the airway, place one hand on forehead and the other hand:
   A. ____ on the soft part of the throat near the chin
   B. ____ on the bony part of the jaw near the chin

5. When giving chest compressions to a child use:
   A. ____ 2 fingers
   B. ____ the heel of one hand

6. Compress an infant's chest:
   A. ____ ½ to 1 inch
   B. ____ 1 to 1½ inches

7. The compression location for an infant is:
   A. ____ well below xiphoid notch
   B. ____ one finger-width above nipple line
   C. ____ one finger-width below nipple line

8. Chest compressions for a child should be given at a rate of:
   A. ____ 60 compressions per minute
   B. ____ 80 compressions per minute
   C. ____ 100 compressions per minute

9. When performing rescue breaths on a child, the head should be positioned in the:
   A. ____ neutral position
   B. ____ above-neutral position

10. Chest compressions are best performed on:
    A. ____ a hard, flat surface
    B. ____ a soft, flat surface

11. Perform chest compressions:
    A. ____ with a quick, thrusting motion
    B. ____ with a smooth and regular motion

Choking

Choose the best answer.

1. An infant is choking. She is conscious but cannot cough or cry. You should:
   A. ____ leave the child alone and watch closely
   B. ____ give 5 back blows and 5 chest thrusts
   C. ____ give 5 abdominal thrusts

2. A child who seems to be choking *can* speak. You should:
   A. ____ leave the child alone and watch closely
   B. ____ give 5 back blows and 5 chest thrusts
   C. ____ give 5 abdominal thrusts

3. To dislodge an object from a conscious, choking child, you should:
   A. ____ give 5 back blows
   B. ____ do a finger sweep
   C. ____ give 5 abdominal thrusts

4. Use your finger to remove an object from an unconscious infant's or child's mouth:
   A. ____ when back blows and chest thrusts fail
   B. ____ only if you can see the object

4

Shock

■ Shock ■ Severe Allergic Reaction ■
■ Fainting ■

Shock

Shock refers to a failure somewhere in the circulatory system that prevents it from pumping blood in sufficient amounts to all body parts. The circulatory system has three parts: a working pump (the heart), a network of pipes (the blood vessels), and an adequate amount of fluid pumped through the pipes (the blood). Damage to any of these parts can disrupt the circulation of blood and produce the condition known as shock.

Some degree of shock occurs with all injuries. In minor injuries, the body is able to recover on its own. In more serious injuries, the body's attempts to correct the shock process do not work, and death can result if emergency medical help is not provided.

The most common form of shock in children results from blood or fluid loss, either outside the body, such as from an open wound, or inside the body where wounds you cannot see are bleeding. Other examples of injuries that disrupt the circulatory system and can cause shock are serious burns, head or spinal injury, broken bones, severe pain, poisoning, drug overdoses, dehydration, or a near-drowning accident. In adults, shock can accompany heart attacks and strokes. Shock can also occur with less serious injuries than these that, by themselves, are not fatal. Always watch for shock.

Shock is most likely to occur in the first hour following an injury. Symptoms can be immediate or can progress over a period of several minutes. Regardless of which part of the circulatory system is disturbed, signs and symptoms of shock as well as treatment for shock are always the same. You should always treat a seriously injured child for shock, even if there initially is no sign of it.

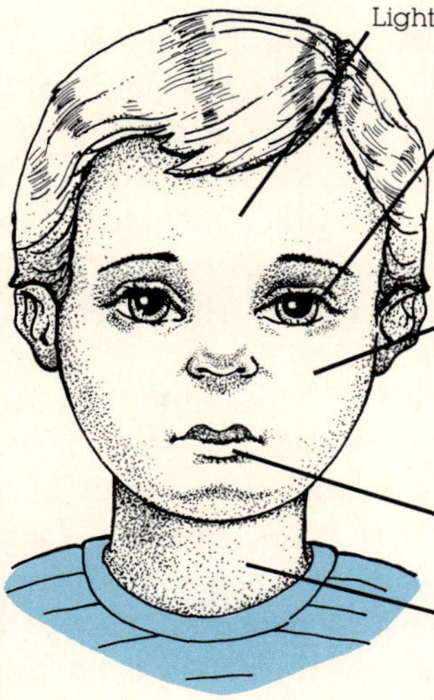

Signs and symptoms of shock

Signs and Symptoms

- Pale skin color. A blue or gray discoloration around the nose and mouth, as well as a blue coloring of the nailbeds shows that too little blood and oxygen are reaching these parts of the body.
- Cool and moist skin. The warm blood is concentrated in the vital organs deep inside the body and not in the blood vessels on the surface.
- Rapid, weak pulse. The heart is trying to compensate for the reduced amount of circulating blood and oxygen.
- Feeling light-headed, confused, or anxious. The brain is not getting enough oxygen.
- Weakness.
- Shallow and rapid breathing.
- Eyes dull and sunken.
- Dilated pupils.
- Sweating.
- Thirst.
- Nausea and vomiting.

First Aid

Guarding against shock by treating a child for it, with or without symptoms, is the safest way to proceed when caring for a child who has had a serious injury. A first aider can slow the progress of shock and even prevent it from occurring by taking the correct steps immediately.

- Check for consciousness by calling the child's name. Any child who is found unconscious after a violent injury must be treated as if a spinal injury has occurred. See Spinal Injuries, Chapter 10.
- Check and monitor the airway, breathing, and circulation and treat accordingly.
- Send someone to call for emergency medical help.
- Control any obvious external bleeding. See Bleeding, Chapter 5.
- Position the child for shock according to the symptoms the child describes or the injuries you find:

1. ***Standard shock position.*** Lay the child flat on his or her back, using blankets or jackets to raise the feet 8 to 12 inches. This helps to increase the flow of blood to the heart and brain. Do not raise the legs any higher because it will affect the breathing by pushing the abdominal organs against the diaphragm.

2. ***Spinal injury.*** Leave the injured child in the position in which he or she is found. NEVER MOVE AN UNCONSCIOUS CHILD EXCEPT TO SAVE A LIFE. If you must move a child with a suspected spinal injury because the location is life threatening, such as lying beside a burning car, use a technique found in the Skill Scan, Emergency Moves, in Chapter 10. If you must reposition a child who is vomiting while lying face up or is in need of CPR, roll the head, neck, and body as one unit. See the Skill Scan, Rolling an Unconsious Child, in Chapter 10.

3. ***Breathing difficulty.*** Raise the head and shoulders or have a younger child sit on an adult's lap.

4. ***Unsure of injuries.*** Keep the child flat on the back without raising the legs.

5. ***Nausea and vomiting.*** If the child complains of nausea or if the child vomits, position the child on the left side by rolling the head, neck, and spine as one unit. See the Skill Scan, Rolling an Unconscious Child, in Chapter 10.

- Cover the child with a blanket or jacket to prevent heat loss. Preventing heat loss, not creating additional warmth, is important in treating shock. Allowing a child to become too warm draws the blood to the skin and away from the vital organs. Also, place a blanket under the child's body to insulate the child from the ground and further reduce heat loss.
- Give nothing to eat or drink. If the child vomits and chokes and the vomitus enters the lungs, a life-threatening condition can develop. Additionally, the child should have an empty stomach in the event that surgery is needed.

Severe Allergic Reaction (Anaphylactic Shock)

Children who suffer allergies to such common agents as pollen, molds, dust, animal fur, or certain foods learn that avoidance is the best way to prevent the unpleasant reaction that their bodies produce. Most common allergic reactions can be brought under control by removing the cause from the child's environment or diet.

However, severe allergic reaction to some eaten or injected substances can be fatal if not reversed within minutes after the reaction begins. This is called anaphylactic shock. It occurs suddenly, usually within seconds or minutes after coming in contact with the allergen (allergic substance).

Anaphylactic shock is unexpected because, initially, neither the child nor parent is aware of the child's extreme allergy to a substance that is harmless to most people. It can occur in a child who receives a dose of a medication such as penicillin or tetanus antitoxin or after eating a food such as shellfish or nuts. The child can also eat a prepared food without knowing that it contains an ingredient to which the child is highly allergic. Stings from an insect of the hymenoptera order which includes bees, wasps (including hornets and yellow jackets), and ants can also cause anaphylactic shock. See Insect Stings, Chapter 7.

A child must be exposed to the allergen at least once in order for this extreme sensitivity to develop. The first exposure does not cause an allergic, or anaphylactic, reaction. It does, however, cause excessive amounts of an antibody named IgE to be produced in the blood. When the allergen next enters the body and comes in contact with the IgE antibody, a series of dangerous internal reactions begin, known collectively as anaphylactic shock. If this allergic reaction is severe, and if epinephrine, the medication that counteracts the anaphylactic reaction, is not available, death can occur within minutes.

Signs and Symptoms

Any of the following can occur immediately or within several minutes following exposure to the allergic substance:

- Sudden sense of uneasiness and anxiety
- Skin flushed
- Hives, a generalized rash of red, raised, blotchy areas on the skin that causes itching
- Swelling of any part of the body, but especially face, lips, and tongue
- Difficulty or noisy breathing due to swelling in the throat, which can block the airway
- Difficulty swallowing
- Tightness in the chest
- Bluish or grayish skin color
- Seizures
- Loss of consciousness
- Cardiovascular collapse, a heartbeat so weak that blood cannot circulate

First Aid

- Check airway, breathing, and circulation. Begin CPR, if necessary.
- Send someone to call for emergency medical help.
- Epinephrine, the medication that reverses the anaphylactic reaction, must be administered immediately. Epinephrine can be given by an emergency medical technician, parent, or it can be given by child care providers, but *only* if they have been trained in how to administer the medication and have written permission from the child's health care provider. Frequently, more than one dose of epinephrine is necessary to reverse an anaphylactic reaction.
- Have the child seen immediately in an emergency medical facility.

Children who have had an extreme reaction to a specific allergen, such as a bee sting, should have kept with the first aid supplies in the child care center an allergic emergency self-treatment kit (also known as an anaphylactic kit or insect sting kit) containing the epinephrine injection. This is not a routine item in all first aid kits, but rather a prescription drug intended specifically for the allergic child in an emergency. It contains an easy-to-use mechanism that administers the correct dose of the drug when it is needed.

Sometimes the signs and symptoms of anaphylactic shock develop slowly over several minutes or hours after the exposure. This is also a dangerous reaction. The child should be seen by a health care provider as soon as the reaction is recognized.

If the child experiences any of the signs and symptoms of anaphylactic shock, it is necessary to identify the substance that caused the reaction. It is important to prevent a second reaction because it could be more severe. This child should always wear a medical alert necklace or bracelet that identifies the allergy to rescuers. These products are available through many drugstores. As an additional precaution, a parent might be advised to remain in the health care provider's office or hospital for at least 30 minutes after the child receives a medication known to cause anaphylactic shock.

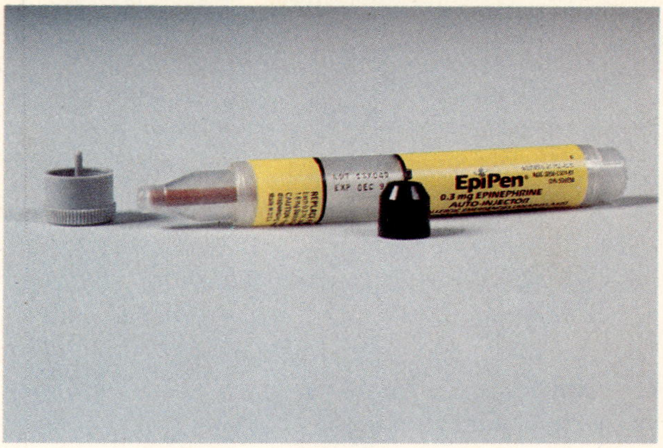

Allergic emergency self-treatment kit

Fainting

Fainting is a mild form of shock. It is a sudden and temporary loss of consciousness due to a brief lack of blood and oxygen to the brain. Fainting is not caused by an injury. It is a nervous system reaction to fear, hunger, pain, or a strong emotional upset. Occasionally, prolonged standing in unusually hot weather will cause fainting.

Signs and Symptoms

Warning signs and symptoms that a child is about to faint include:

- Lightheadedness and dizziness
- Seeing spots or unusual images
- Nausea
- Pale skin color
- Sweating

First Aid

If the child is on the verge of fainting:

- Lay the child down on the back to prevent falling.

- Elevate the legs 8 to 12 inches to increase the supply of blood to the brain, possibly avoiding fainting altogether.
- Apply a cool, wet cloth to the face.

If the child has already fainted:

- Lay the child on the back and elevate the legs 8 to 12 inches.
- Open the airway and check to be sure the child is breathing.
- Check for injuries that might have occurred from falling.
- Loosen tight clothing.
- Apply a cool, wet cloth to the face.
- If vomiting begins, roll the child onto the left side to prevent choking or vomitus entering the lungs.
- Give nothing to eat or drink until the child is well enough to continue with a normal routine.
- Do not use smelling salts or ammonia because they irritate the lining of the nose and breathing passageways.
- Notify the child's parent of the incident.

A child who has fainted recovers quickly, often in 1 to 2 minutes and seldom longer than 5 minutes. Fainting is generally not serious and, in children can usually be traced to a triggering event. You should call for emergency medical help if the child fails to recover from fainting and remains unconscious. The child should be seen by a health care provider if there are repeated attacks of fainting for no apparent reason.

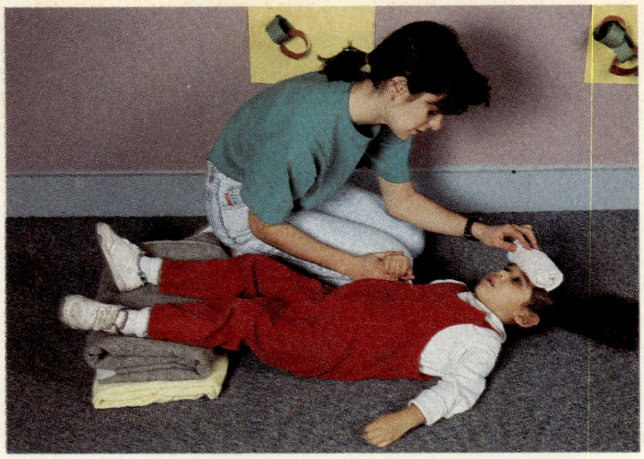

Positioning and care for a child who has fainted.

Some young children cause themselves to faint by holding their breath. These breath-holding spells are often caused by frustration or anger, and sometimes fear. Commonly, uncontrolled crying is followed by breath-holding until the child loses consciousness. The child will begin to breathe spontaneously once becoming unconscious, and will regain consciousness within several seconds. There is no specific treatment, and the episodes disappear as the child matures. The parent might want to discuss the problem with a health care provider for reassurance.

■ SHOCK ■

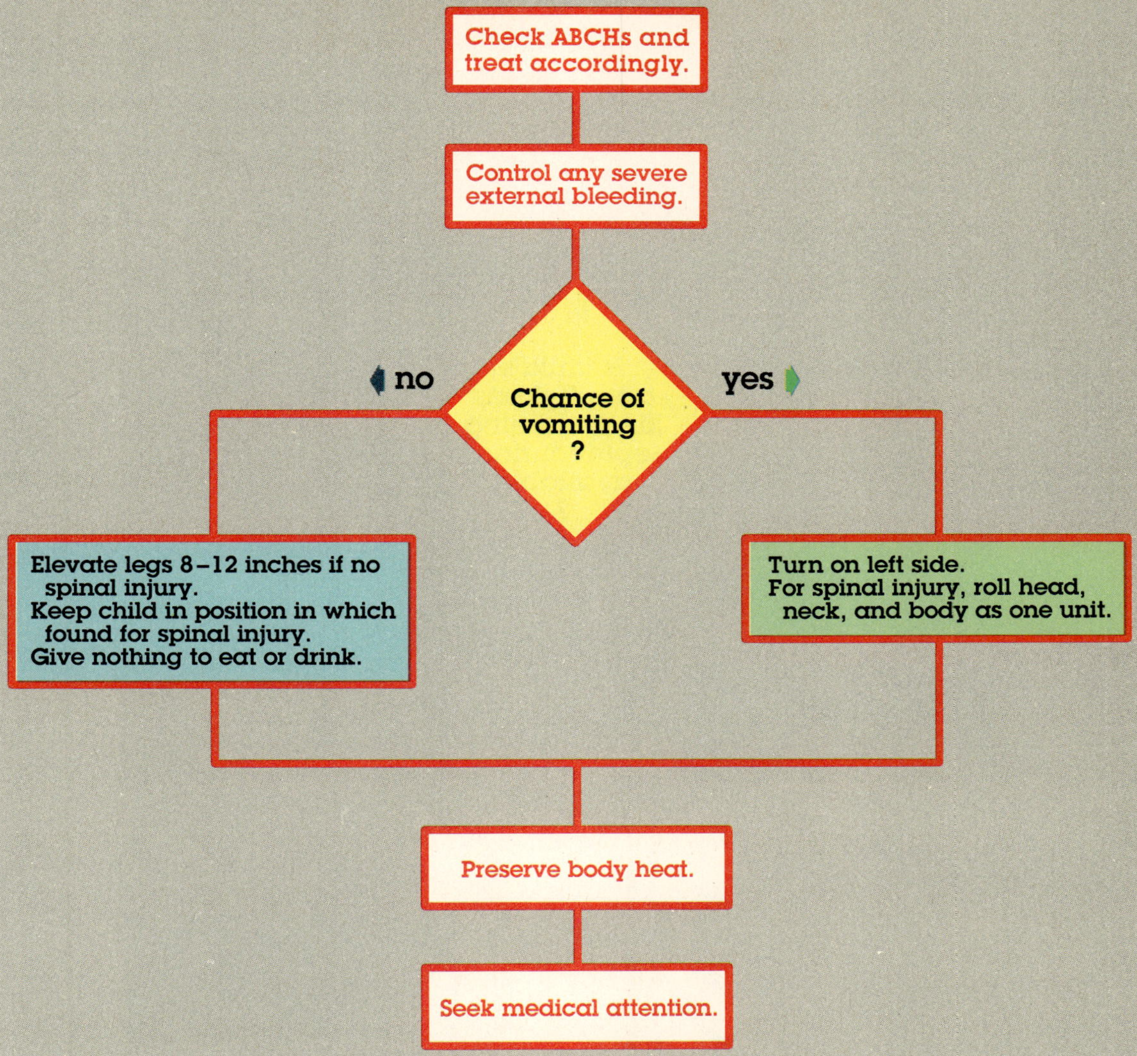

Check ABCHs and treat accordingly.
Control any severe external bleeding.
Chance of vomiting ?
no
Elevate legs 8–12 inches if no spinal injury.
Keep child in position in which found for spinal injury.
Give nothing to eat or drink.
yes
Turn on left side.
For spinal injury, roll head, neck, and body as one unit.
Preserve body heat.
Seek medical attention.

■ SEVERE ALLERGIC REACTION ■
(Anaphylactic Shock)

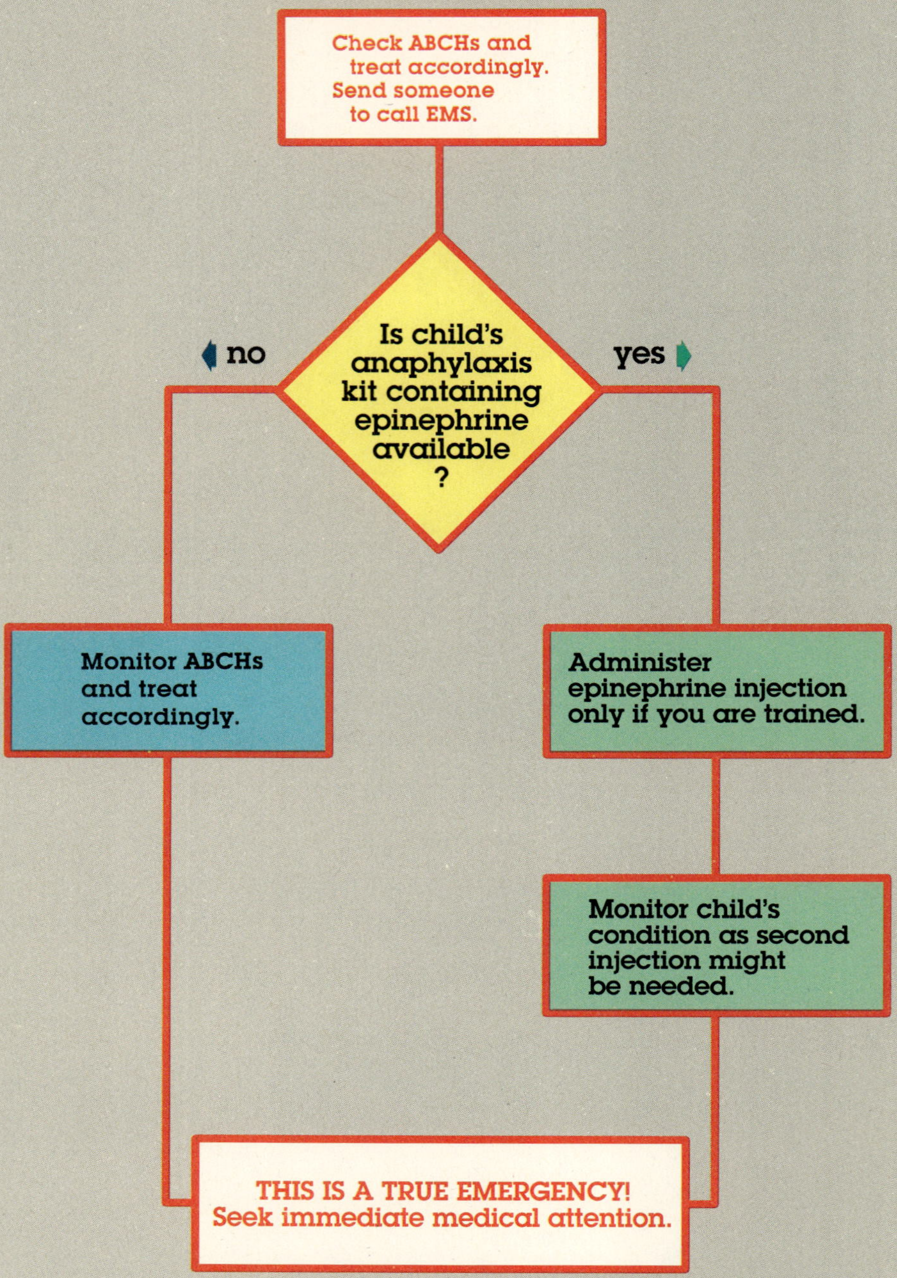

■ FAINTING ■

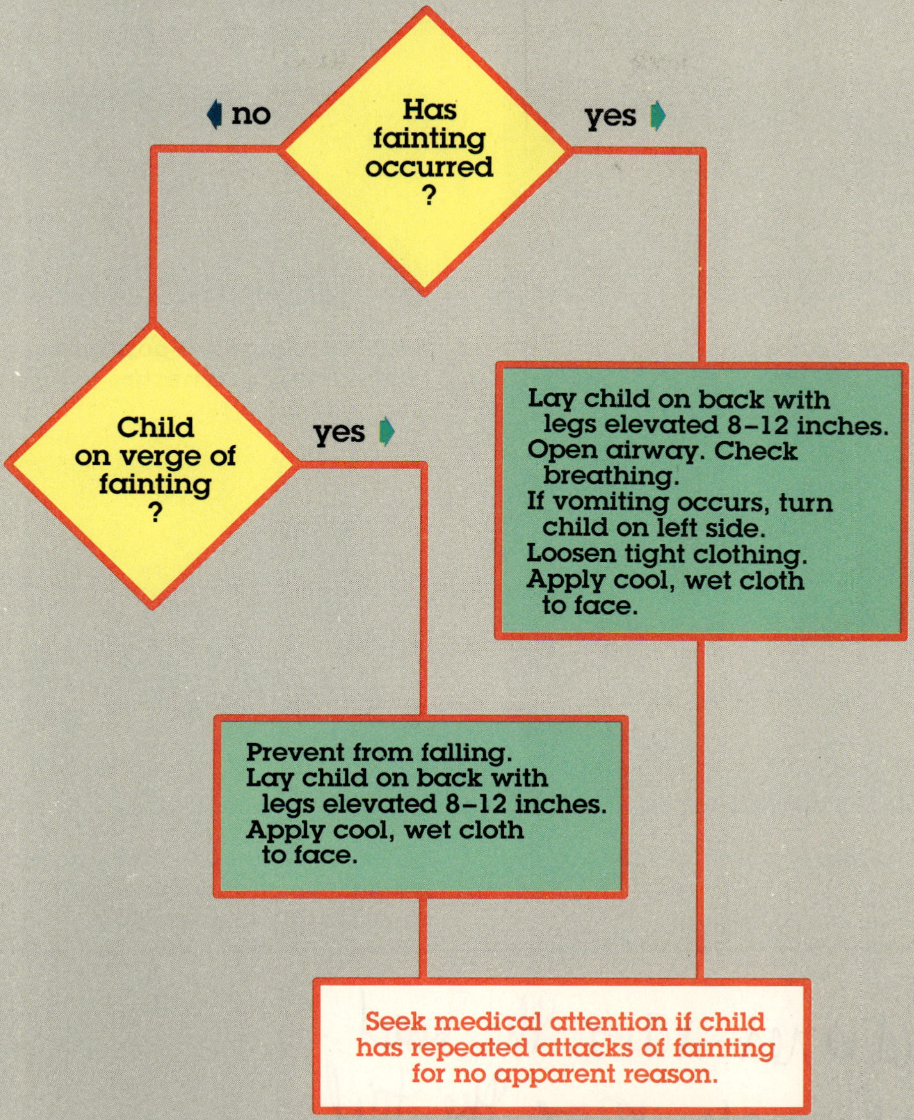
no
Has fainting occurred ?
yes
Child on verge of fainting ?
yes
Lay child on back with legs elevated 8–12 inches.
Open airway. Check breathing.
If vomiting occurs, turn child on left side.
Loosen tight clothing.
Apply cool, wet cloth to face.
Prevent from falling.
Lay child on back with legs elevated 8–12 inches.
Apply cool, wet cloth to face.
Seek medical attention if child has repeated attacks of fainting for no apparent reason.

SKILL SCAN: Positioning the Shock Victim

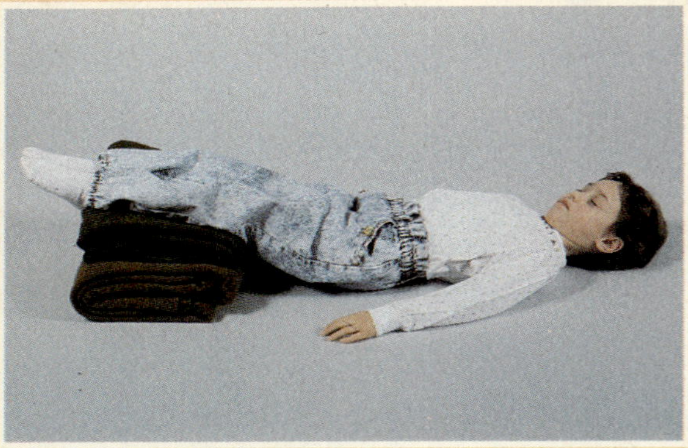

Standard shock position.

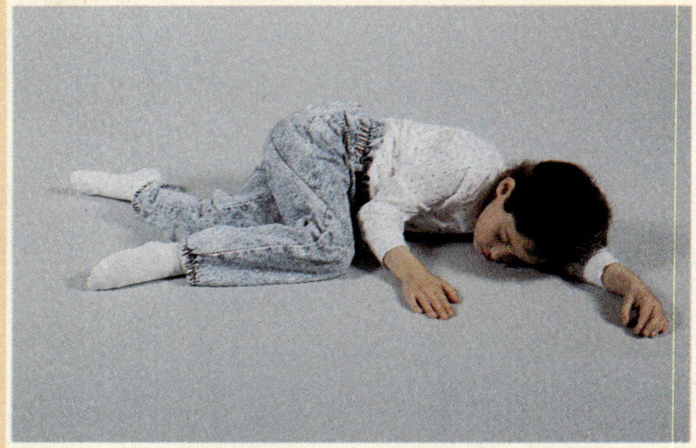

Avoid changing the position for a suspected spinal injury or if unsure of injuries.

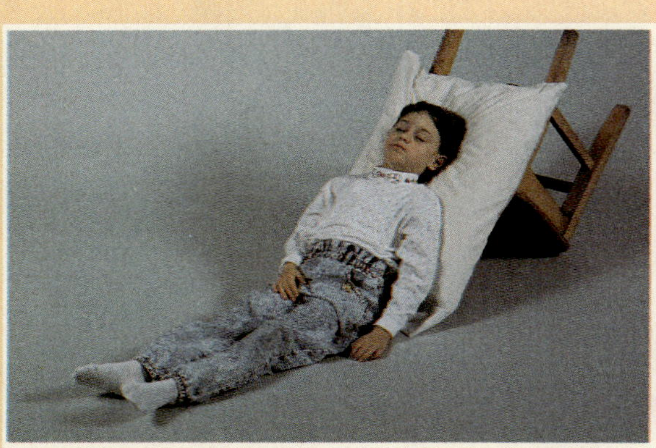

Raise the head and shoulders for breathing difficulties.

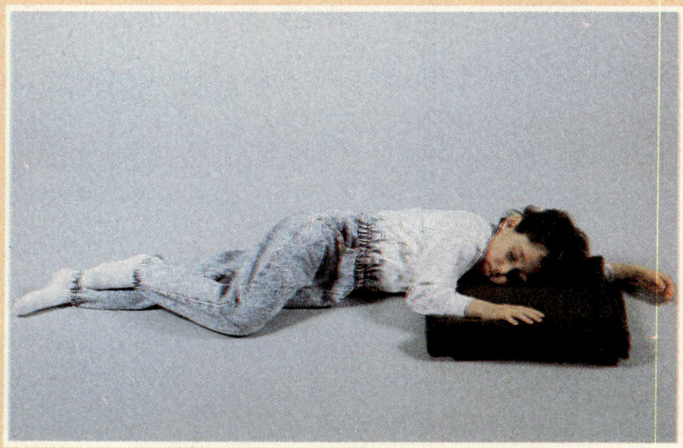

Recovery position—keeps airway open and is safest position for vomiting. Use only if no spinal injury is suspected.

if head is red - raise the head
if head is pale - raise the tail

Shock

Mark each statement true (T) or false (F).

1. ____ Shock results when parts of the body do not receive enough blood.
2. ____ Shock is a concern only in life-threatening injuries.

Complete the following statement.

When a child experiences shock, usually the:

1. ____ **A.** skin is pale.
   B. skin is flushed.
2. ____ **A.** skin is dry.
   B. skin is moist.
3. ____ **A.** skin is hot.
   B. skin is cool.
4. ____ **A.** pupils are dilated.
   B. pupils are constricted.
5. ____ **A.** child feels hungry.
   B. child feels nauseous.
6. ____ **A.** breathing and pulse are rapid.
   B. breathing and pulse are slow.

Check the correct action.

A child begins to show signs of shock. Which of the following would you do?

1. ____ Give fluids to the child.
2. ____ Help a conscious child walk around to aid blood flow to the heart.
3. ____ Place a conscious child on his back and elevate the feet and legs, if no spinal injury is suspected.
4. ____ Elevate the head of a child having difficulty breathing.
5. ____ Use several blankets or jackets to warm up the child.

Match the position with the condition/injury.

Write *A, B, C,* or *D* to show the best position for a child with the condition or injury listed below.

Best position

A. Child on left side
B. Child flat on back with legs elevated 8 to 12 inches
C. Leave as found
D. Elevate the head and shoulders

Condition or injury

1. ____ Vomiting
2. ____ Unconscious
3. ____ Difficulty breathing
4. ____ Suspected spinal injuries
5. ____ Fainting

Severe Allergic Reaction (Anaphylactic Shock)

Check the causes of anaphylactic shock in sensitive people.

1. ____ Sting by bee
2. ____ Eating nuts
3. ____ Taking penicillin

Check the signs and symptoms of anaphylactic shock.

1. ____ Coughing and/or wheezing
2. ____ Breathing difficulty
3. ____ Bleeding from nose
4. ____ Intense itching and hives
5. ____ Fever
6. ____ Difficulty swallowing

Mark each statement true (T) or false (F) regarding severe allergic reactions.

1. ____ Although the child appears in distress, these reactions are not life threatening.
2. ____ The only really effective treatment for severe allergic reaction is an immediate injection of epinephrine.
3. ____ Some severe allergic reactions can be severe enough to require CPR.
4. ____ More than one dose of epinephrine might be needed.
5. ____ Epinephrine is only available with a physician's prescription.
6. ____ Mild symptoms of anaphylactic shock that appear slowly pose no risk to the child.

Fainting

Mark each statement true (T) or false (F).

1. ____ Lack of oxygen to the brain causes fainting.
2. ____ Recovery within five minutes usually occurs after a fainting episode.
3. ____ A person might report feeling dizzy or seeing spots just before fainting.
4. ____ When a child's face becomes red and dry, fainting might occur.

Mark each action yes (Y) or no (N).

What should you do for a child turning pale who complains about feeling dizzy?

1. ____ Prevent the child from falling.
2. ____ Place a cool wet cloth on the face.
3. ____ Place the child in a semisitting position.

Choose the best answer.

What should you do for a child who suddenly complains of dizziness and falls to the floor?

1. ____ **A.** Open the airway and check for breathing.
   B. Deliver abdominal thrusts.
2. ____ **A.** Give sips of clear fluid.
   B. Wipe the face with a cool, wet cloth.
3. ____ **A.** Lie the child flat on back with legs elevated 8-12 inches.
   B. Elevate head and shoulders.

5

Bleeding and Wounds

■ External Bleeding ■ Internal Bleeding ■ Abrasions ■ Lacerations ■
■ Puncture Wounds ■ Avulsions and Amputations ■ Animal Bites ■ Human Bites ■

Bleeding

When a blood vessel of any size is broken, there is bleeding. If the skin is broken, the bleeding is external and obvious. If the skin is not broken, the bleeding is internal and might not be immediately apparent.

The severity of an injury can be determined, in part, by the amount of bleeding and the time it takes to get it under control. This depends on the depth of the injury and the type of blood vessels that are damaged.

The most severe bleeding is from the arteries, the largest and deepest vessels in the body. Arteries carry blood away from the heart to all parts of the body under the strong pressure exerted by each heartbeat. Bright red arterial blood spurts from the wound with each beat of the heart and can be difficult to control—even life threatening. Injury to the arteries is uncommon because they are located deep within the body and are well protected.

Bleeding from veins is slower than from arteries because the blood is under less pressure. This blood is dark red in color. Blood loss from a vein can be significant, but because of the lower pressure, a bleeding vein can be easier to control.

Barriers between You and Blood

A covering that provides a protective shield between one person's blood and the skin of another is called a barrier. Barriers also protect a child with an open wound from contaminants on your hands. Examples of barriers include:

- Disposable rubber or latex gloves
- A plastic bag
- Several thick layers of gauze pads
- A large clean dish towel
- A folded cloth diaper

Additionally, plastic wrap placed over the gauze or cloth covering increases the effectiveness of these barriers.

Smaller blood vessels throughout the body are called capillaries. There are thousands of tiny capillaries throughout the surface of the skin. When broken, their oozing is the most easily controlled.

Some parts of the body have better circulation than others. The abundance of blood vessels in the head and face provide excellent circulation to this area, whereas such areas as hands, toes, and ears have fewer vessels and less circulation.

External Bleeding

Many children, as well as adults, become anxious at the sight of blood. In most situations, bleeding can be controlled in 5 to 10 minutes with proper first aid.

First Aid

- In cases of severe bleeding, check for consciousness by calling the child's name. Check and monitor the airway, breathing, and circulation, and treat accordingly.
- Send someone to call for emergency medical help, if needed.
- Stop the bleeding by using the following steps in the order given:

Step 1. Apply ***direct pressure.*** Most external bleeding can be controlled by direct pressure over the injury.

a. Cover the injury with several gauze pads, a cloth, or the cleanest covering available. Apply firm, direct pressure against this dressing to reduce the blood flow to the injured area. Direct pressure does not interrupt blood flow to the areas surrounding the bleeding wound. Keep the pad or cloth in place for 5 to 10 minutes without peeking. It will be easier to see the extent of the injury after the bleeding has slowed or stopped. As a barrier between you and the child's blood, wear disposable rubber or latex gloves, or use extra layers of gauze or cloth.

b. Add more gauze pads or cloths on top of the first dressing if it becomes soaked with blood.

■ BLEEDING ■

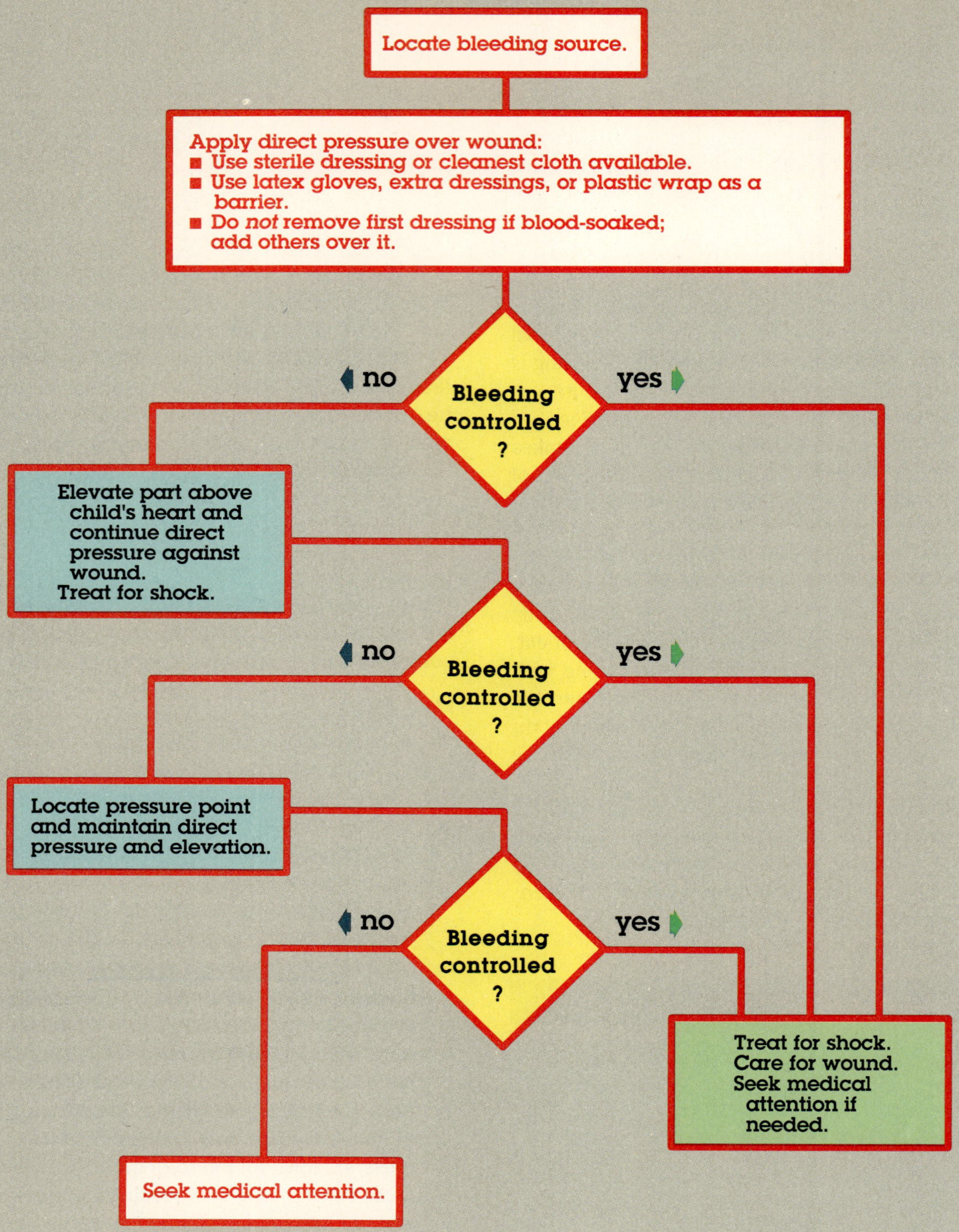
Locate bleeding source.
Apply direct pressure over wound:
■ Use sterile dressing or cleanest cloth available.
■ Use latex gloves, extra dressings, or plastic wrap as a barrier.
■ Do *not* remove first dressing if blood-soaked; add others over it.
no
Bleeding controlled ?
yes
Elevate part above child's heart and continue direct pressure against wound.
Treat for shock.
no
Bleeding controlled ?
yes
Locate pressure point and maintain direct pressure and elevation.
no
Bleeding controlled ?
yes
Treat for shock.
Care for wound.
Seek medical attention if needed.
Seek medical attention.

Do not remove the original dressing because the bleeding vessels will clot more quickly if undisturbed. *Clotting* is the process that thickens the blood at the injury to gradually stop the bleeding, seal the wound, and begin to heal it. It takes 3 to 5 minutes for clotting to begin, once the heavy flow of blood is reduced.

Step 2. ***Elevate*** the injured body part without releasing the direct pressure. This measure uses gravity to slow the flow of blood and to promote clotting, but it is not effective alone. It is most effective if the injured area is raised above the level of the heart. However, do not elevate if a fracture is suspected or if movement causes additional pain.

Step 3. After bleeding has stopped, maintain pressure with a ***pressure bandage.*** A pressure bandage is made by placing several gauze pads over the injury and securing them in place with a rolled gauze bandage, wrapped snugly and covering the dressing and wound area completely. A pressure bandage keeps firm pressure on the bleeding wound while allowing you freedom to attend to other injuries.

- Treat for shock. See Shock, Chapter 4.

Pressure Points

Pressure points are used only when direct pressure and elevation alone cannot control severe bleeding or when direct pressure cannot be applied to a bleeding wound due to a protruding broken bone or an embedded object, such as a piece of glass.

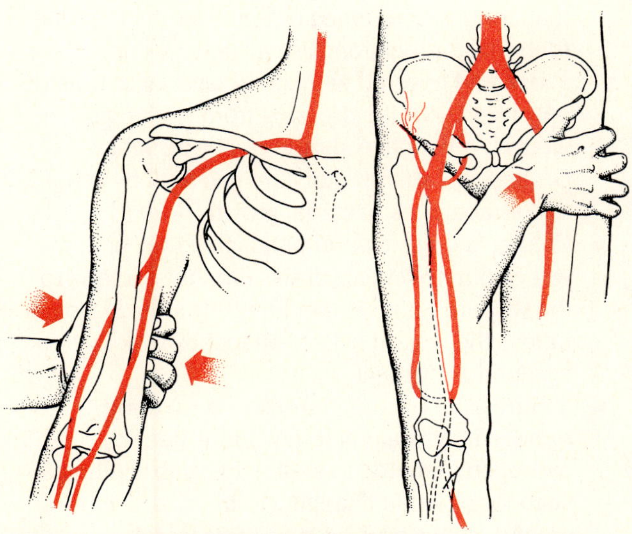

Brachial and femoral pressure point locations

Locating a Pressure Point

A pressure point is located between the injury and the heart where a main artery passes over a bone. Compressing the artery against the bone slows the flow of blood to the bleeding limb.

The most frequently used pressure points are the brachial and femoral, found on both sides of the body. Locate the brachial pressure point by placing your fingertips inside the upper arm, halfway between the elbow and armpit, in the groove between the muscles. Squeeze the arm firmly between the thumb and fingertips, keeping the fingers flat. Locate the femoral pressure point by placing the heel of your hand at the middle of the groin. Apply firm and steady pressure. See the Skill Scan, Controlling Bleeding.

Tourniquets

A tourniquet cuts off the circulation to the entire injured limb and is used to stop massive, life-threatening bleeding. However, future amputation of the injured limb is very likely following the use of a tourniquet. Because of this, tourniquets are rarely used. Do not attempt to apply a tourniquet and discourage others from doing so. With the first aid skills of direct pressure, elevation, and pressure points, you can manage even a severe bleeding emergency until more skilled help arrives.

Internal Bleeding

Internal bleeding occurs when blood vessels inside the body are broken but the skin over the injury remains intact.

Signs and Symptoms

When giving first aid for a severe blow or crushing injury such as in a motor vehicle accident, look for the following signs and symptoms of internal bleeding:

- Rapid pulse
- Cold, moist skin
- Nausea, or vomiting of red blood or blood that looks like coffee grounds
- Painful, tender, rigid abdomen
- Bruises anywhere on body
- Dilated pupils
- Anxiety and restlessness
- Thirst

First Aid

- Send someone to call for emergency medical help.
- Check and monitor airway, breathing, and circulation, and treat accordingly.
- Treat for shock. Serious internal bleeding is always accompanied by shock. If you do not suspect a spinal injury, raise the child's legs 8 to 12 inches and cover the child with a blanket or jacket to prevent heat loss. If a spinal injury is suspected, keep the child lying flat.
- If vomiting occurs, position the child on the side to prevent choking. If a spinal injury is suspected, roll the head, neck, and body as one unit.
- Give nothing to eat or drink.

Bruises

A bruise is minor internal bleeding in a soft tissue area of the body caused by a forceful blow. Bruises often accompany the good natured fun of active children engaged in vigorous play.

The skin bruises when blood vessels and other cells break. This causes immediate redness and sometimes swelling. Later the area turns blue or purple. As the blood is absorbed over the next few days the area turns yellow and then fades.

Apply ice wrapped in a cloth against the skin. Elevate the arm or leg if the bruise is large. If the bruise is unusually swollen or painful, the bone might be broken. Contact the child's health care provider.

Wounds

A wound is an injury that causes a break in the surface of the skin. Bleeding from a wound can be mild or severe, depending on the size, depth, and location of the wound.

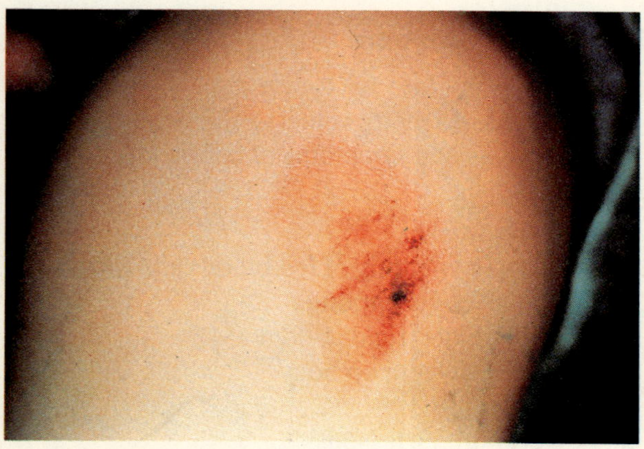

Abrasion

Abrasions

An abrasion is a scrape, or partial loss of the skin surface, such as a skinned elbow or knee that is accompanied by a small amount of bleeding or oozing of clear fluid. An abrasion is usually a minor wound, but it can be painful if it covers a large area or is located near a joint where it restricts movement.

First Aid

- Wear disposable gloves to wash the wound and surrounding area. Use soap and warm water, even if there is little or no bleeding. Take care to remove all dirt and debris. Hydrogen peroxide (available over the counter in a 3 percent solution) helps to clean the wound by loosening blood and dirt particles, although it does not kill bacteria. It does not sting and can be poured on liberally. Rinse the wound well and dry it with a sterile gauze pad.
- An antibacterial spray, cream, or ointment can be applied but is not necessary. Know your center's policy about the use of these products. Avoid old remedies such as Mercurochrome™, Merthiolate™, and iodine. These products can sting and irritate the skin and some can cause allergic reactions.
- *Dressings* should be sterile, or free of all microorganisms, and are applied directly against wounds. *Bandages* cover the dressings to hold them in place. A roll of wrapped gauze makes a good bandage because it can be used on any part of the body, including at the joints. Secure gauze wrap with tape. See Skill Scan, Bandaging, in this chapter.
- Leave a small, clean wound uncovered whenever possible.
- Use a dressing and bandage to cover a wound that continues to bleed or needs protection due to its size or location. Use a "nonstick" pad or a gauze pad covered with a thin layer of petroleum jelly to prevent the dressing from sticking to the wound. A bandage should not be airtight because it can trap moisture given off by the skin and encourages bacterial growth.
- Change a dressing and bandage if they become wet or dirty. Wetness draws dirt and bacteria to the wound. Remove them entirely after 24 hours unless the wound's location makes it likely to be bumped or stressed.
- If a dressing becomes stuck to the wound, remove it by soaking it in warm water or hydrogen peroxide to soften the scab. Pulling a scab loose while changing a dressing can be painful, slows healing, and increases the likelihood of infection.

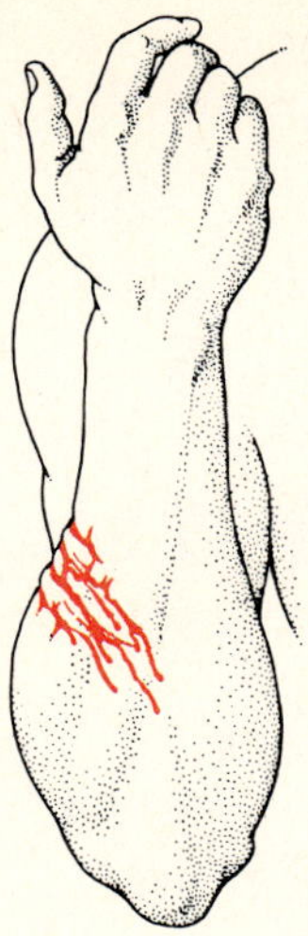

Laceration

Lacerations

A laceration is a deep wound with jagged, irregular edges that bleed freely. The amount of bleeding depends upon the size, depth, and location of the wound. A deep laceration can damage the underlying muscles, nerves, and tendons.

First Aid

- Remove any clothing covering the wound.
- Wear disposable gloves and use direct pressure and elevation, as needed, to control bleeding.
- Clean a superficial laceration with soap and water. Take care to remove all dirt and debris. Hydrogen peroxide (available over the counter in a 3 percent solution) can help to loosen blood and dirt particles, although it does not kill bacteria. It does not sting and can be poured on liberally. Rinse the wound well and dry it with a sterile gauze pad.
- Assess the need for suturing, or stitches. To do this, gently try to separate the edges of the laceration using gloved fingers. If the edges can be easily separated, if the laceration is deep or jagged, or if it is located on the face, it might need to be closed with stitches. The need for suturing is not always easy to assess. Call the child's parent if in doubt as to whether a laceration needs suturing. Apply a sterile dressing and bandage to protect the wound from contamination, if needed.
- A deep or large laceration with edges that are clearly separated will need suturing. Do not attempt to clean these more serious wounds because cleaning can damage torn edges. The laceration will be thoroughly cleaned by a health care provider before suturing. Cover the laceration with a sterile dressing and bandage to protect the wound. Ask the child's parent to contact the child's health care provider.

Suturing

Deep wounds need to be sutured, or stitched, to prevent infection and to promote faster healing with less scarring. The size of the wound as well as the location on the body help to determine whether sutures are necessary. The need for sutures should be evaluated by a health care provider within 4 to 6 hours after the injury. If more time is allowed to pass, the separate edges of the wound will begin to heal on their own and cannot mend together. The wound will heal more slowly, increasing the likelihood of infection and scarring.

Incisions

An incision is a cut with smooth edges that bleeds freely. "Incision" is a medical term referring to an intentional cut and is most often used in a controlled, sterile, surgical setting. See Lacerations.

Puncture Wounds

A puncture wound is an injury from a sharp object that pierces the skin and penetrates the underlying tissue. The entrance wound is usually small. Puncture wounds have a high rate of infection because they generally do not bleed and do not benefit from the cleansing effect that bleeding provides. Additionally, puncture wounds are sometimes so deep that air does not reach them and bacteria can become sealed inside. Many strains of bacteria including tetanus thrive under such conditions.

Puncture wounds vary in severity from minor wounds caused by a splinter, staple, safety pin, thumbtack, or nail to more severe wounds from sharp scissors or an arrow.

First Aid

- Do not remove an object if it is deeply embedded. Secure it in place and have the child seen immediately in an emergency medical facility. See the sections on abdominal injuries, chest injuries, and eye injuries for specific treatment of deep puncture wounds.
- Remove objects that are barely penetrating or loosely hanging with clean fingers. Tweezers are effective for removing small splinters. Never dig beneath the child's skin to remove a splinter.
- Clean minor puncture wounds with soap and

■ AMPUTATION ■

Control bleeding.

Care for severed part:
1. Wrap part in dry sterile gauze or clean cloth.
2. Put wrapped part in waterproof container (plastic bag, cup, etc.).
3. Place wrapped part and container on bed of ice; do *not* submerge in ice or cold water.

Seek medical attention.

warm water. A small amount of bleeding can be encouraged by gently squeezing the area to force a little bleeding while washing. This is good because it helps to clean the wound.

- Notify the child's parent if the puncture wound is deep and the child needs to be seen by a health care provider.

Wound Care Follow-Up

Any wound, even one that has received the most careful treatment, can become infected after an injury. Many small wounds develop superficial infections in the course of healing that the body's defenses can handle alone. Occasionally, however, a wound develops a more serious infection, and medical treatment becomes necessary.

Observe a healing wound daily for signs of a developing infection. Try to keep all bandages clean and dry. This will reduce the risk of infection.

Signs and Symptoms

- Pain and tenderness
- Swelling
- Pus
- Skin warm to the touch around the wound
- Redness around the wound or red streaks leading away from the wound
- Fever

Avulsions and Amputations

An avulsion is a partial tearing of body tissue. An amputation is the complete severing of a body part. Both injuries can involve damage to the skin, muscles, tendons, nerves, bones, and blood vessels. It is sometimes possible for an avulsed or amputated body part to be successfully repaired if it receives proper first aid and is surgically reattached within a few hours after the injury. Examples of injuries that can result in an avulsion or amputation are an animal bite that tears a child's nose and cheek or a finger slammed in a heavy door.

First Aid

- Send someone to call for emergency medical help.
- Wear disposable gloves and use direct pressure, elevation, and pressure points, as needed, to control bleeding.
- Treat for shock.
- Rinse the amputated part but do not attempt to clean it. Avoid touching torn edges. Cleaning and excessive handling might damage the torn tissues. Wrap the amputated part in dry gauze or other available dry clean cloth. Place on bed of ice but avoid burying it.

Tetanus

Tetanus is a grave disease that causes strong, painful spasms in the back, arms, legs, and jaw—hence its other name, "lockjaw." The disease is usually fatal. Fortunately, however, because of widespread immunization, most residents of the United States are immune to the disease; in this country there are only about 100 deaths from tetanus each year, far below the world average.

Tetanus bacteria live in soil, dust, and human and animal feces. It is usually introduced into the human body by a sharp object that pierces the skin, but they can enter through any opening in the skin that becomes contaminated with material containing the bacteria. Puncture wounds, because they can be deep and are difficult to clean, are the most likely wounds to become infected with the tetanus bacteria. Furthermore, puncture wounds close and the tetanus bacteria are trapped inside where they thrive in an environment with little or no oxygen. In this environment the bacteria produce a toxin that attacks the central nervous system and brain.

Tetanus can be completely prevented through immunization. Immunization enables the immune system to manufacture its own antitoxin against a future exposure to tetanus. Children should receive a series of five tetanus immunization injections by the age of 6. They should receive a booster in the early adolescent years, and then every 10 years thereafter. Immunizations are the best defense against tetanus.

Animal Bites

Dogs are responsible for approximately 60 to 90 percent of all animal bites in the United States each year. Of the 1.5 million serious dog bites reported annually, approximately 80 percent of these bites involve preschool or school-age children. Often, children own or know the dog that bites them. Frequently, bites are provoked by the child's teasing or mistreating the animal. See Dog Safety, Chapter 13. Cats are less likely to bite than dogs, but cat bites are more likely to become infected. Wild animals, such as raccoons, skunks, chipmunks, and squirrels are also known to bite.

If an animal bite breaks the child's skin, infection can occur. The most dangerous infection is rabies, a viral disease. The rabies virus is present in the saliva of an infected animal and is transmitted to a child through a bite wound. The disease affects the brain and nervous system and eventually causes death unless the child receives immediate preventive treatment in the form of a vaccine given in a series of injections.

Any warm-blooded animal can carry rabies. However, the animals most commonly infected are raccoons, bats, skunks, foxes, and coyotes. According to the Centers for Disease Control, more than 80 percent of rabies cases in the United States occur in skunks, raccoons, and bats. A bite from a stray cat or dog is also of concern because these animals have not been immunized. If a child is bitten by one of the animals thought to carry rabies, it must be assumed that the animal has rabies, and the child should receive the rabies vaccine.

Household dogs and cats are generally considered rabies-free in many metropolitan areas. Nevertheless, you should check with the animal's owner if a child is bitten to be sure that the animal's immunizations are up to date. Small animals that are popular in child care centers such as hamsters, gerbils, and guinea pigs are generally healthy and do not carry rabies because they are not exposed to the wild.

Many of the animals known to carry rabies are nocturnal. Should you see one of these animals, assume that it is sick or hungry because it otherwise would not be wandering during the day. Stay away from the animal and call the animal control officer in your community to report your concern and the animal's location.

First Aid

- Wearing disposable gloves, wash the wound with soap and warm water unless the wound is bleeding heavily. A small amount of bleeding while washing helps to remove the bacteria from the tissue.
- Use direct pressure, as needed, to control bleeding.
- Animal bites that break the skin should be examined by a health care provider. Cover the wound with a sterile dressing and bandage. Encourage the parent to contact the child's health care provider.
- Animal bites that do not break the skin should be washed with soap and water and left uncovered. Notify the parent at the end of the day.

Human Bites

Biting occasionally occurs among small children who have not yet learned socially acceptable behavior for meeting their needs. Many of these bites are minor and more of an emotional upset than a physical injury. However, the human mouth contains a large number of bacteria, some of which can cause infection if introduced into another's blood through a bite. The likelihood of infection from a human bite is greater than from an animal bite.

First Aid

- Wearing disposable gloves, thoroughly wash the wound with soap and warm water. Bites that break the skin, however small, introduce bacteria into the blood. Bites that do not break the skin are not serious.
- Notify the child's parent immediately if the bite breaks the skin. The child might need a tetanus shot or antibiotics.
- If the skin is not broken, you may wait until the end of the school day to notify the parent.

Repeated biting is unacceptable behavior in a child care center. The problem should be dealt with on a case-by-case basis.

■ ANIMAL BITES ■

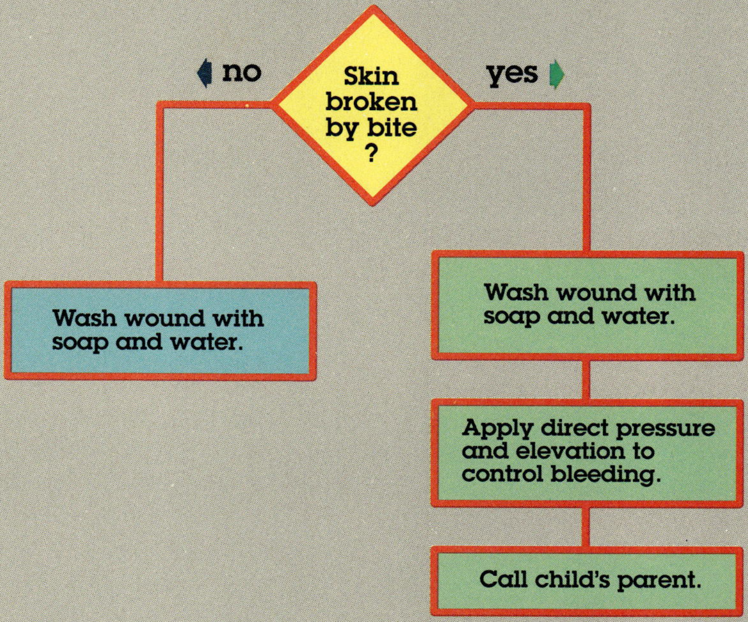

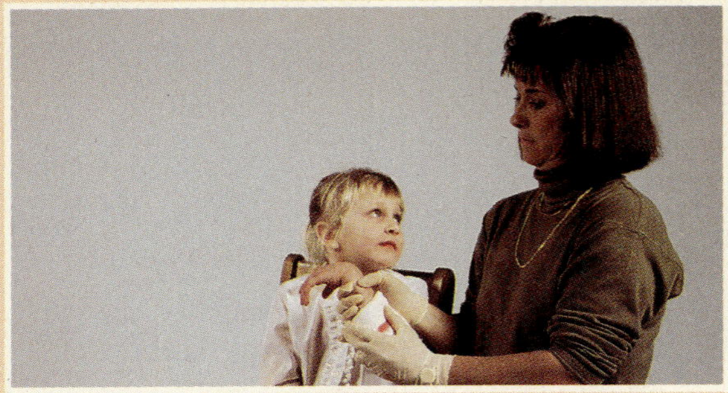

1. Direct pressure using dressing.

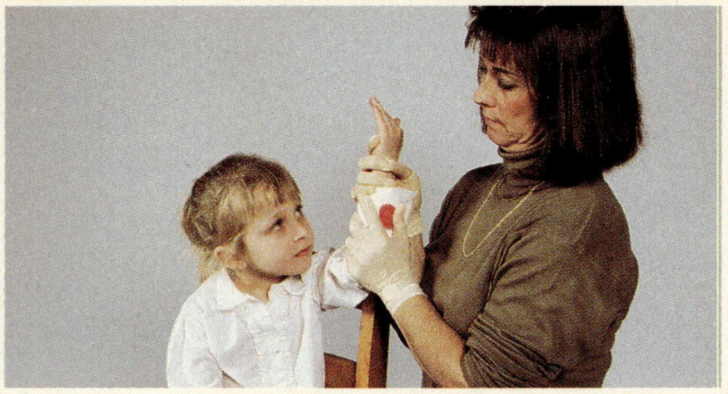

2. Combine direct pressure and elevation.

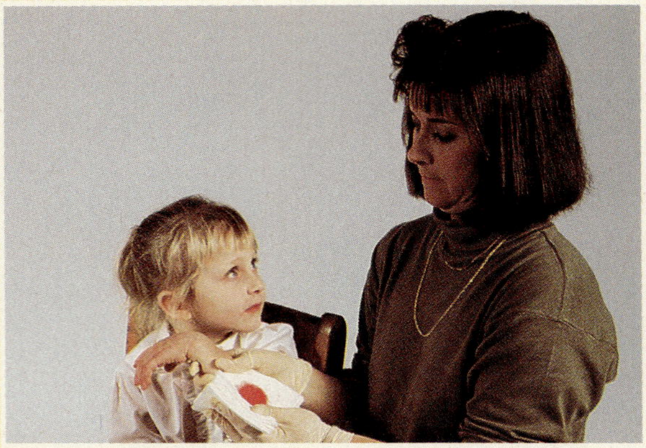

3. Reinforce blood-soaked dressing with more gauze.

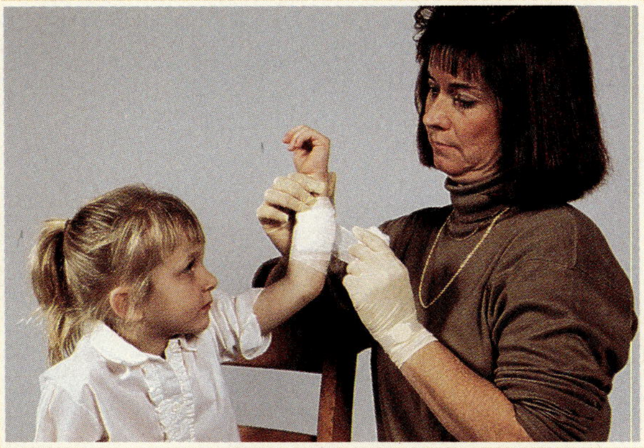

4. Pressure bandage.

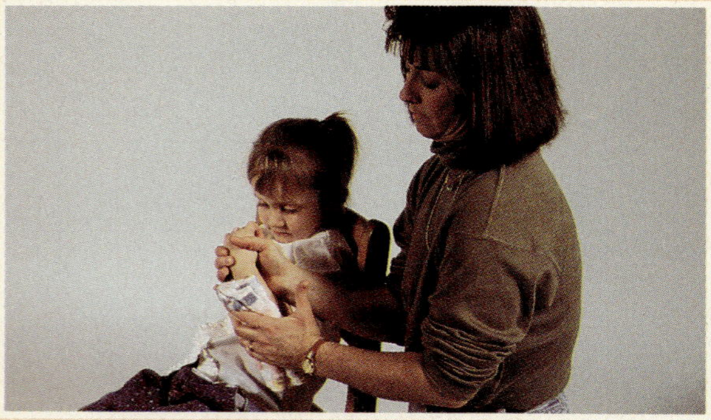

5. Direct pressure using thick barrier when gloves not available.

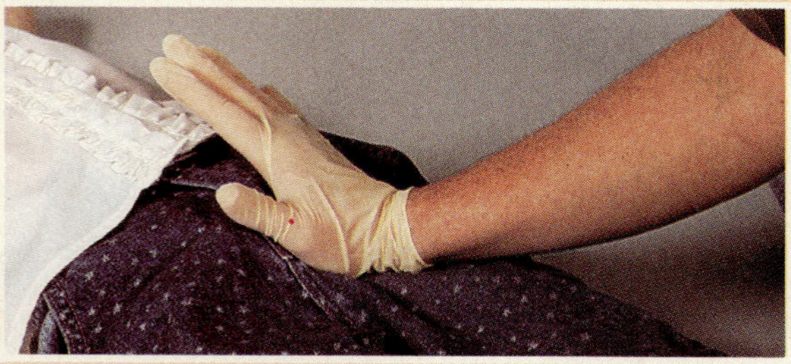

7. Femoral pressure point.

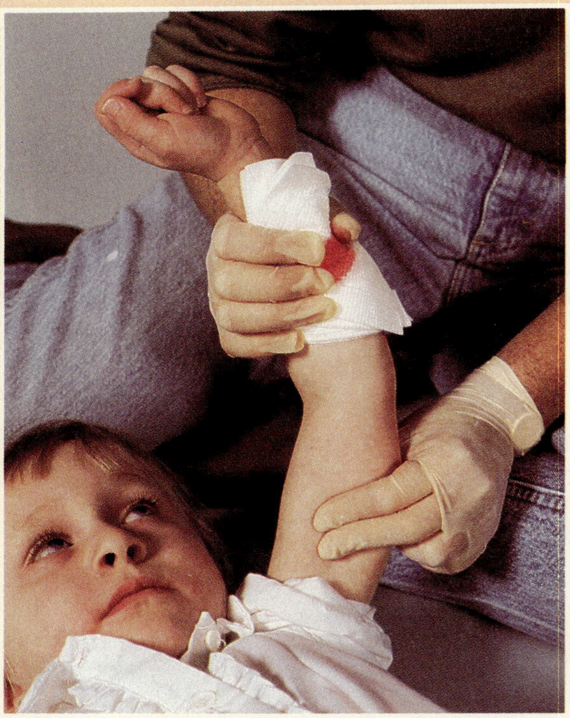

6. Brachial pressure point.

A Figure-of-Eight bandage secures a dressing in place on an arm or leg.

Dressing and bandaging a hand wound.

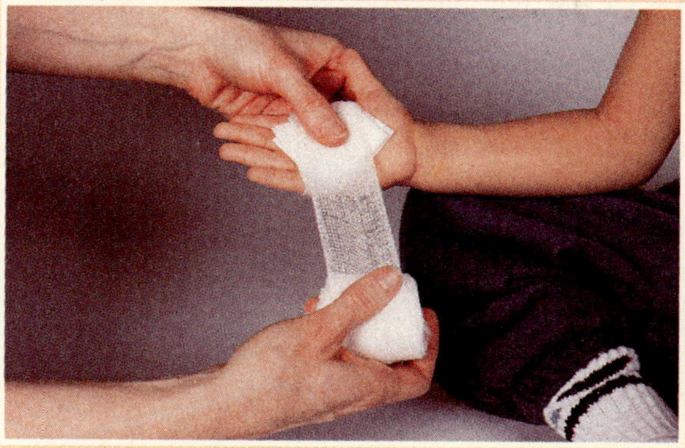

1.

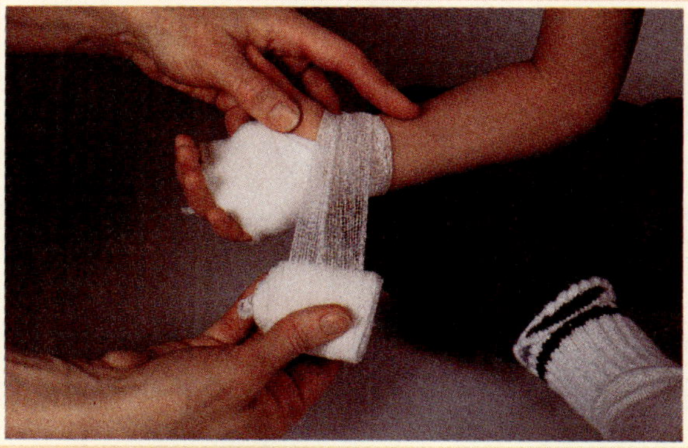

2.

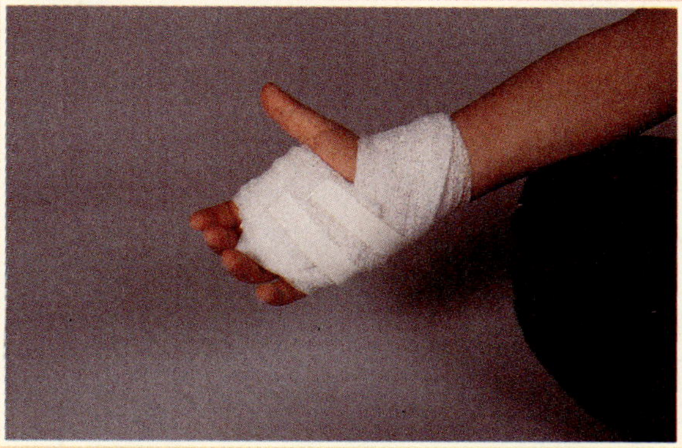

3.

Dressing and bandaging a forearm wound.

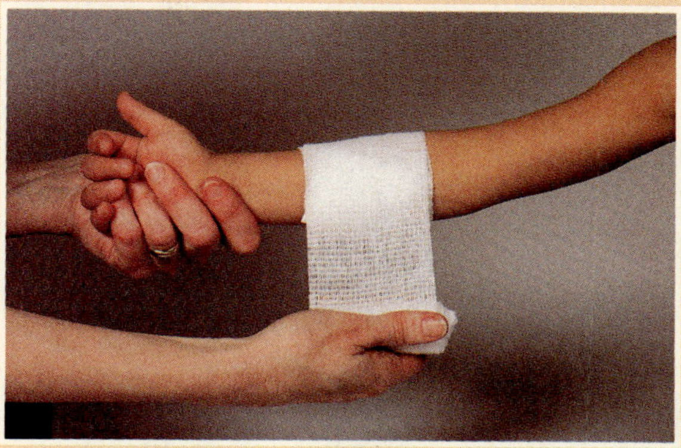

1.

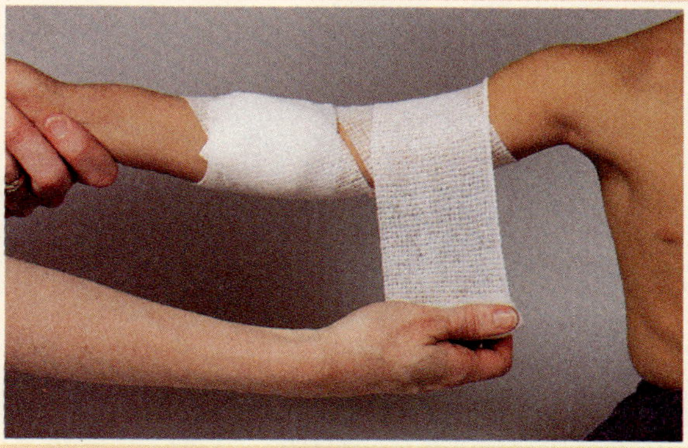

2.

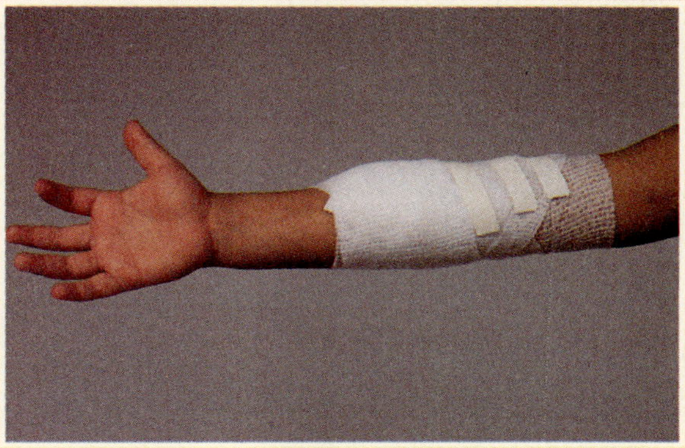

3.

Dressing and bandaging a foot wound.

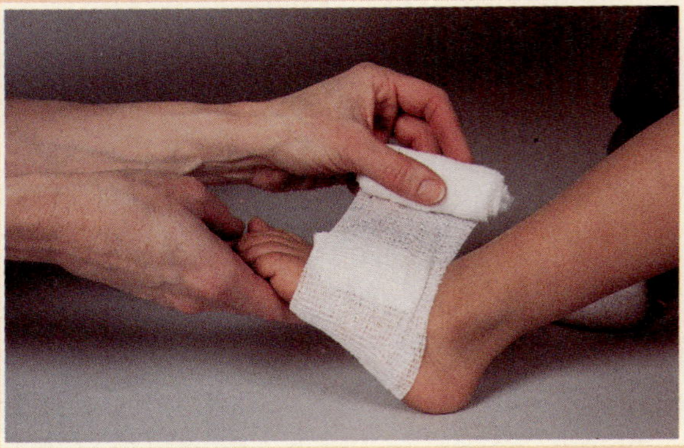

1.

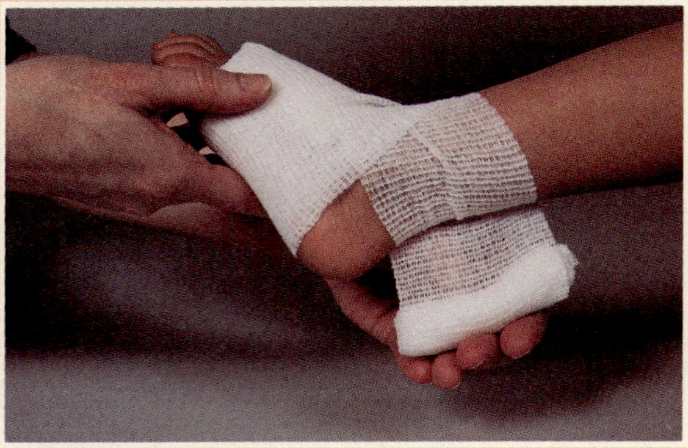

2.

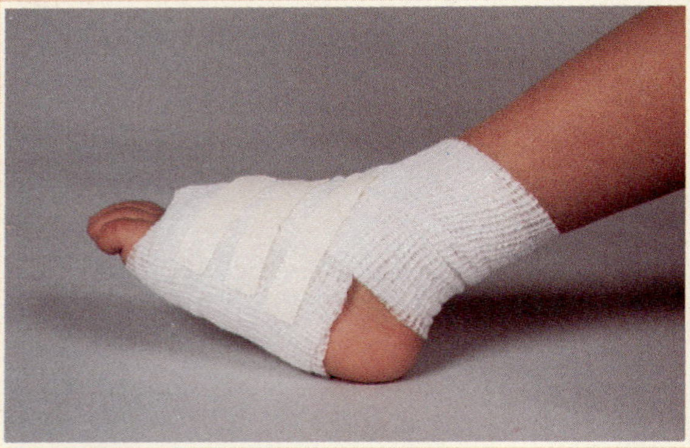

3.

Dressing and bandaging a head wound using a rolled gauze bandage.

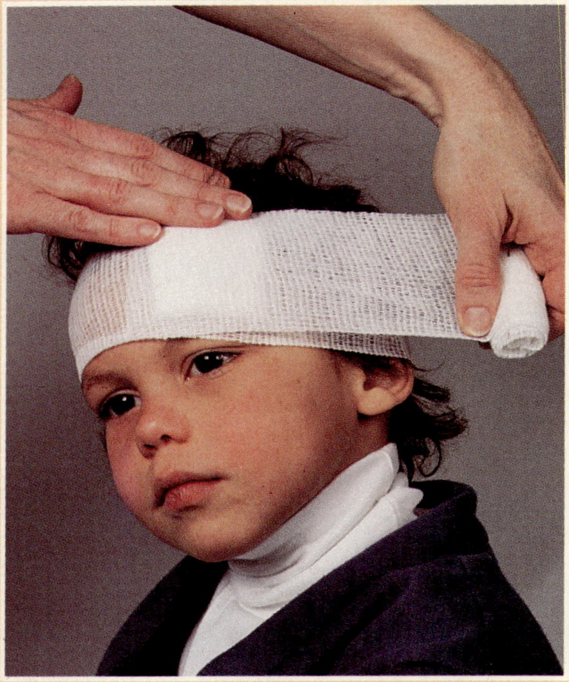

1.

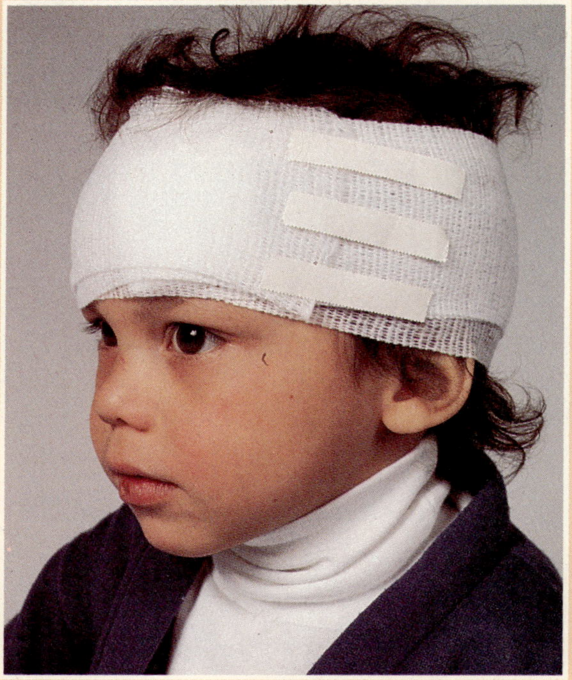

2.

Bleeding and Wounds

Mark each statement true (T) or false (F).

1. ____ Loss of blood occurs only in external bleeding.
2. ____ Internal bleeding occurs when blood vessels beneath the skin are broken.
3. ____ Bleeding from veins is usually fast and in spurts.
4. ____ Arterial bleeding is usually more serious than venous bleeding.
5. ____ A first aider should wear disposable latex or rubber gloves when treating a bleeding wound.

Check (√) which of the following action(s) should be taken to control bleeding when blood is flowing freely from a wound.

1. ____ Place firm, direct pressure on the wound.
2. ____ If the arm is elevated to control bleeding, release the direct pressure.
3. ____ Use a pressure point alone if direct pressure fails to stop the bleeding.

Mark each statement true (T) or false (F).

1. ____ Hydrogen peroxide is helpful in cleaning a wound.
2. ____ Apply an airtight bandage over a minor wound to prevent infection.
3. ____ Sutures can be placed as long as 24 hours after an injury occurs.
4. ____ Dressings and bandages must be changed if they become wet or dirty.
5. ____ Wounds are sutured primarily to reduce infection and scarring.
6. ____ There is a difference between a dressing and a bandage.

Choose the best answer regarding types of wounds.

1. ____ **Skinned elbows and knees are examples of which type of wound?**
   A. Incisions
   B. Avulsions
   C. Lacerations
   D. Abrasions
2. ____ **Which type of wound has a jagged, irregular edge?**
   A. Incision
   B. Laceration
   C. Bruise
   D. Puncture wound
3. ____ **Which type of wound is caused by a sharp, pointed object such as a nail or splinter?**
   A. Abrasion
   B. Avulsion
   C. Puncture
   D. Laceration
4. ____ **Which of the following is most susceptible to tetanus?**
   A. Laceration
   B. Amputation
   C. Incision
   D. Puncture
5. ____ **Which of the following describes bleeding from a vein?**
   A. Spurting
   B. Slow and even stream

Choose the best answer regarding dressings.

1. ____ **Use of a sterile dressing on a laceration will:**
   A. kill any bacteria present in the wound.
   B. reduce further contamination of the wound.
   C. prevent shock.
2. ____ **If bleeding soaks through a dressing, the first aider should:**
   A. remove the blood-soaked dressing and replace it with another dressing.
   B. leave the dressing in place and add another dressing on top of it.

Mark each statement yes (Y) or no (N).

Prevent infection by:

1. ____ Immediately washing a wound with soap and water.
2. ____ Covering an open wound with an airtight dressing and bandage.

Tetanus

Mark each statement true (T) or false (F).

1. ____ One dose of tetanus vaccine provides adequate defense against tetanus for a lifetime.
2. ____ The type of wound most susceptible to tetanus is a puncture wound because the bacteria can live inside the wound without oxygen.

Human and Animal Bites

Mark each statement true (T) or false (F).

1. ____ Animal bites that break the skin should be treated by a health care provider.
2. ____ Unless the wound is bleeding heavily, wash the wound first with soap and warm water.
3. ____ Family pets are the leading rabies carriers.
4. ____ Both warm-blooded and cold-blooded animals can carry rabies.
5. ____ A wound from an animal bite is more likely to become infected than a wound from a human bite.

6

Specific Body Area Injuries

■ Head Injuries ■ Eye Injuries ■ Nosebleeds ■ Dental Injuries ■ Chest Injuries ■ Abdominal Injuries ■ Removal of Foreign Objects ■ Blisters ■ Splinters ■ Bleeding Under a Fingernail ■ Nail Avulsion ■

Head Injuries

Head injuries are common during the childhood years. They can be superficial, with bruising and swelling of the skin, such as a goose egg, or severe enough to cause permanent internal brain damage or death. The Centers for Disease Control estimates that falls account for more than half of all head injuries in children under the age of 5. Among children ages 5 to 9, head injuries are caused equally by sports, falls, and motor vehicle accidents.

> - Almost 30 percent of all childhood injury deaths result from head injuries.
> - Each year, an estimated 29,000 children suffer permanent disability from moderate or severe head injury.
>
> *Statistics taken from the Centers for Disease Control:* Childhood Injuries in the United States, *June 1990.*

Because head injuries are such a common occurrence, parents and child care providers must be able to assess the severity of a head injury as well as to provide first aid.

Bump on the head

During the first few years of life when young children are learning to crawl, climb, and walk, small bumps on the head are an everyday occurrence. Because there is little fat and other soft tissue surrounding the skull to absorb the blood and other fluids released from such an injury, this fluid collects under the skin in one bulging area known as a goose egg. Keep in mind that a child with a minor bump on the head will not lose consciousness. Apply ice wrapped in a cloth to decrease swelling and observe for signs and symptoms of internal head injury. See Internal Head Injury.

Scalp Wound

The severity of a cut, or wound on the head can be deceiving because the head has a rich supply of blood vessels so that even minor wounds tend to bleed heavily. Because of this rich supply of blood, cuts on the head rarely become infected.

Control bleeding from these wounds by applying light pressure directly on the wound and assess the need for sutures. See Sutures, Chapter 5. Bleeding should stop with 5–10 minutes of direct pressure. Apply ice wrapped in a cloth to decrease swelling and observe for signs and symptoms of internal head injury.

Internal Head Injury

Internal head injury refers to damage within the skull. A **skull fracture** is a break or crack in the skull bone. **Concussions** and **contusions** are conditions that result from a violent jarring of the brain. In all of these injuries, damage can result from the increased pressure caused by the bleeding and swelling that often occurs.

Since the bones of the skull cannot expand to accommodate bleeding and swelling, pressure is exerted against the brain tissue resulting in some or all of the following signs and symptoms:

Signs and Symptoms

- Unconsciousness. Any child who loses consciousness for more than 5 to 10 seconds immediately following a head injury should be examined in an emergency medical facility immediately. A child might appear stunned for several seconds following a head injury, but this is not the same as unconsciousness.
- Pupils of unequal size. The small, black, round centers of the child's eyes should be of equal size and should become smaller when exposed to light.
- Seizure (convulsion).
- Skull depression. A depressed skull fracture is most often seen in infants because their skull bones are especially fragile.
- Clear fluid (spinal fluid) dripping from the nose or collecting in the ear(s).
- Unusual sleepiness. Sleeping will not worsen the child's condition. The worry is that a sleeping

child cannot be observed for changes in behavior and level of consciousness.

- Confusion or dizziness. A child can be upset after a head injury but should know where he or she is and what happened.
- Severe headache lasting more than several hours. Never give any pain medication, including acetaminophen or aspirin, to a child who has suffered a head injury unless instructed to do so by a health care provider.
- Unusual swelling of an infant's soft spot, the fontanel, located on the top of the head.
- Difficulty with speech or vision.
- Difficulty with walking.
- Vomiting more than once.
- Pale, sweaty appearance.

Even if there is no visible skull injury, there might still be an internal head injury. The signs and symptoms in the preceding list are much better indicators than cuts or bruises on the skull.

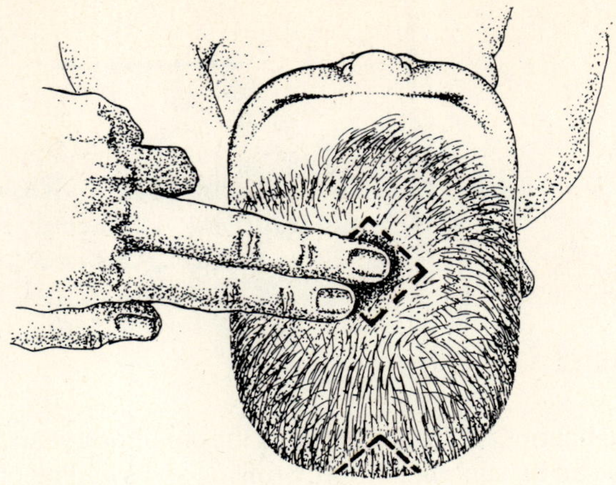

Location of infant fontanels (soft spots)

First Aid

- Check for consciousness by calling the child's name. Check and monitor the airway, breathing, and circulation and treat accordingly. Any child who loses consciousness after a violent head injury must be treated as if a spinal injury has occurred. NEVER MOVE AN UNCONSCIOUS CHILD EXCEPT TO SAVE A LIFE. See Spinal Injuries, Chapter 10.
- Send someone to call for emergency medical help, if needed.
- If the child is breathing but unconscious, keep the child in the position in which found. Immobilize the head, neck, and body by padding them with towels, blankets, or jackets, without changing the child's position.
- Cover the child to prevent heat loss.

If the child is conscious and breathing and you do **not** *suspect a spinal injury, continue with the following steps:*

- Control bleeding by applying light pressure directly on the wound and assess the need for sutures. See Sutures, Chapter 5. If there is a skull depression, apply light pressure to the bony area surrounding the wound.
- Apply ice or a cold pack to the injury to decrease swelling that can occur. Wrap the ice or cold pack in a cloth to protect the skin.
- Give nothing to eat or drink until the child is well enough to continue a normal routine.
- Observe the child for signs and symptoms of an internal head injury. Any child who suffers a head injury, no matter how minor, should be observed for delayed symptoms for 48 to 72 hours following the injury. It is important for child care providers to let parents know if a head injury occurs so they can watch the child at home. If the child shows any signs or symptoms of internal head injury, the child's health care provider should be contacted immediately.

Infants have soft spots, called fontanels, under the skin of the scalp where the skull bones have not yet grown together. They are especially vulnerable to head injuries because the brain is not well protected in these areas. Therefore, any infant who receives a blow to the head should be examined by a health care provider even if initially there are no signs of internal injury. You should continue to look for swelling of the fontanels for 48 to 72 hours following the injury.

A child who does not lose consciousness and who quickly returns to normal activity is probably fine. You should continue to be alert, however, for drowsiness, vomiting, headache, or any of the signs of a more serious injury. If you are uncertain of a child's condition, whether or not unconsciousness has occurred, contact the child's health care provider by phone.

Eye Injuries

Penetrating Injuries

Almost all penetrating eye injuries are obvious. You should suspect penetration whenever you see an eyelid laceration or cut. Sometimes first aiders concentrate on the eyelid injury and neglect the underlying eye injury. A penetrating injury requires immediate ophthalmological attention.

Cold Pack Alternatives

Some ways to apply cold to an injured area to reduce swelling after an injury include:

1. Crushed ice in a baggie.
2. Wet washcloth placed in a baggie and kept in the refrigerator.
3. Commercial "snap pack" ice packs.
4. Frozen vegetables and other frozen foods.
5. Popsicle placed directly on the skin when treating an injury inside the mouth.

Never place cold packs directly against a child's skin. Always wrap the cold pack in a cloth to protect the skin.

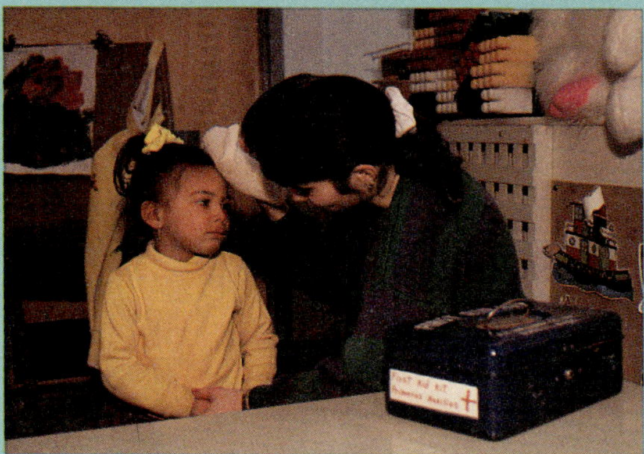

Applying cold to an injured area to reduce swelling

- Do NOT remove foreign objects stuck in the eye.
- Protect the injured eye with a paper cup to keep the object from being pushed deeper into the eye. Rest the cup on several thick gauze pads and tape into place.
- Because both eyes move in unison, covering the uninjured eye will protect the injured eye from further movement and damage.
- Keep the child flat on the back.
- Have the child seen in an emergency medical facility immediately.

Blow to the Eye*

Gently place a cold pack on the bones around the injured eye for 10 to 15 minutes to reduce pain and swelling. A black eye or blurred vision could mean internal eye damage and indicates that the child should be seen as soon as possible by a health care provider.

**Source: Adapted from the American Academy of Ophthalmologists.*

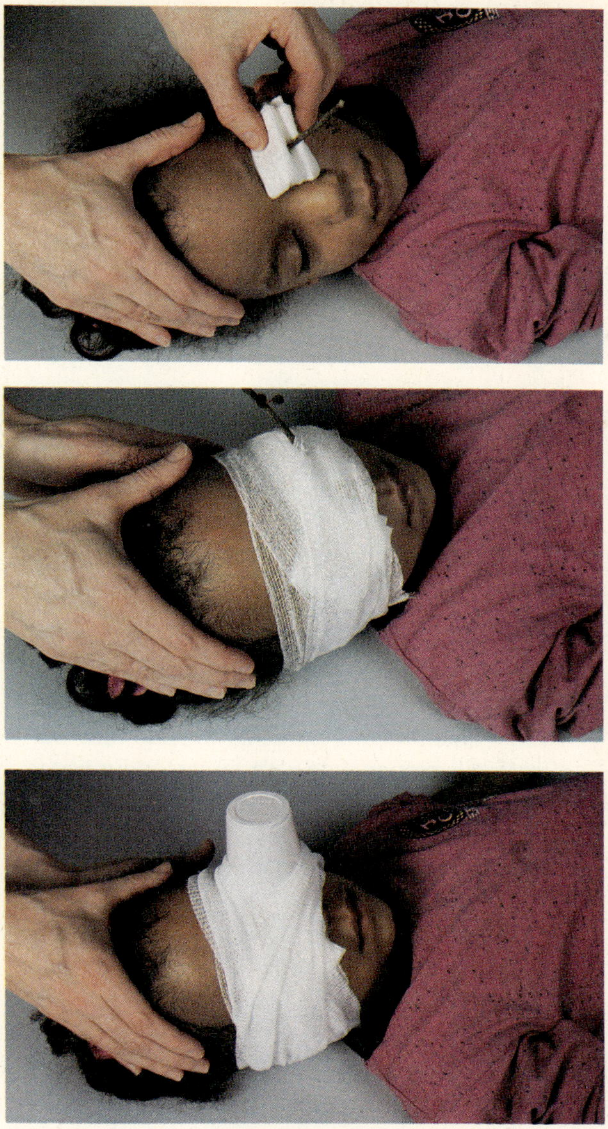

Bandaging an eye using a paper cup

Avulsion of the Eye

An extremely violent blow to the face can cause an eye to be partially torn from its socket. This is called an avulsion.

- Do not attempt to push the eye back into the socket.
- Cover the injured eye loosely with a sterile dressing that has been moistened with clean water. Then cover the eye with a paper cup and follow the same first aid procedure as for a penetrating injury.
- Because both eyes move in unison, covering the uninjured eye will protect the injured eye from further movement and damage.

Cuts of the Eye and Lid*

- Do not attempt to flush the eye with water.
- Do not apply pressure to the injured eye or eyelid.
- Cover both eyes with gauze pads and bandage lightly.
- Keep the child in a semisitting position.
- Have the child seen by a health care provider.

Chemical Injury*

A chemical burn in an eye requires immediate first aid treatment to prevent damage to the cornea. An eye that appears only slightly red at first might later develop deep inflammation and tissue damage, depending on the chemical and the length of exposure before treatment starts.

- Flush the chemical from the eye with warm water immediately. Position the child's head over a sink with the affected side down to prevent contaminating the other eye. Holding the injured eye open with your fingers, pour water from an unbreakable cup or pitcher into the eye for 15 minutes. Always wash from the inside of the eye toward the outside. You may need to wrap a young child in a large towel to hold the child still.
- Have someone call the poison control center immediately.
- Loosely bandage both eyes. This will protect the injured eye from further movement and damage because both eyes move in unison. Secure the pads with strips of gauze, as illustrated.

**Source: Adapted from the American Academy of Ophthalmologists.*

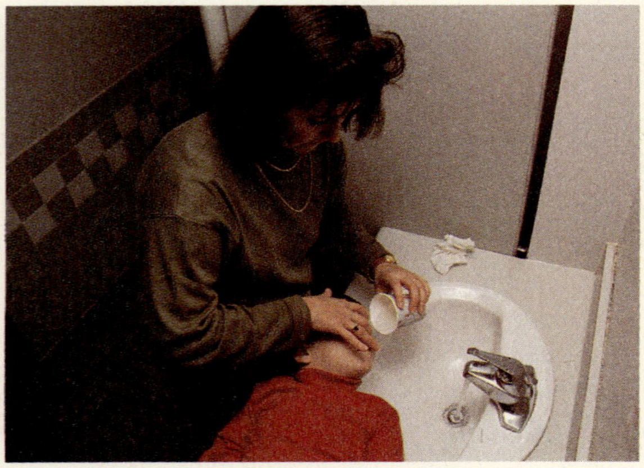

Flushing a chemical from an eye with warm water

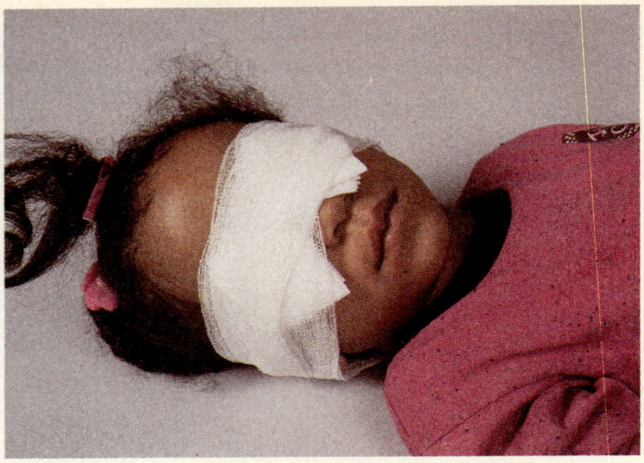

Bandaging both eyes

- Take the child for further medical treatment if instructed to do so by the poison control center.

Foreign Object

Bits of sand, dirt, insects, and eye lashes are examples of foreign objects that commonly get caught in a child's eye causing discomfort and watering eyes. Discourage a child from rubbing the eyes because this motion can scratch the cornea, the transparent outer covering of the eyeball. A corneal scratch not only damages the cornea but can also introduce infection.

- Pull down the child's lower eyelid and look at the inner surface while the child looks up. A speck of dirt or a bug can usually be removed with the corner of a clean, white cotton handkerchief. Do not use cotton swabs or tissues because they can deposit their own fibers in the eye. If you cannot see the object, it might be under the upper lid. Gently grasp the upper lid and pull it out and down over the lower eyelid. Flush the eye with warm water if you still cannot find the object and the child continues to be uncomfortable.

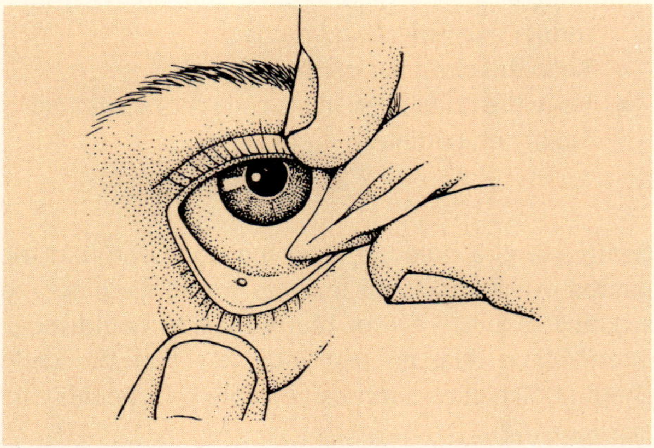

Removing a small floating object with the corner of a clean, white cotton handkerchief

■ HEAD INJURY ■

Check ABCHs and treat accordingly.

Is head bleeding?

- **yes** → If skull fracture suspected, apply pressure only to the surrounding bony area; otherwise apply light pressure directly on wound.
- **no** → (continue)

Is child unconscious?

- **no** →
  - Elevate head and shoulders slightly. If spinal injury suspected, keep child in position found.
  - Apply cold pack to injury. Observe for signs and symptoms of internal head injury.
  - Seek medical attention if:
    - ■ Unconsciousness occurred temporarily
    - ■ Child needs sutures
    - ■ Any of the signs and symptoms of internal head injury appear
- **yes** →
  - Check ABCHs and treat accordingly. Keep child in position found.
  - Seek medical attention immediately.

■ EYE INJURIES ■

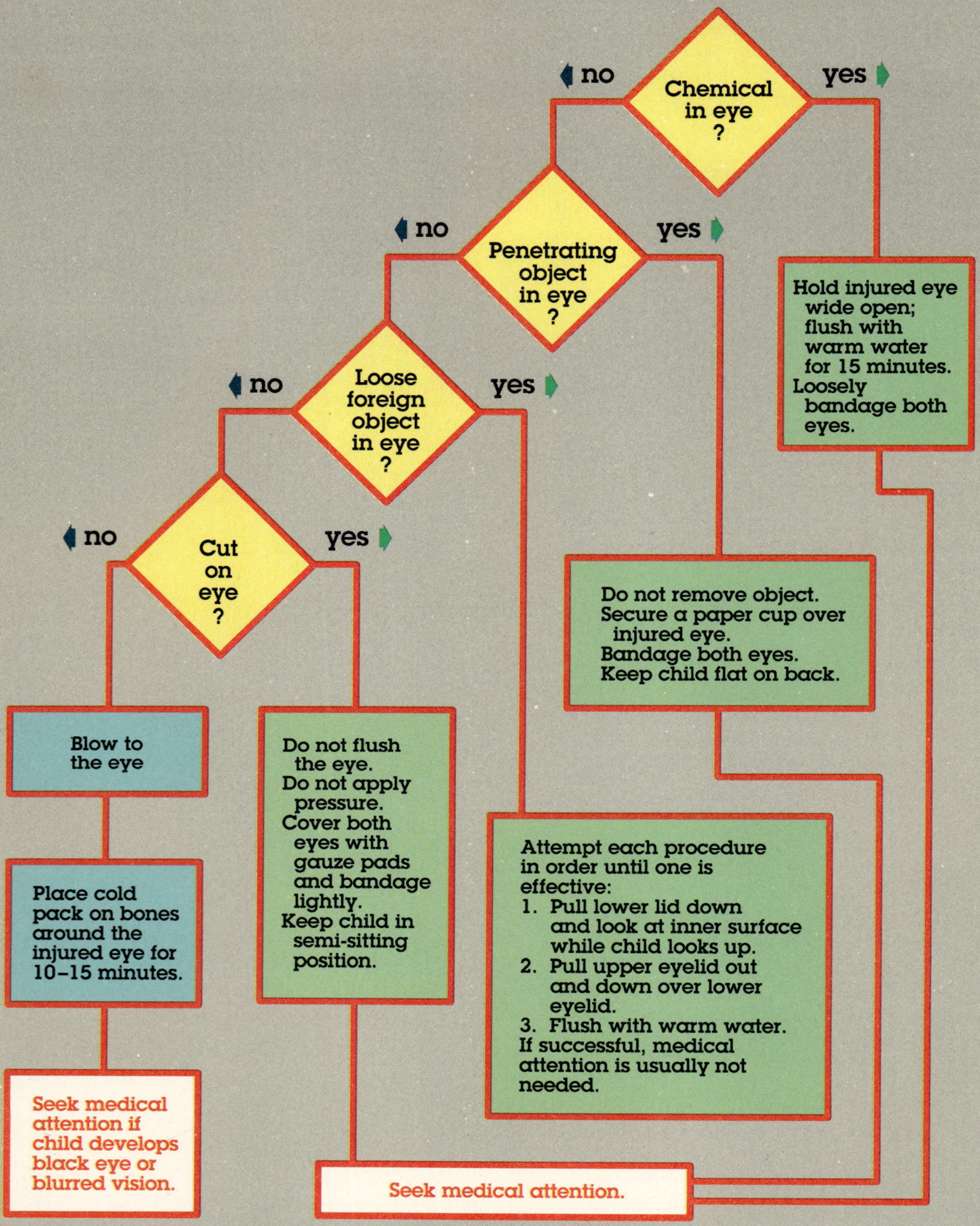

- Have the child seen by a health care provider if the eye continues to be red, watering, or painful longer than 10 to 15 minutes after treatment. The foreign body might have scratched the surface of the eye, and this injury cannot be detected without special instruments.

Nosebleeds

Nosebleeds are generally more annoying than serious, especially in young children. It is the sometimes abrupt appearance of a nosebleed that alarms adults. A bump to the nose can cause a nosebleed, but so can crying, laughing, running hard, and picking at the nose. Bleeding can seem heavier than it actually is; a tissue that appears very bloody might contain only a tiny amount of blood. However, all nosebleeds should be reported to parents by child care providers. If the child received a direct, forceful blow to the nose, suspect a fracture.

First Aid

Most nosebleeds stop on their own as the capillaries clot off.

- With your thumb and index finger, pinch the nostrils together below the bridge, on the soft part of the nose. Squeeze for 10 minutes, without letting go to check the progress.
- Tilt the head forward so that the blood will run out of the nose rather than down the throat. Blood is very irritating to the stomach and can cause the child to feel nauseated and vomit.
- Have the child seen by a health care provider if the bleeding cannot be controlled. Parents should discuss frequent, unprovoked nosebleeds with their health care provider.

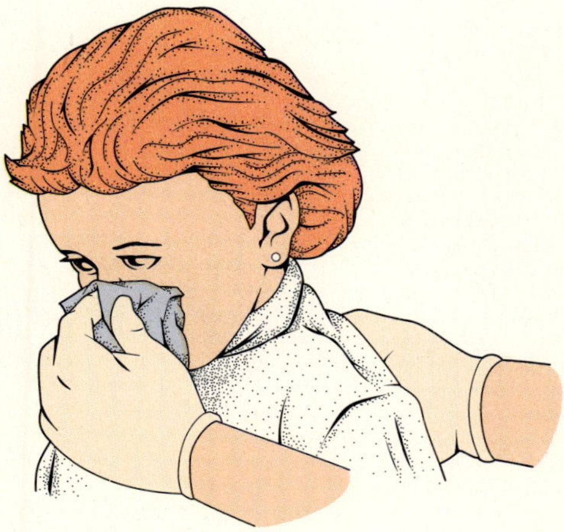

Nosebleed

Care after a Nosebleed

1. Encourage child not to pick or rub the nose.
2. Keep the nostrils moist by applying a little petroleum jelly just inside the nostrils twice a day.
3. Use a cool mist vaporizer in the child's sleeping area when air is dry during the winter months.

Dental Injuries

The following first aid procedures provide temporary relief for dental emergencies, but it is important to consult with a dentist as soon as possible.

Knocked-Out Tooth

In the United States, more than 2 million teeth are accidentally knocked out each year. More than 90 percent of them can be saved with proper treatment.

- When a permanent tooth is completely knocked out, save it and have the child seen by a dentist within 30 minutes. With proper first aid procedures the tooth can be successfully reimplanted in the socket. Time is of the essence!
- A knocked-out primary or baby tooth can also be reimplanted if the child is seen by a dentist within 30 minutes. Although the child will eventually lose this tooth, it will act as a space-saver until the adult tooth erupts.
- Do not put the tooth in mouthwash or alcohol, or scrub it. Do not touch the root of the tooth.
- Place the tooth in a cup of whole milk. Avoid low-fat or powdered milk, or milk byproducts such as yogurt.
- Some experts recommend that the tooth be placed in the child's mouth to keep it moist until dental treatment is available. This method is risky in young children because the tooth can accidentally be swallowed.
- A partially knocked out tooth can be pushed into place without rinsing the tooth. Have the child seen by the dentist so the tooth can be stabilized.

Broken Tooth

A child who breaks a tooth should be seen by a dentist immediately because the break can extend down to the root of the tooth. In minor cases, a dentist will simply file off sharp edges to prevent the child from

■ NOSEBLEEDS ■

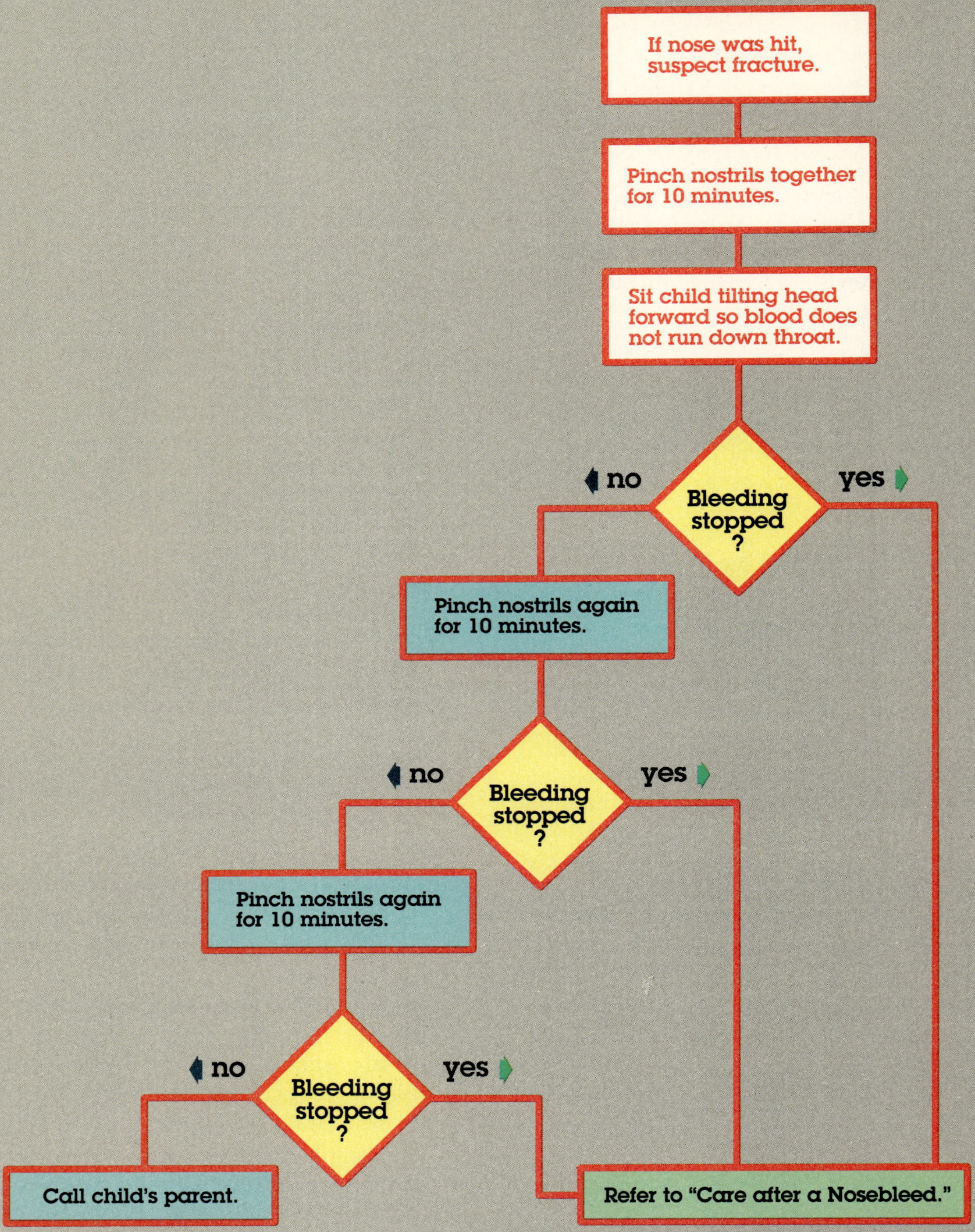
If nose was hit, suspect fracture.
Pinch nostrils together for 10 minutes.
Sit child tilting head forward so blood does not run down throat.
Bleeding stopped?
no
yes
Pinch nostrils again for 10 minutes.
Bleeding stopped?
no
yes
Pinch nostrils again for 10 minutes.
Bleeding stopped?
no
yes
Call child's parent.
Refer to "Care after a Nosebleed."

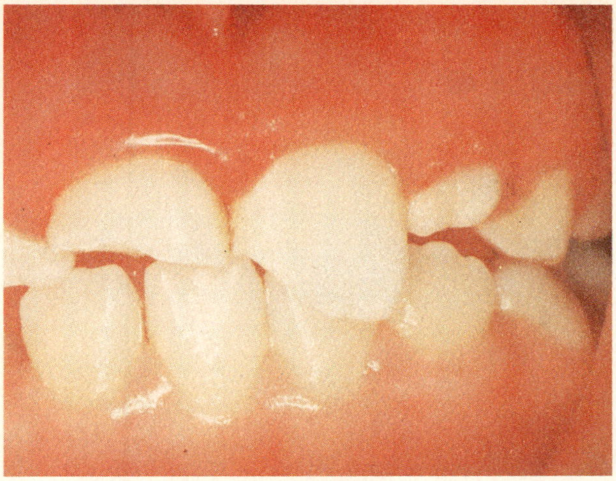

Broken teeth
Source: Courtesy of William B. Chan, DMD, Tufts University, School of Dental Medicine.

cutting the lip or tongue. In severe cases the tooth might need more extensive dental work.

- Rinse mouth with warm water.
- Apply ice or a cold pack to decrease any swelling that might occur. Wrap the cold pack in a cloth to protect the skin.

Jaw Fracture

If you suspect a jaw fracture due to a blow to the jaw, immobilize the child's jaw by wrapping a cloth under the jaw and tying it at the top of the head. Have the child seen in an emergency medical facility.

Bitten Tongue or Lip

Although this is a common injury of young children, damage is often difficult to assess. The mouth has a very rich supply of blood, and cuts tend to bleed heavily. The amount of bleeding, however, is deceiving because when blood mixes with saliva there appears to be more blood than there actually is. Stitches are seldom used when treating cuts of the mouth. The lips, gums, and the skin inside the mouth (mucous membranes) are very delicate and not easy to suture.

First Aid

- Rinse the child's mouth gently with warm water.
- Apply pressure with a piece of gauze or a clean cloth to stop the bleeding. Decrease the swelling by applying ice wrapped in a clean cloth to protect the skin.
- Keep the child in a sitting position.
- Call the child's parent and have the child seen by the health care provider if either of the following occur:

  1. A deep cut extends from the lip to the skin surrounding the lips. This cut will probably need stitches.

  2. A gaping cut on the tongue with persistent bleeding.

Toothache

If a child complains of a toothache, the child's parent should be notified and arrangements should be made to have the child seen by a dentist as soon as possible.

- Rinse out the child's mouth with warm water to remove any food.
- With parental permission, you may place a cotton ball saturated with oil of clove onto the problem tooth to relieve some discomfort. Know your center's policies.
- Also, with written parental permission, aspirin or acetaminophen may be given to provide some relief. Aspirin should never be placed directly on the tooth as it might burn the delicate tissue of the gums.

Objects Wedged between Teeth

Occasionally children will complain of food caught between the teeth. Most often these particles can be removed by gripping the object with a piece of sterile gauze or clean dry tissue. If this is unsuccessful, you might have to help the child to use a piece of dental floss. Never use sharp pointed objects such as tooth picks to remove something trapped between the teeth.

Chest Injuries

Although most childhood chest injuries consist of minor scrapes and bruises, more serious chest injuries have the potential to damage the underlying organs of the heart, lungs, and deep blood vessels within the chest wall.

Chest injuries can be open or closed. A closed chest injury is usually the result of a forceful blow to the chest wall. A forceful blow can cause bruising or break ribs which can then pierce or tear internal organs. An open chest injury is caused by an object that penetrates the chest wall and then passes through to the underlying organs. As children become older, the risk of serious chest injury increases as they begin to ride bicycles, compete in contact sports, and generally

■ DENTAL INJURIES ■

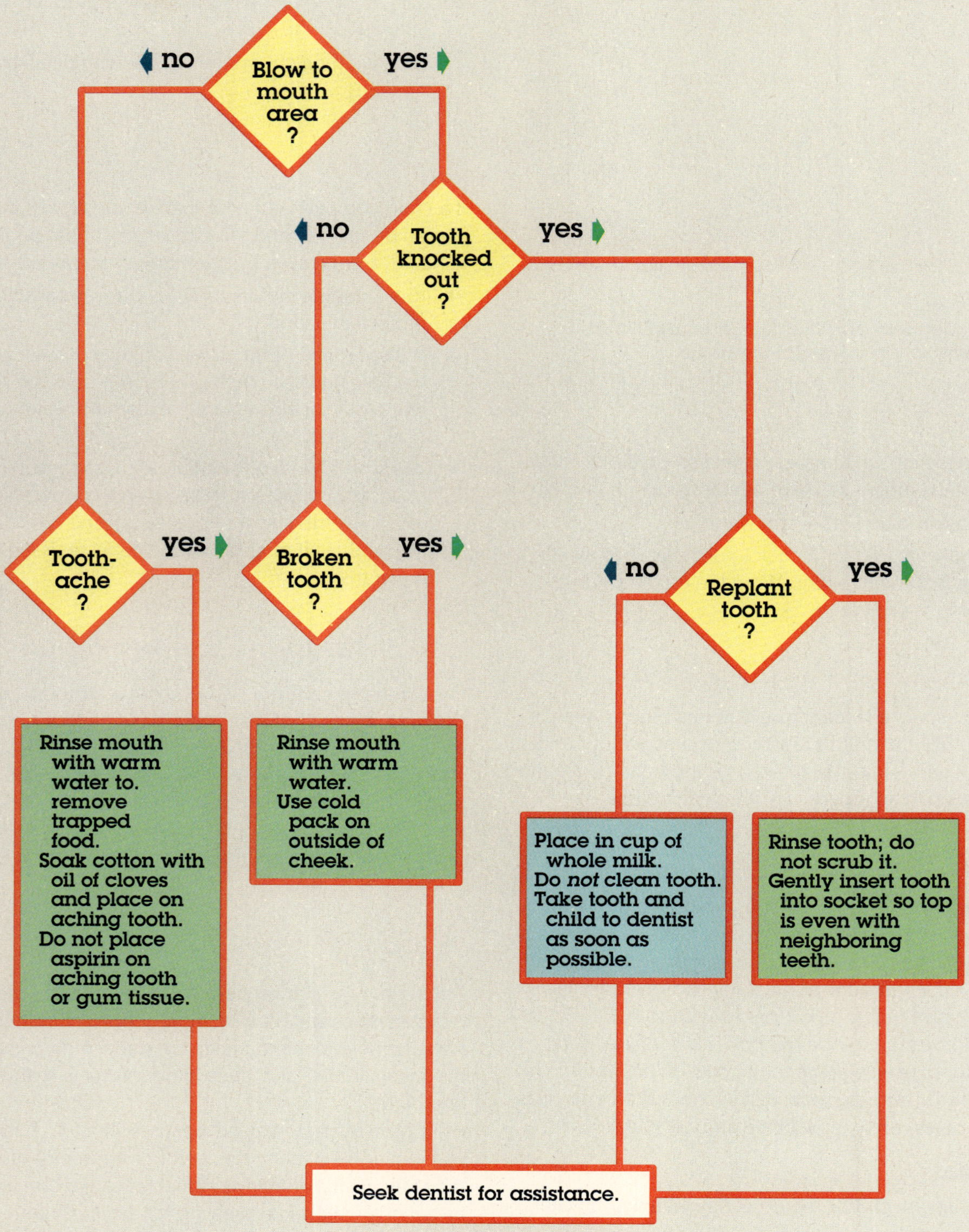

become more active. Older children are in control of their own seat belts and might not use them. Additionally, seat belts offer less protection than the car seats younger children use.

If the heart or major blood vessels are damaged, internal bleeding will occur and the child will need immediate surgery to repair this life-threatening damage. A first aider can do little besides calling for emergency medical help and treating for shock.

A puncture or tear of the lungs can also occur with any chest injury. This, too, is life threatening but there are first aid measures you can take while waiting for emergency medical help.

Signs and Symptoms

- Pain at the site of the injury.
- Blue or gray discoloration around lips and nose. This happens when the child is having trouble breathing.
- Rapid shallow breathing. This is a result of the uninjured lung having to do the work of two lungs.
- Failure of either one or both sides of the chest to expand normally when the child inhales.
- Shock. This can be caused by pain as well as blood loss.
- Coughing up blood.

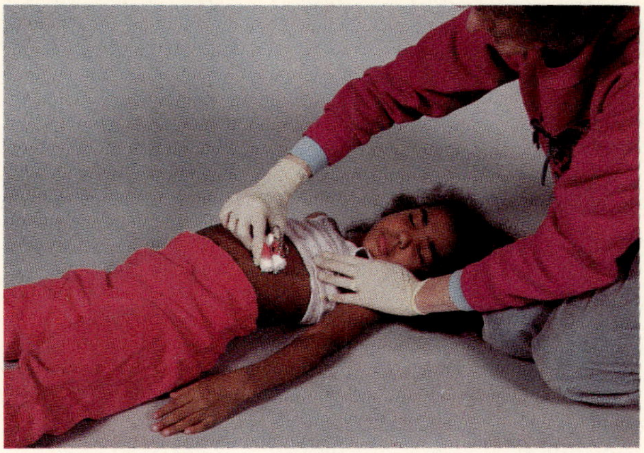

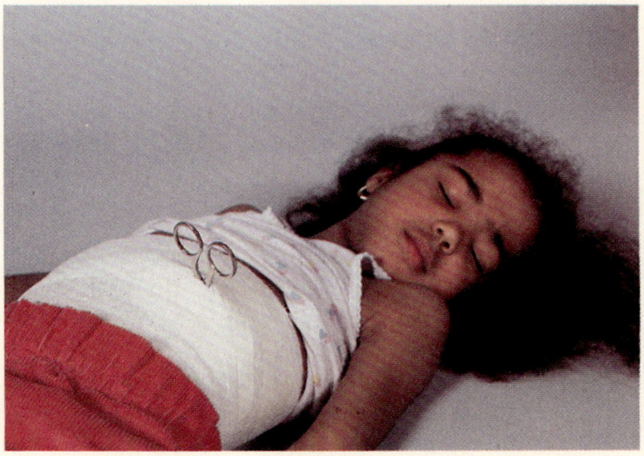

Stabilizing an object that has penetrated the chest wall

Penetrating Chest Wound

This type of wound must be closed quickly to prevent outside air from entering the chest cavity. The lungs might or might not be punctured.

First Aid

- Monitor the airway, breathing, and circulation and treat accordingly.
- Send someone to call for emergency medical help.
- Do not remove the penetrating object because this can result in further bleeding. Secure the object with a large bulky dressing, as illustrated.
- Observe for signs of air leaking from chest wound making a sucking sound. If air is permitted to leak through the wound opening, it can cause the lung to collapse and shift all the internal organs away from their natural location, making it difficult for the remaining lung to function properly.
- Place a large dressing coated with petroleum jelly, if available, against the open chest wound after the child has exhaled. Several layers of plastic wrap are a good alternative. This will prevent the movement of air through the wound. If the penetrating object is still in place, wrap the dressing around the object as best you can.

Fractured Ribs

Rib fractures are common injuries that can be the result of a sports injury or a bicycle accident. They are usually painful. A child who has fractured a rib will have difficulty taking deep breaths, coughing, and laughing. Additionally, the child will tend to splint the injured side of the chest with the upper arms to prevent movement.

First Aid

- Observe for signs of lung damage. If the injury was forceful the fractured ribs could puncture or tear internal organs.
- Send someone to call for emergency medical help if the child is in pain or shows signs of internal damage to the lungs.

- Have the child rest in a semisitting position and support the damaged ribs with a pillow or jacket.
- If the child is comfortable and shows no signs of internal damage to the lungs, ask the child's parent to take the child to the health care provider.

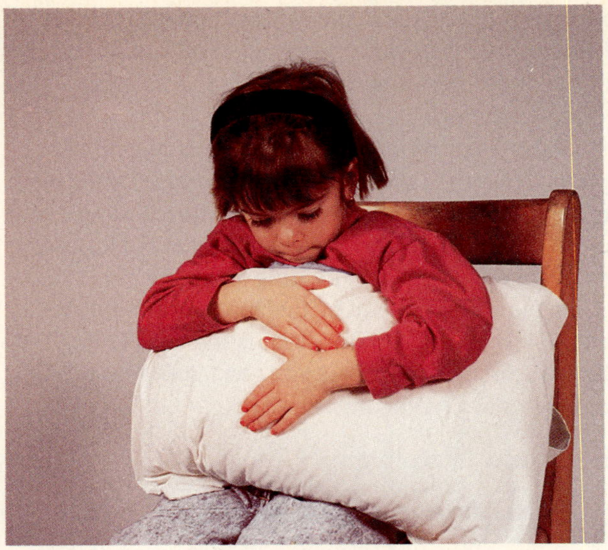

Supporting broken ribs with a pillow

Abdominal Injuries

Abdominal injuries can be open or closed. Open injuries occur when a foreign object enters the abdomen, resulting in external bleeding. Closed injuries are caused by a forceful blow. There is no open wound or bleeding on the outside of the body but there can be internal injury and bleeding. Damage to hollow organs, such as the stomach and intestines, will cause them to rupture and spill their contents into the abdominal cavity. Damage to solid organs, such as the liver and pancreas, will cause severe bleeding.

Signs and Symptoms

- Pain in the abdomen. Pain can be sharp or cramping and cause the child to draw the legs up to the chest.
- Nausea and vomiting. This will be present immediately after an abdominal injury.
- Open abdominal wound or a large bruise.
- Hard, rigid abdomen.
- Blood in the urine or stool.

Blunt Injury

A blunt injury is a closed wound resulting from a forceful blow such as a hit from a baseball bat or a fall from a climbing structure onto a hard object.

- Treat for shock. See Shock, Chapter 4.
- Send someone to call for emergency medical help.
- Place the child on the side to prevent choking if vomiting occurs.
- Give nothing to eat or drink.

Penetrating Injuries

A penetrating injury is an open wound caused by a sharp penetrating object. Do not remove any penetrating objects because this can result in further bleeding. Secure the object in place with a large bulky dressing as illustrated for penetrating chest injury. Treat as you would for a blunt abdominal injury.

Removal of Foreign Objects

It is common practice to keep small objects out of the reach of young children because of the risk of choking. We should also be aware that children sometimes put tiny objects in the nose and ears as well as swallow them. Examples are beads, buttons, bits of food, plant parts, and pencil-top erasers. Some children have a history of such behavior.

Ears

You might suspect that there is a foreign body in a child's ear canal if the child pays unusual attention to the ear but does not appear to be in pain. The child might also tell you that there is something in the ear. If you can see the object, do not try to remove it yourself. It is easy to damage the ear by using cotton swabs or tweezers. The child should be seen by a health care provider who will remove the object from the ear with special tweezers or flush the ear with a special solution to dislodge the object. This can be done easily by a health care provider in a clinic or office.

■ CHEST INJURIES ■

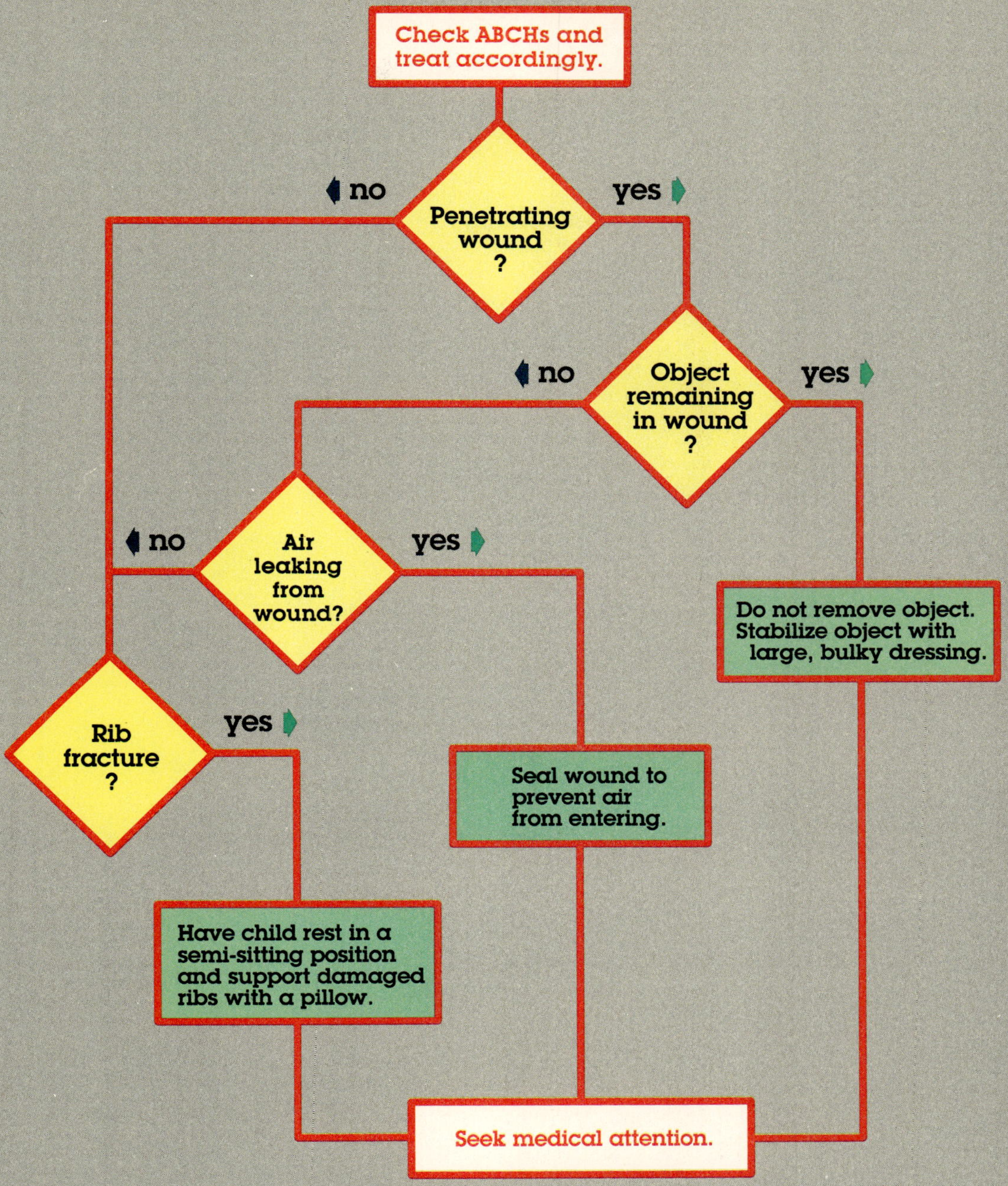

■ ABDOMINAL INJURIES ■

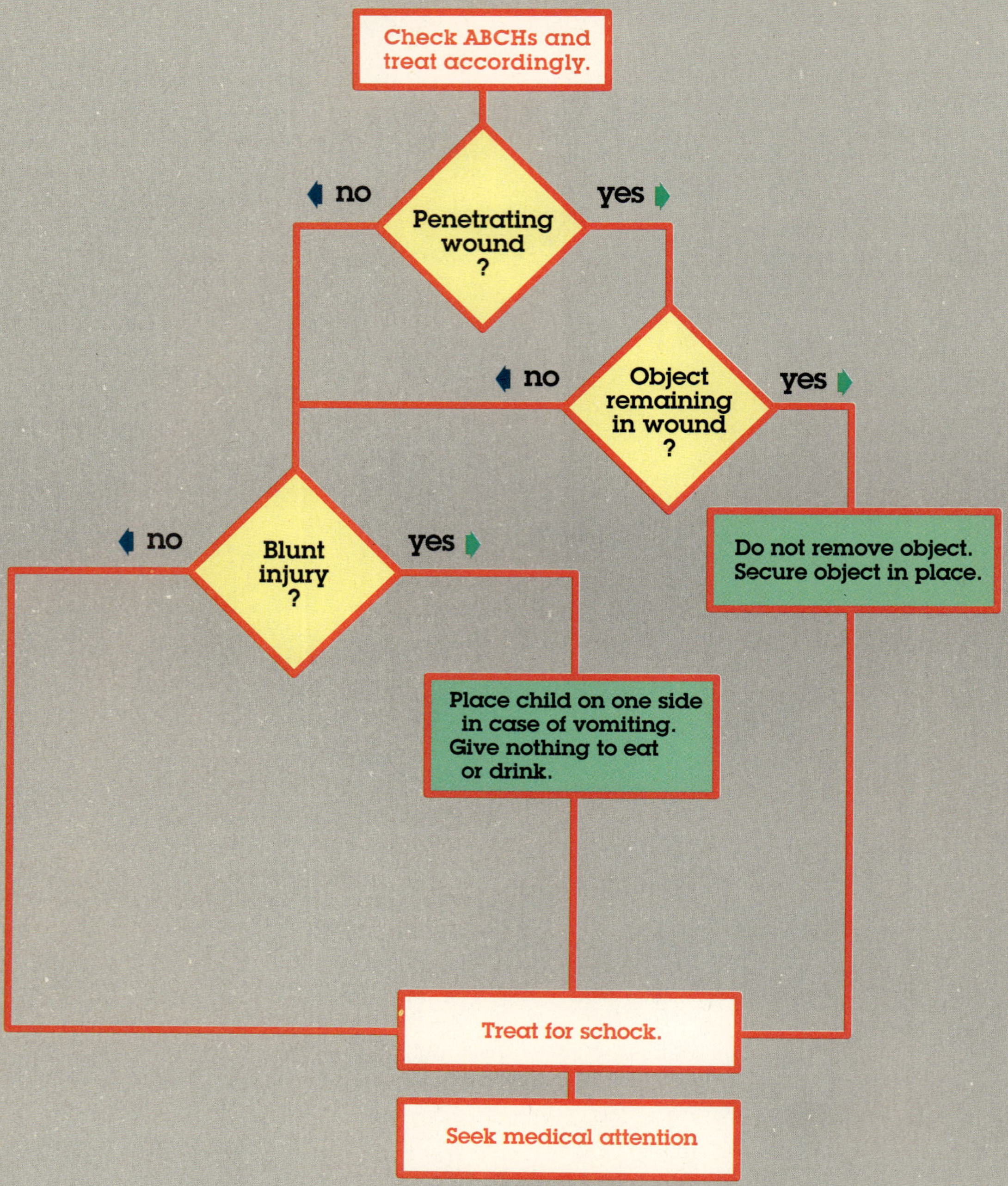

Nose

A foreign object in the nose might smell foul and cause a one-sided runny nose within a few hours. The child might pick at the nose if the object is annoying or interferes with nose breathing. It is not unusual for a child to have a foreign object caught in the nose for several days before telling a parent or provider.

A child may try to expel a foreign object by gently and repeatedly blowing the nose, but only if old enough to have mastered this skill. If this fails, do not attempt to remove the object yourself. The moist environment of the nose allows some objects to expand, and you will only make removal more difficult for a health care provider if you push it farther in. All clinics and health care providers have special tweezers that can remove most of these objects easily.

Swallowed Objects

A foreign object that becomes caught in the throat, interferes with swallowing or breathing, or causes unconsciousness due to airway blockage is a serious emergency requiring immediate action. The techniques are discussed in the Conscious Choking Child section in Chapter 3.

Except for poisons and sharp items, an object swallowed by a child will pass through the system without problems in 3 to 4 days. Examples of such normally harmless objects are buttons, small toy pieces, and crayons. Child care providers should notify the child's parent about the swallowed object. The parent might want to call the health care provider if there is any question about the danger of the swallowed object. Your local poison control center can also be a good source of information. Watch for the swallowed object to appear in the child's stool over the next few days. Providers should notify the parent if it passes and be certain that the parent notifies you. Never give a laxative. Any abdominal pain during these few days is a concern and the child will need medical attention.

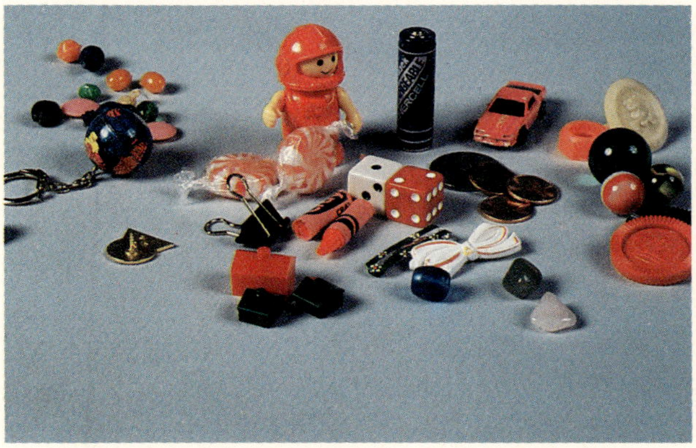

Children sometimes swallow tiny objects or put them in their noses or ears

Blisters

A blister is a collection of fluid in a "bubble" under the outer layer of skin. If not infected, blisters usually heal in 3 to 7 days.

First Aid

- Gently wash blisters with soap and water, and dry thoroughly. Cover with a nonstick plastic-coated gauze pad which allows moisture to escape.
- If a blister ruptures, wash the area with soap and water, and apply a small amount of antibiotic ointment and an adhesive bandage. Check your center's policy about the use of antibiotic ointment.
- Check daily for the following signs of infection: redness, swelling, or pus.

This first aid treatment applies only to blisters that are caused by friction. Blisters that are a result of frostbite, a burn, or contact with a poisonous plant are treated differently. See Frostbite, Chapter 9; Burns, Chapter 8; and Poison Ivy, Oak, and Sumac, Chapter 7.

Splinters

If a splinter becomes lodged under the surface of the skin or beneath a child's fingernail, remove it by grasping the end of the splinter with a pair of clean tweezers and pulling it out the way it came in. If the splinter breaks off or is deeply embedded, it should be covered with an adhesive bandage and left for the parent to remove at home. Most splinters are not serious. Digging with a needle or tweezers will only cause more discomfort and might not be successful. Warm water soaks at home can help to remove a splinter, and most splinters will work themselves out in several days. Check all wooden playground equipment and climbing structures several times a year for areas that are splintering and need to be sanded.

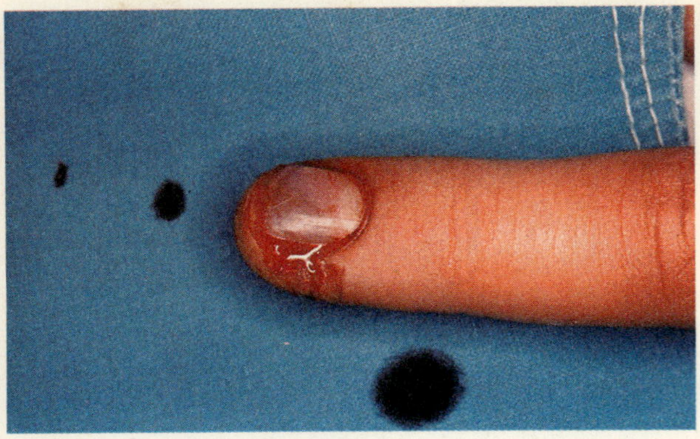

Finger slammed by door

Bleeding Under a Fingernail

A child who accidentally catches a finger in a closing drawer or door or who receives a direct blow to the tip of one of the fingers might experience bleeding under one or more fingernails. The accumulation of blood causes pressure under the nail and can be quite painful. This pressure is easily relieved by making a hole in the surface of the nail. It is a quick and simple procedure, but it should be done by a parent trained in this technique or the child's health care provider.

Nail Avulsion

A fingernail that is partially torn loose is called an avulsion. Secure the damaged nail in place with an adhesive bandage. If part or all of the nail is completely torn away, apply an adhesive bandage coated with an antibiotic ointment. Check your center's policy about the use of this product. Do not trim the loose nail. If a child is very uncomfortable, the parent should call the child's health care provider. A new nail will appear in about one month.

Head Injuries

Check the signs and symptoms of an internal head injury.

1. ____ Skull depression
2. ____ Clear fluid dripping from nose or collecting in ear(s)
3. ____ Pupils of unequal size
4. ____ Vomiting more than once
5. ____ Fever
6. ____ Confusion or dizziness

Mark each sign yes (Y) or no (N).

After a head injury, which signs indicate a need for medical attention?

1. ____ Vomiting, beginning 24 hours after the injury
2. ____ Headache lasting more than several hours
3. ____ Seizure or convulsion

Eye Injuries

Mark each action yes (Y) or no (N).

Which represents proper first aid for an embedded object in the eye?

1. ____ Using a sterile or clean cloth to remove the object
2. ____ Using a paper cup to cover the eye without touching the object
3. ____ Covering the injured eye but allowing the child to see by leaving the uninjured eye uncovered

Mark each action yes (Y) or no (N).

If a child falls on a pavement, lacerating the skin of the eyelid and possibly scratching the eye, a first aider should do the following:

1. ____ Apply a dressing tightly over the injured eye.
2. ____ Have the child lie flat.
3. ____ Loosely apply a dressing over the injured eye.
4. ____ Loosely apply a dressing over both eyes.

Mark each statement true (T) or false (F).

1. ____ Hitting the eye can cause a black eye or blurred vision.
2. ____ A health care provider should see a child with blurred vision.
3. ____ First aid for a blow to the eye includes applying a cold pack wrapped in ice to protect the skin, for 10 to 15 minutes.

Choose the best answer.

1. ____ A child has accidentally sprayed a cleaning product into both eyes. What should you do first?
   - **A.** Cover both eyes with dressings and immediately obtain medical care.
   - **B.** Hold eyes open and flush them with water for 15 minutes.
   - **C.** Allow tears to flush out the cleaning product.
   - **D.** Hold eyes open and flush them with water for 5 minutes.

Nosebleeds

Choose the best techniques for controlling most nosebleeds.

1. ____ **A.** Have the child sit down.
   B. Have the child lie down.
2. ____ **A.** Have the child tilt his head slightly forward.
   B. Have the child tilt his head slightly backward.
3. ____ **A.** Pinch both nostrils for 2 to 3 minutes.
   B. Pinch both nostrils for 10 minutes.

Dental Injuries

Mark answers true (T) or false (F).

1. ____ Use dental floss rather than a toothpick to remove an object stuck between teeth.
2. ____ A broken tooth should be filed down by a dentist to prevent cutting the lip or tongue.
3. ____ Place a tooth that was knocked out in mouthwash or alcohol to preserve it.

Chest Injuries

Mark each statement yes (Y) or no (N).

Which of the following actions serve as effective immediate first aid for a sucking chest wound?

A. ____ Remove a penetrating object from the chest.

B. ____ Apply a sterile or clean dressing loosely over the wound.

C. ____ Leave the wound uncovered.

D. ____ Tape a piece of plastic wrap tightly over the wound.

Abdominal Injuries

Choose the best answer.

Which is proper first aid for a blow to the abdomen in which you suspect internal injuries?

1. ____ **A.** Place the child on the back to relieve abdominal pressure.
   B. Place the child on the side.
2. ____ **A.** Give the child ice chips or sips of water to drink.
   B. Give the child nothing to eat or drink.

Which is proper first aid for an abdominal wound resulting from a penetrating object?

3. ____ **A.** Remove the penetrating object.
   B. Secure the object in place with a large bulky dressing.

1-800-682-9211
Poison Control

7

Poisoning

■ Swallowed Poisons ■ Poisonous Plants ■
■ Poison Ivy, Oak, and Sumac ■ Insect Stings and Bites ■

A poison is a substance that when swallowed, absorbed, injected, or inhaled in a relatively small amount can cause damage to body tissues and organs and can sometimes cause death.

Poisoning is one of the most common emergencies experienced by children under the age of 5. Swallowed poisons account for the vast majority of these emergencies. Deaths from swallowed poisons have decreased in the last two decades largely because the public is better educated in poison prevention strategies and effective treatment is more available, thanks to the advice of local poison control centers.

Unfortunately, poisonings still remain a major cause of emergency care and hospital admission. For every poisoning death among children under age 5, 80,000 to 90,000 nonfatal cases receive emergency medical treatment and 20,000 children need hospitalization.

Accidents often happen when adults are tired or preoccupied, when children have been left alone, even momentarily, and when proper storage of a poison is forgotten or proper disposal has been interrupted. Most accidental poisonings of children can be prevented by safe use and proper storage of household products and medicines. Make a habit of good poison prevention. Treating a swallowed poison injury can be terrible. Storing chemicals correctly takes only a few minutes.

Your responsibility checklist includes the following:

1. Eliminate careless storage of poisons. Keep all chemical substances including household products and all garage and basement chemicals out of the reach of children. Store them in locked cabinets or on high shelves. Lock medicine cabinets. Purchase corrosive chemicals, such as

Swallowed Poisons

Any substance that a child swallows other than food can cause harm in a large enough dose. Many of the products we use every day to clean our homes, treat our illnesses, maintain our yards, and pursue our hobbies are highly toxic and potentially fatal. Be especially cautious with the storage of household cleaners and all chemicals customarily stored in garages and basements. They can have tragic consequences when swallowed. In general, the poisonous substances that are the most devastating to children are pesticides, medications, alcoholic beverages, and petroleum products, such as gasoline.

Preventing a Swallowed Poisoning

Young children are curious by nature. Colored plastic containers, colorful pills, and never-before-seen items invite the child to explore. Taste is the first sense toddlers and many preschoolers use when investigating something new, whether it is a toy, food, chemical, or plant.

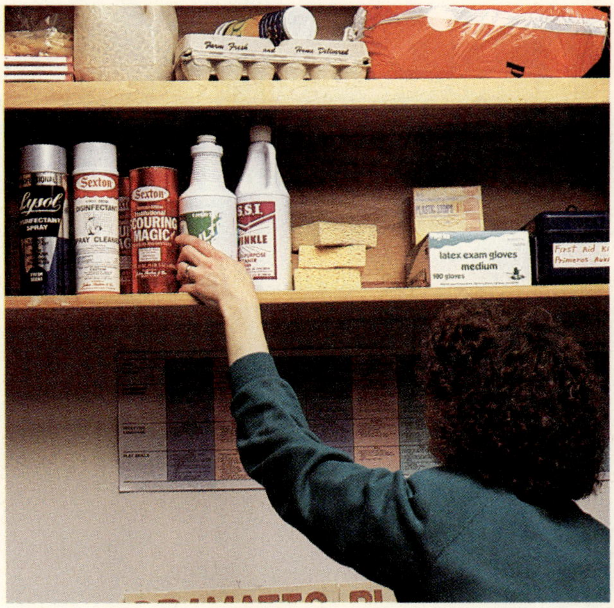

Store poisons out of the reach of children

Some Common Household Poisons

Acetaminophen
Aftershave lotion
Alcohol rub
Alcoholic beverages
Ammonia
Antifreeze
Antihistamines
Aspirin
Bathroom cleaning products
Bleach, liquid or powder
Boric acid
Button-size batteries
Charcoal lighter fluid
Cigarettes
Corn and wart remover
Cosmetics
Deodorant
Diabetic urine test tablets
Dishwasher powders
Dishwashing liquids
Drain cleaners
Fabric softeners
Fireworks
Flea powder
Floor and furniture waxes and polishes
Gasoline
Grease remover
Hair dyes and permanents
Hair straighteners
Hydrogen peroxide
Ibuprofen
Insecticides
Kerosene
Laundry detergents
Lighter fluid
Lime
Lye
Matches
Mothballs
Mouthwash
Nail polish
Oven cleaners
Paintbrush cleaners
Paint removers
Perfume
Plants and plant food
Plastic and rubber cements
Rug cleaners
Rust remover
Scouring powder
Shampoo
Shoe polish
Silver polish
Spot removers
Sunscreen products
Toilet cleaners
Turpentine
Varnish
Weight reduction pills
Windshield washer fluid
Wood preservatives

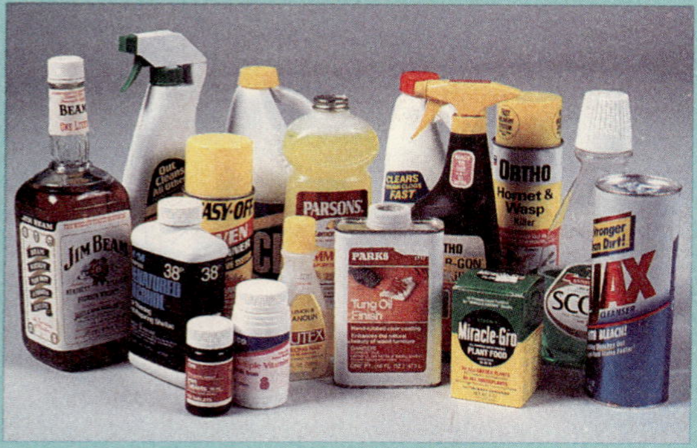

Common poisonous household products

drain cleaner, in one-time-use quantities whenever possible.

2. Conduct a child-level inspection of every room in your child care center or home to see what dangers you can find.

3. Avoid interruption when using a poisonous product. If you must leave your work area, put the chemical safely away or carry it with you.

4. Do not store household products with food. The differences between them might not be apparent to a young child.

5. Purchase products with child-resistant safety caps whenever possible. Although much safer, these containers are not completely child-proof. Children watch and imitate adult behavior, and some children can master the task of getting the lids off. Also, the lids do not work unless they are completely closed. Accidental poisonings commonly occur with vitamins and acetaminophen, both of which come in child-resistant containers.

6. Keep products in their original containers. If a poisonous substance is swallowed, correct identification is critical for proper emergency treatment. Do not reuse empty containers such as soft drink bottles, juice bottles, paper cups, and empty food containers.

7. To avoid accidental poisonings with medicines, follow these rules:

- Remember that nonprescription medicines are not less dangerous than prescription medicines. Both can be deadly.
- Give prescription medicine only to the child for whom it is intended. What is helpful for one child can harm another.
- Check the medicine label for the dosage each time you give it. The wrong dose of medicine can poison a child. More is not better when giving medicine.
- Only one adult in the child care center should be responsible for administering a child's medicine so that the child does not receive more than one dose.
- Never call medicine "candy" in an effort to get a child to swallow it. This practice invites a later poisoning accident.
- Flush old medicine down the toilet and rinse out the container before discarding it.

8. Look for poison hazards when taking a young child on a field trip or into a home or other building where poison prevention steps might be inadequate.

9. Keep all pocketbooks out of the reach of children.

10. Plants can also contain potentially dangerous chemicals. These rules apply to plants:

- Identify all of the indoor and outdoor plants at your child care center or home. If possible, move poisonous plants out of the reach of children. Refer to the Poisonous Plants section in this chapter for information on nonpoisonous plants to use in and around the center or home.
- Avoid using the December holiday plants, poinsettia, holly, mistletoe, and bittersweet, in your center. Although festive, they are extremely dangerous.
- When outdoors, teach children to keep all plants, including flowers and berries, out of their mouths. Do not share your knowledge of edible wild plants with young children because they are not always able to correctly identify safe plants when the experienced adult is not around.
- Plant food is poisonous. Keep it stored with other poisons.

11. Be sure that the art product packages in your child care center are labeled "AP" for approved product or "CP" for certified product. Some art supplies can be toxic if ingested or inhaled. See table on page 90.

What Poisons Children?

More than 80 percent of the reported exposures involved products and substances found in the following nine categories:

- Medicines and vitamins
- Cleaning substances and chemicals
- Cosmetics and personal care products
- Insecticides/pesticides
- Plants
- Bites/envenomations
- Hydrocarbons (such as gasoline and kerosene)
- Foreign objects
- Alcoholic beverages

Source: American Association of Poison Control Centers, Washington, D.C.

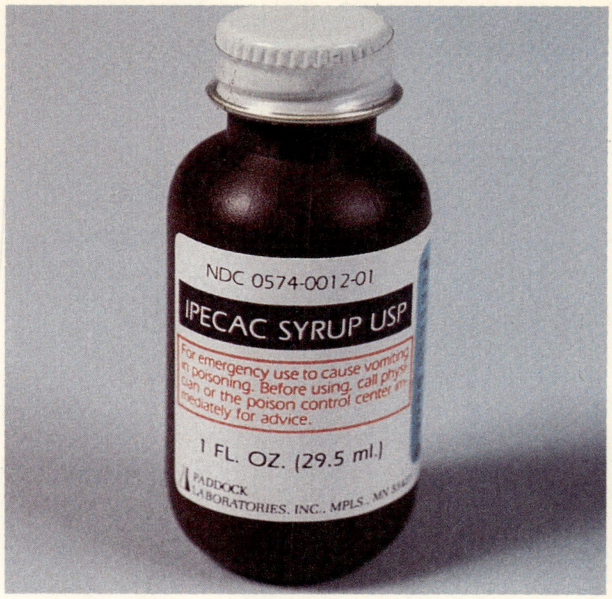

Syrup of ipecac

Be Prepared for a Poison Emergency

Maintaining good poison-prevention standards includes being prepared for a poisoning. Should one occur, the following steps, taken now, will prepare you to respond quickly and appropriately.

1. Keep the telephone number of your local poison control center and rescue ambulance posted at every phone in your center or home.

2. Keep syrup of ipecac in the first aid kit or other handy location, out of children's reach. Ipecac is a plant extract that causes vomiting when swallowed. It is *important* to know that ipecac is used only to treat swallowed poisons that can be safely vomited; with other swallowed poisons, its use can be devastating. Do NOT give it until the poison control center tells you to do so. Ipecac is available without prescription and is the fastest and most effective way to induce vomiting.

3. Call the poison control center whenever you have a question about a chemical or plant.

Managing a Swallowed Poison Emergency

Signs and Symptoms

Early indicators:

- Unusual odors from mouth, or stains on skin or clothes
- Nausea, vomiting, abdominal pain, or cramping

Art Materials: Recommendations for Children Under 12

DO NOT USE	SUBSTITUTES
Dusts and powders	
1. Clay in dry form. Powdered clay, which is easily inhaled, contains free silica and possibly asbestos. Do not sand dry clay pieces or do other dust-producing activities.	1. Order talc-free, premixed clay (e.g., Amaco white clay). Wet mop or sponge surfaces thoroughly after using clay.
2. Ceramic glazes or copper enamels.	2. Use water-based paints instead of glazes. Artwork may be waterproofed with acrylic-based mediums.
3. Cold water, fiber-reactive dyes, or other commercial dyes.	3. Use vegetable and plant dyes (e.g., onionskins, tea, flowers) and food dyes.
4. Instant papier mâché (creates inhalable dust and some may contain asbestos fibers, lead from pigments in colored printing inks, etc.).	4. Make papier mâché from black and white newspaper and library or white paste, or use approved papier mâché.
5. Powdered tempera colors (create inhalable dusts and some tempera colors contain toxic pigments, preservatives, etc.).	5. Use liquid paints or paints the teacher premixes.
6. Pastels, chalks, or dry markers that create dust.	6. Use crayons, oil pastels, or dustless chalks.
Solvents	
1. Solvents (e.g., turpentine, shellac, toluene, rubber cement thinner) and solvent-containing materials (solvent-based inks, alkyd paints, rubber cement).	1. Use water-based products only.
2. Solvent-based silk screen and other printing inks.	2. Use water-based silk screen inks, block printing or stencil inks containing safe pigments.
3. Aerosol sprays.	3. Use water-based paints with brushes or spatter techniques.
4. Epoxy, instant glue, airplane glue, or other solvent-based adhesives.	4. Use white glue, school paste, and preservative-free wheat paste.
5. Permanent felt tip markers which may contain toluene or other toxic solvents.	5. Use only water-based markers.
Toxic metals	
1. Stained glass projects using lead came, solder, flux, etc.	1. Use colored cellophane and black paper to simulate lead.
2. Arsenic, cadmium, chrome, mercury, lead, manganese, or other toxic metals which may occur in pigments, metal filings, metal enamels, ceramic glazes, metal casting, etc.	2. Use approved materials only.
Miscellaneous	
1. Photographic chemicals.	1. Use blueprint paper and make sun grams, or use Polaroid cameras.
2. Casting plaster. Creates dust and casting hands and body parts has resulted in serious burns.	2. Teacher can mix plaster in a separate ventilated area or outdoors for plaster casting.
3. Acid etches and pickling baths.	3. No acceptable substitutes. Should not use techniques employing these chemicals.
4. Scented felt-tip markers. These teach children bad habits about eating and sniffing art materials.	4. Use water-based markers.

This information was excerpted from The Center for Safety in the Art's Datasheet, Children's Art Supplies can be toxic. Further information is available from Art Hazards Information Center, 5 Beekman Street, New York, NY 10038.

- Sudden changes in behavior including fear, irritability, overactivity, and drowsiness
- Painful burns in and around the mouth that might indicate a caustic chemical burn
- Opened container of medicine or other household or garage product

Later indicators:

- Breathing difficulties
- Headache
- Cold, clammy skin
- Weakness and disorientation
- Slurred speech

Poison Control Centers

Poison control centers are a reliable source of information and can provide help for every kind of poisoning emergency. These centers are located throughout the United States and are staffed by registered nurses and pharmacists who have special training in toxicology, the study of poisons. They have access to detailed product information on hundreds of thousands of household products and medications. They also have access to a network of specialists with information about such uncommon poisons as mushrooms and snake venom.

Poison control centers serve emergency medical facilities, community health care providers, and the general public. They are equipped to answer routine questions as well as handle poisoning emergencies. They can determine whether a poisoning can be treated over the telephone or whether the child needs to be seen in an emergency medical facility. If the poisoning can be treated at home, they provide specific directions on what steps to take. In addition, they can help arrange for emergency medical transportation, if necessary.

Everyone in the United States can reach a regional poison control center with either a local phone call or by using an "800" number. Check your telephone book or call telephone information to obtain the number for the poison control center in your area. This number should be posted next to each telephone in your center or home.

- Seizures
- Unconsciousness

The signs that the child exhibits depend on the chemical swallowed and the time that has passed since the incident. Most absorption of the chemical begins when it passes into the small intestine. This can happen in less than 30 minutes.

First Aid

Swallowed poisons are of two types: corrosive poisons that burn tissue, and noncorrosive poisons. Because treatment is entirely different for these two groups of poisons, you MUST call the poison control center and follow their directions. A calm and nonaccusatory approach toward the child is essential when handling this emergency.

- Determine the following information for the poison control center:
  - **Who?** Age and approximate weight of child.
  - **What?** Type or name of the poison swallowed. Bring the container to the phone.
  - **How much?** "A taste," "half of the pills," "half of the liquid."
  - **When?** Approximately how long ago.
  - **Condition?** Conscious, vomiting, burns in mouth, abdominal pain.
- Call your local poison control center immediately. Do not give any fluid—even water—to the

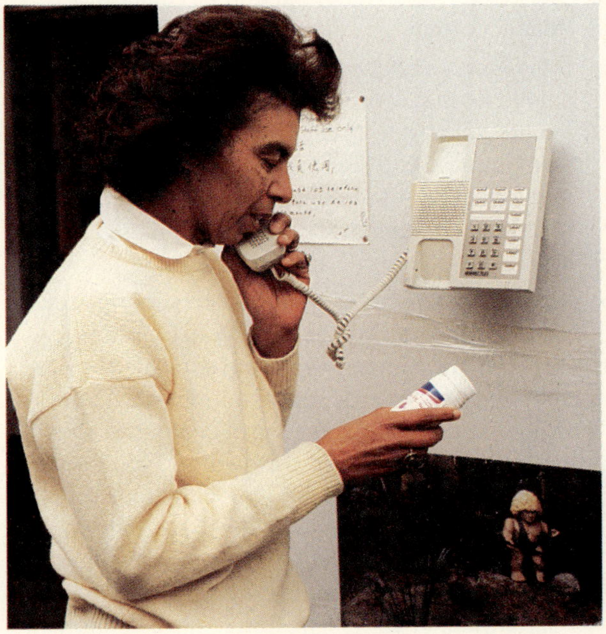

Call your local poison control center immediately if a child swallows a poisonous substance

child. The poison control center staff will determine whether the poisoning can be treated over the telephone or whether the child needs to be seen in an emergency medical facility. In addition, they will help arrange for emergency medical transportation, if necessary. Fortunately, most poisonings can be successfully treated where they occur.

- An unconscious child must be treated in an emergency medical facility immediately. Check airway, breathing, and circulation and treat accordingly. Place the child on the side.

Corrosive Poisons

- Monitor airway, breathing, and circulation and treat accordingly.
- Position the child on the left side to reduce the likelihood of the chemical entering the lungs if vomiting occurs. Corrosive poisons burn when swallowed. They should *not* be intentionally vomited because the throat and mouth will be injured further if exposed to the chemical again.
- Send someone to call for emergency medical help. A child who has swallowed a corrosive substance, whether conscious or unconscious, must be treated in an emergency medical facility immediately. There, the child will be given a drug that will neutralize, or bind, the poison before it enters the intestines. Time is of the essence.

Noncorrosive Poisons

- Monitor airway, breathing, and circulation and treat accordingly.
- If the child is *unconscious,* position on the left side to keep the airway open and, if vomiting occurs, allow it to drain from the mouth. Do not give ipecac. Send someone to call for emergency medical help. An unconscious child must be treated in an emergency medical facility immediately.
- If the child is *conscious,* the poison control center might instruct you to give syrup of ipecac. Because not all noncorrosive chemicals require treatment with ipecac, never administer it to a child unless the poison control center has specifically told you to do so. They will tell you the correct dose and what fluid the child may drink. Most children will vomit within 15 to 20 minutes. The additional fluid in the stomach, as well as walking or other movement, might speed the action of the ipecac. The poison control center will also advise whether the child needs further medical treatment.
- If the child needs to be seen in an emergency medical facility, take the labelled container of poison, as well as a container with any vomitus, along with the child.

Special points about treating a swallowed poison emergency:

1. Always call the poison control center first. It is the most knowledgeable source for emergency help.

2. Never give antidotes listed on the product containers. These antidotes are often incorrect.

3. Never induce vomiting unless told to do so by the poison control center. Giving ipecac for a corrosive poison can be devastating.

4. Never induce vomiting if the child is drowsy or unconscious. The child might choke on the vomitus or the vomitus might enter the lungs.

5. Do not attempt to dilute the poison by offering fluids before calling the poison control center. The presence of fluid in the stomach causes some chemicals to be dissolved quickly and, therefore, speeds absorption.

6. Never induce vomiting if there are burns and/or blisters present in and around the mouth from a corrosive chemical. A corrosive chemical that burns the throat when swallowed will burn again when it is vomited.

According to the American Association of Poison Control Centers:

- Nearly 90 percent of poisonings are accidental. Some of these poisonings, however, result from improper use of a medicine, such as when both parents give a drug to the child unaware that the other had already done so, or one parent gives a very large dose thinking that more is better. Nine percent are intentional, and 1 percent are due to adverse reactions from drugs or food.
- Poisonings occur in the following ways:

Swallowed	77%
Topical, or skin absorption	7%
Ophthalmic, or through the eye	6%
Inhalation of gases and fumes	6%
Bites and stings	3%
Other	1%

- Seventy-five percent of poison exposure incidents can be treated where they occur.

Source: American Association of Poison Control Centers, Washington, D.C.

■ SWALLOWED POISON ■

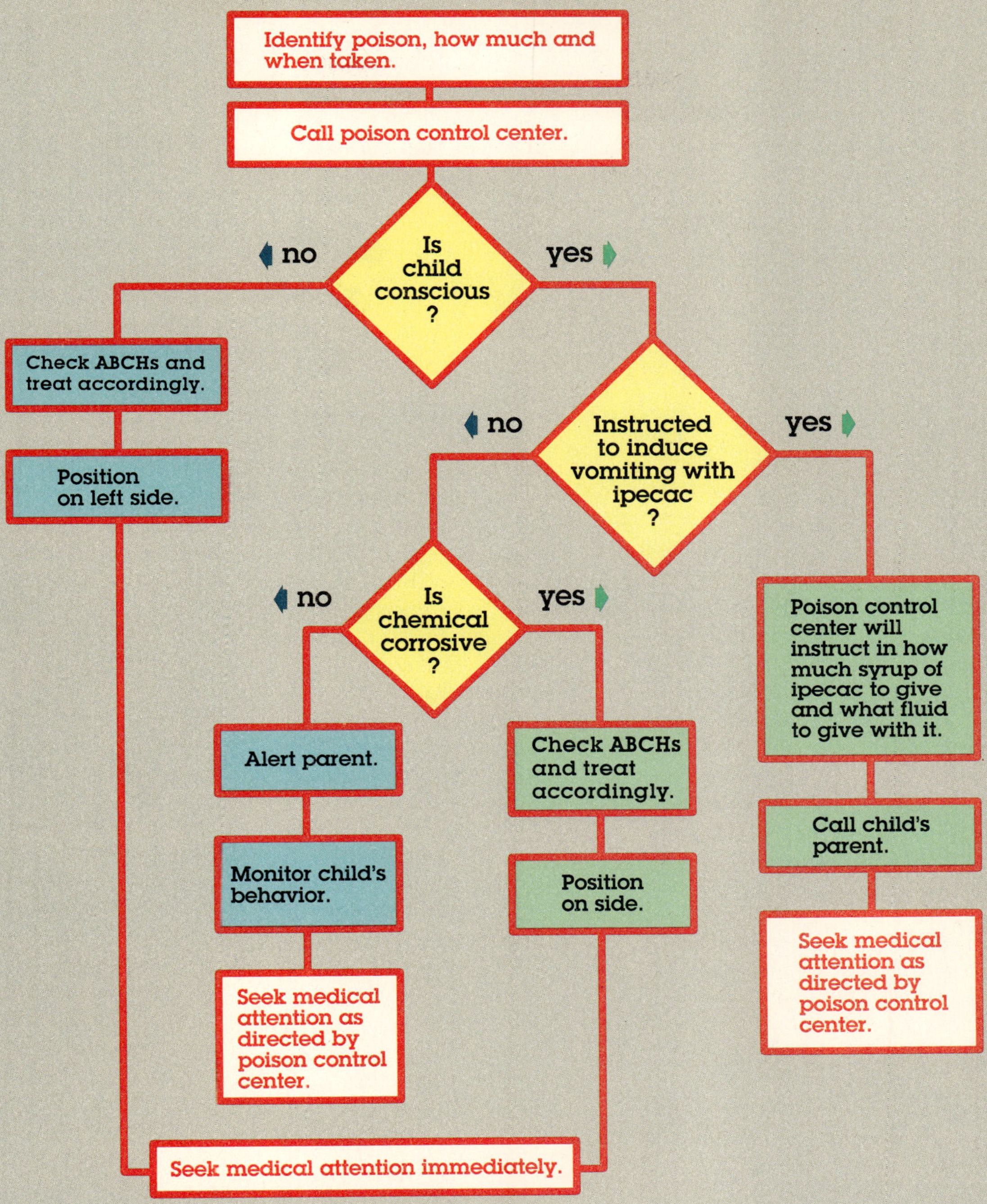

Poisonous Plants

The following list provides the names of some of the more common indoor and outdoor poisonous plants. Though the toxicity varies, ingesting, or swallowing, any amount of these plants is dangerous.

Acorn
Aloe vera
Amaryllis
Anthurium
Arrowhead
Autumn crocus
Avocado leaves
Azalea
Baneberry
Belladonna
Bird-of-paradise
Bittersweet
Black locust
Bleeding heart
Boston ivy
Boxwood
Buckeye
Buttercup
Caladium
Calla lily
Caper spurge
Carnation
Castor bean
China berry
Chrysanthemum
Crown of thorns
Cyclamen

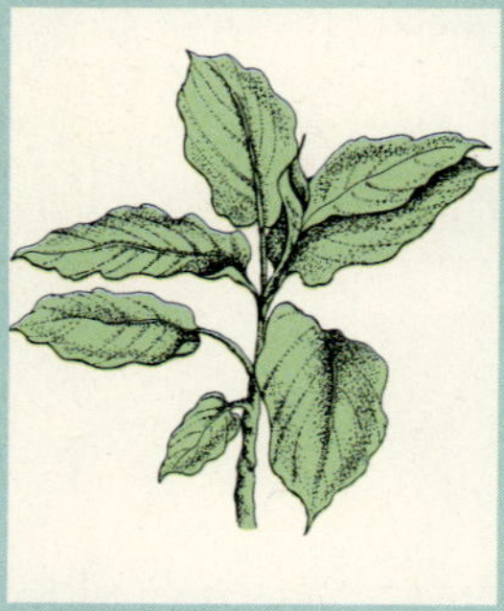

Dieffenbachia

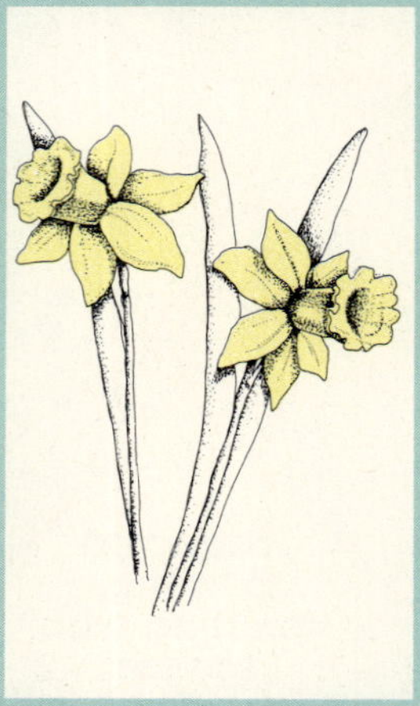

Daffodil

Daffodil bulb
Daisy
Daphne
Delphinium
Dieffenbachia
Dumb cane
Elephant ear
English ivy
Four o'clock
Foxglove
Glory lily
Golden chain tree
Ground ivy
Holly
Hyacinth
Hydrangea
Iris
Jack-in-the-pulpit

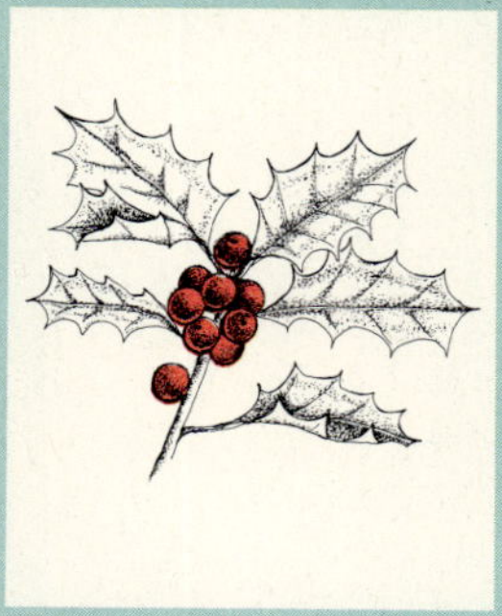

Holly

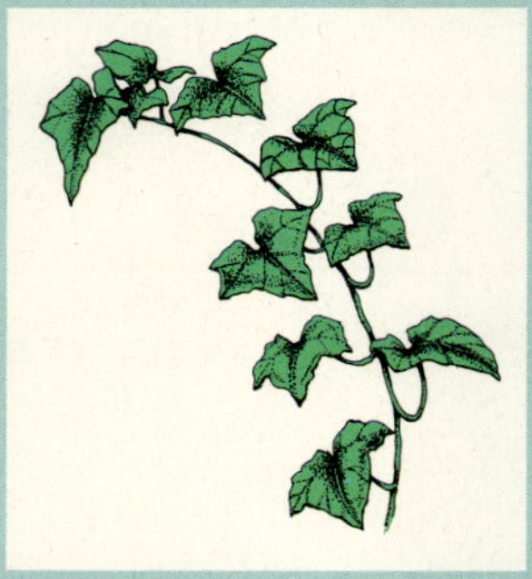

Ivy

Jerusalem cherry
Jessamine
Jimson weed
(Thorn apple)
Juniper
Lantana
Larkspur
Marijuana
Mistletoe
Morning glory
Mountain laurel
Mushrooms
Narcissus
Nightshade
Ohio buckeye
Oleander
Periwinkle
Philodendron
Pits of apricot,
cherry, peach
and plum
Poinsettia
Poison hemlock
Poison ivy
Poison oak
Poison sumac

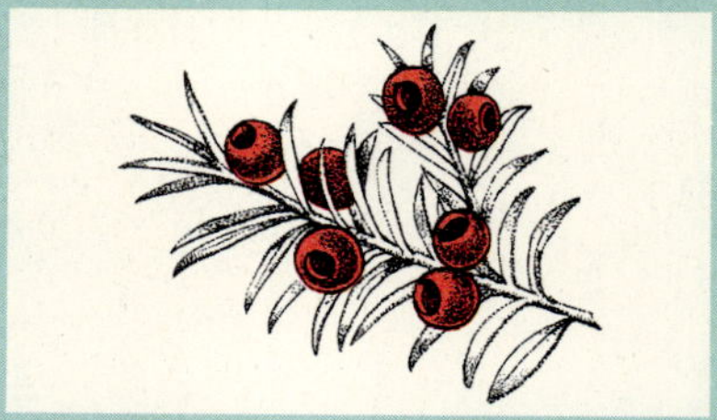

Yew

Privet
Rhododendron
Rhubarb
Rubber vine
Shamrocks
Skunk cabbage
Sweet pea
Tobacco
Tomato leaves
Tulip bulbs
Water hemlock
Wisteria
Yew

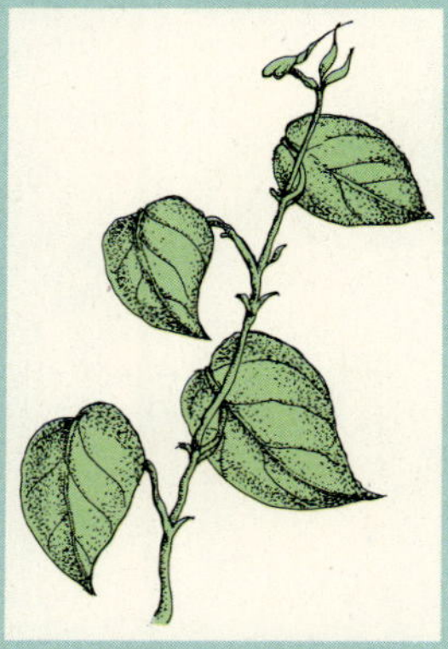

Philodendron

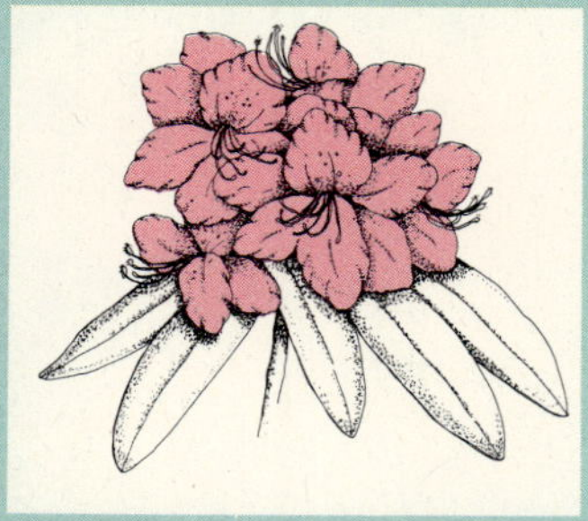

Rhododendron

7. Do not waste time using old remedies to cause vomiting such as swallowing salt water or trying to stick a spoon or fingers in the back of the mouth.

8. Syrup of ipecac expires after a few years. Check the expiration date on the bottle of ipecac in your first aid kit.

9. Activated charcoal is not recommended for use in the child care center or home. Activated charcoal is effective in treating some poisonings because it binds to the poison within the digestive system, preventing it from being absorbed. However, because it is difficult to give to a child, it should be administered in an emergency medical facility.

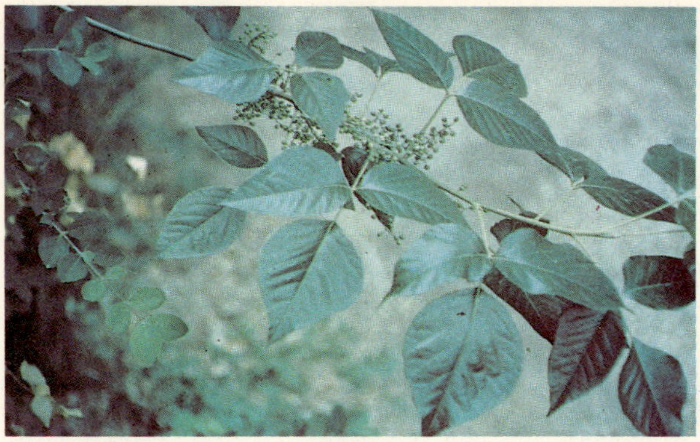

Poison Ivy

Poisonous Plants

Like many adults, most young children know little about toxic plants and cannot be relied on to recognize and avoid them. Because many toddlers and preschoolers use their senses of touch and taste when investigating something new, it is not unusual for children to touch and mouth leaves, berries, and flowers. Plants can be harmful in different ways. Poisonings can occur from swallowing the plant, absorbing the toxins through the skin, or inhaling the fumes from a fire that contains the poisonous plant. There are thousands of poisonous plants and no "sure-fire" way to tell a nontoxic plant from a toxic one.

Some poisonous plants cause only minor stomach irritation; others can cause abdominal cramping, breathing difficulties, and even death.

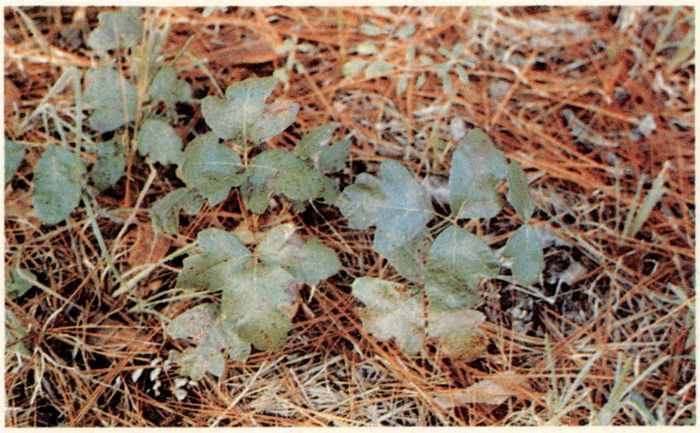

Poison oak

First Aid

Should a child eat any part of a plant, take the child and a sample of the plant to the telephone and call the poison control center. They will instruct you in what to do.

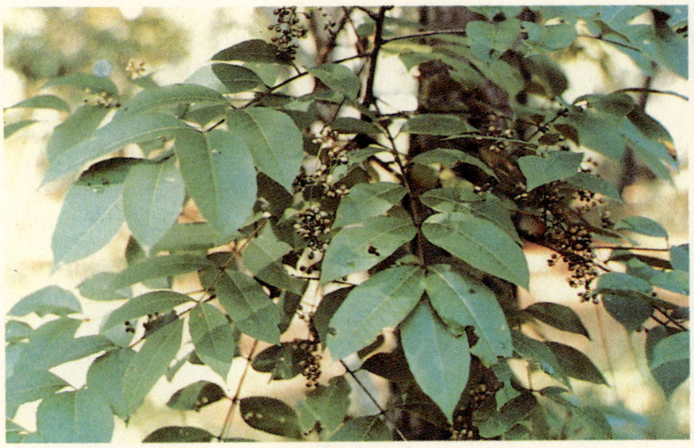

Poison sumac

Poison Ivy, Oak, and Sumac

A small number of plants cause an allergic reaction when they contact the skin. The best known are poison ivy, poison oak, and poison sumac, all of which are found throughout the United States. Exposure to the oil of these plants causes a delayed allergic reaction in the form of a rash that varies in severity. Several hours to 2 days is the usual time between contact with the plant and the eruption of the rash. A child can be exposed to the poison ivy oil directly by touching the leaves, stem, or roots, or indirectly by touching exposed tools, clothes, pets, or any other article touched by the plant. Smoke from a brush fire containing the burning plant will carry this oil in tiny droplets to the skin and into the nose, throat, and lungs. Contact with poison ivy can happen during any season of the year.

Unfortunately, most people cannot recognize these plants so they can neither avoid them nor treat themselves immediately after exposure, which sometimes lessens the reaction. To help everyone avoid poison ivy, oak, and sumac, teach the children in your care the short rhyme, "Leaves of three—LET THEM BE!"

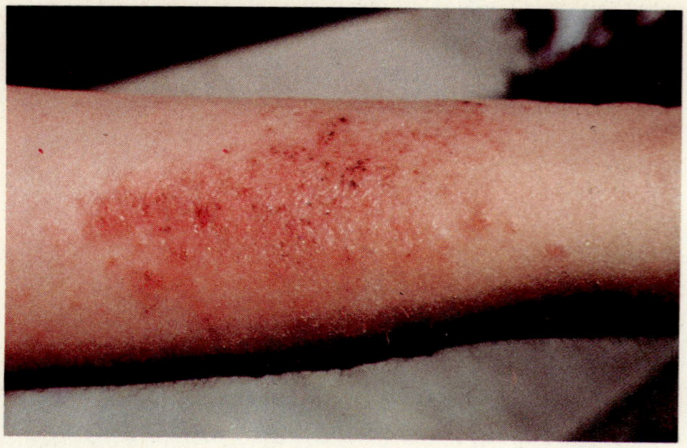

Poison ivy rash

Signs and Symptoms

Poison ivy, oak, and sumac symptoms can vary in intensity from a mild case with itching and redness of the skin to a severe case with redness, itching, blisters, and a generalized swelling of the entire area. Sometimes a severe rash is accompanied by a secondary infection of the skin causing the infected area to look yellow from pus accumulation.

First Aid

If you suspect that a child in your care has been exposed to one of these plants, follow these steps:

- Immediately wash the exposed areas of the body with a mild soap and plenty of water to flush the area and rinse the plant oil away. Sometimes the severity of the rash can be lessened if washing occurs within the first 5 minutes after exposure.
- Do not use pretreated towelettes or any wiping motion because that will spread the oil and the rash.
- Notify the parent when the child is picked up about the exposure and treatment. Should the child have a moderate to severe reaction, it is possible that he will be at home for a few days due to intense itching and burning and general discomfort.

Home Care Treatment

- Baking soda can be used frequently either as a bath or as a paste. Calamine lotion also reduces itching and promotes drying of the blisters.
- Cortisone medicines in strengths prescribed by the health care provider in either pills or ointments will help speed recovery. Antibiotics will be given if the area becomes infected.
- Wash all belongings that might have come in contact with the plant immediately in hot water and detergent. If the child is known to have a severe reaction to poison ivy, wash the clothes twice. Also scrub everything that accompanied the child through the poison ivy including shoes, toys, tools, and pets. These are the carriers of the oil that can continue to spread poison ivy for weeks to unsuspecting people who touch these items where the oil adheres and remains potent.

Nonpoisonous Plants

The following plants are generally considered to be nontoxic. However, it is always possible for an individual to have an allergic reaction from ingesting a part of one of these plants.

African violet
Aluminum plant
Asparagus fern
Baby's breath or baby's tears
Bachelor buttons
Begonia
Boston fern
Cacti (certain varieties)
Christmas cactus
Coleus
Corn plant
Crape myrtle
Creeping Jenny
Crocus
Dahlia
Dandelion
Dogwood
Dracaena
Easter lily
Forget-me-not
Forsythia
Fuschia
Gardenia
Geranium
Gloxinia
Hibiscus
Honeysuckle
Hoya
Impatiens
Jade plant
Kalanchoe
Lipstick plant
Monkey plant
Norfolk pine
Orchid
Pansy
Petunia
Phlox
Prayer plant
Purple passion
Rose
Rubber plant
Sedum
Sensitive plant
Snapdragon
Spider plant
Swedish ivy
Tiger lily
Umbrella plant
Umbrella tree
Venus's flytrap
Violet
Wandering Jew
Wax plant
Weeping fig
Weeping willow
Yucca
Zebra plant
Zinnia

- To prevent infection, scrub fingernails with a hard brush, trim fingernails short, and discourage scratching.

The child may return to your child care center before the rash is fully healed. Expect some breaking and weeping blisters. There is no poison ivy oil in this fluid nor anywhere else on the healing skin. Poison ivy cannot be spread from coming in contact with the healing rash. Be certain that all staff know this often misunderstood fact.

Insect Stings and Bites

Bites from such insects as mosquitoes, gnats, fleas, and flies seldom require any medical attention.

Stings from the Hymenoptera order of insects, which includes bees, wasps (including hornets, yellow jackets, polistes, and mud daubers), and ants, are more painful and can be dangerous. These insects inject venom under the skin that can produce a severe allergic reaction. See Severe Allergic Reaction, Chapter 4. Fortunately, such reactions are not common. Approximately 1 percent of all children are severely allergic to insect stings. Treatment that reduces sensitivity to the venom is available for these children. Parents should discuss this with their child's health care provider.

In some children, a sting from a Hymenoptera insect causes the body to produce a large quantity of the specific antibody that attacks the insect venom. This internal reaction is not detectable and causes no outward signs of future sensitivity. When the child is stung again, the reaction between the insect venom and the antibody causes a series of damaging internal reactions evidenced by severe allergic symptoms that can be life threatening if medical treatment is not immediately available.

Signs and Symptoms

Because of the pain associated with Hymenoptera stings, and the uncertainty of allergy in a child, such injuries always deserve your care and concern.

Nonallergic reaction. Although a painful surprise to a child, this reaction is not serious.

- Immediate stinging pain
- Redness around site
- Skin warm to touch
- Swelling for a few hours

Allergic reaction. Allergic reactions can be mild or severe and can progress slowly or rapidly.

Initial signs and symptoms include:

- Sudden sense of uneasiness and anxiety
- Skin flushed
- Hives, a generalized rash of red, raised, blotchy areas on the skin that causes itching
- Swelling, sometimes severe, at the sight and elsewhere, especially face, lips, or tongue
- "Tickle" in throat
- Difficulty or noisy breathing due to swelling in the throat, which can block the airway
- Difficulty swallowing.

Life-threatening signs and symptoms include:

- Tightness in the chest
- Bluish or grayish skin color
- Seizures
- Loss of consciousness
- Cardiovascular collapse, a heartbeat so weak that blood cannot circulate

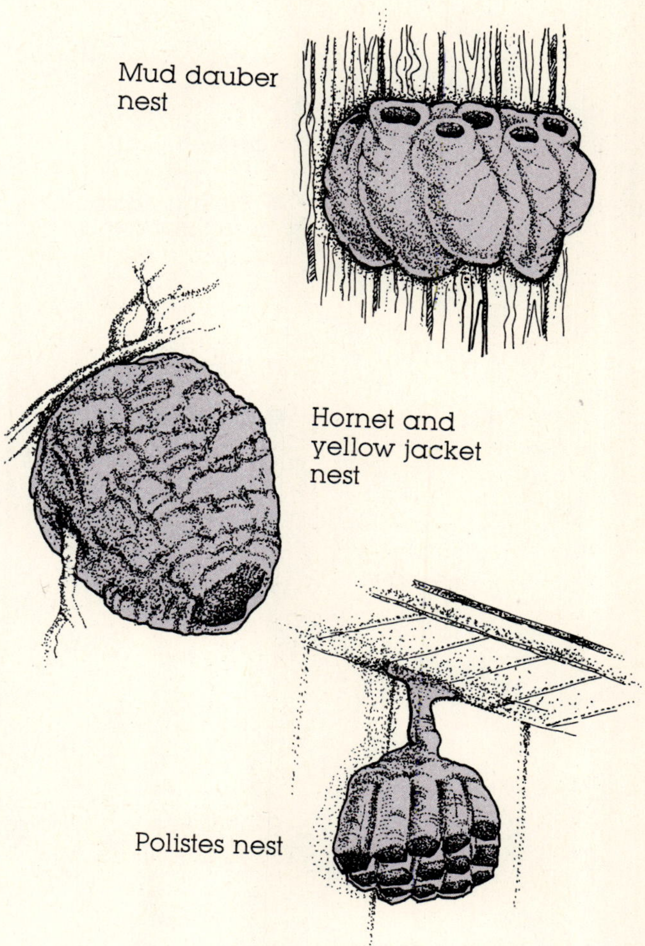

Adapted from: American Academy of Allergy and Immunology.

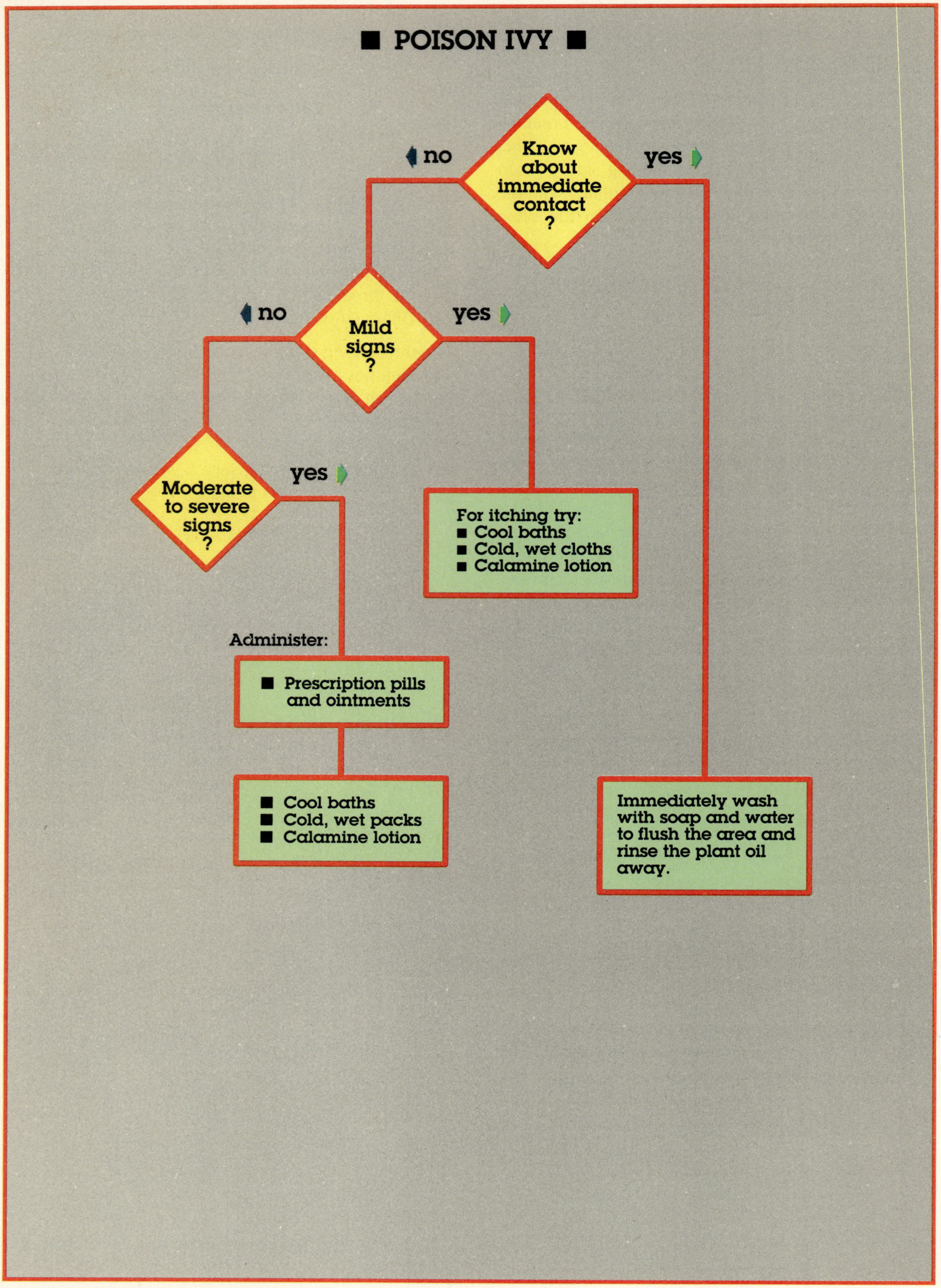
■ POISON IVY ■
Know about immediate contact ?
no
yes
Mild signs ?
no
yes
Moderate to severe signs ?
yes
For itching try:
■ Cool baths
■ Cold, wet cloths
■ Calamine lotion
Administer:
■ Prescription pills and ointments
■ Cool baths
■ Cold, wet packs
■ Calamine lotion
Immediately wash with soap and water to flush the area and rinse the plant oil away.

First Aid for Nonallergic Reactions

- Examine the sting site for a stinger left in the skin. Only honey bees leave the stinger with venom sac attached. It must be removed because it continues to inject venom for 2 or 3 minutes longer if left in the skin. Do not squeeze the stinger sac with fingers or tweezers because this will inject more venom. Instead, gently scrape it away from the site with a fingernail.
- Wash with soap and water.
- Apply a cold pack wrapped in a cloth to protect the skin for 15 to 20 minutes. This will slow the absorption of venom and relieve pain.
- Apply a baking soda and water paste to the site to reduce the stinging pain. Baking soda neutralizes the acidic venom.
- Apply calamine lotion to the sting site to help control itching. Know your center's policy about the use of this product.
- Keep the child sitting quietly while holding the cold pack against the sting site. This allows you to observe the child for 30 minutes for any signs of an allergic reaction. A child who exhibits even mild signs of an allergic reaction should be examined by a health care provider.

First Aid for Allergic Reactions

- Send someone to call for emergency medical help.
- If the child is unconscious, open the airway, check for breathing and circulation, and begin CPR if necessary. Swelling in the throat will interfere with rescue breaths.
- If the child has an allergic emergency kit at the center, the medication can be administered immediately, but *only* by an adult who has been instructed in its use. A second dose of medication might be necessary while waiting for emergency medical help to arrive.
- Position the child so that the sting site is lower than the heart.
- Treat for shock.

Avoiding Insect Stings

There are ways for children and staff to reduce the chance of being stung while outdoors. These are especially important for the allergic child.

- A nonallergic adult should destroy any nests that appear around the building. Check under eaves and windowsills.
- Check other locations where children play for nests such as old tree stumps, auto tires that are part of a playground, holes in the ground, and around rotting wood.
- Allergic children should not play outside alone during the months when stinging insects are active.
- Sneakers are safer than sandals for allergic children.
- Clothing for allergic children should not have bright floral prints. Colors such as white or khaki are best. Avoid loose-fitting clothes because they can trap a stinging insect.
- Avoid perfumes, hairsprays, or other products with scents that might make the child attractive to insects.
- When eating outdoors, be aware that stinging insects are attracted to foods and can enter soft drink cans. These foods especially attract insects: tuna, peanut butter and jelly sandwiches, watermelon, and melting ice cream.
- Avoid garbage cans and dumpsters because they attract insects.
- If an insect is near you, do not swat or run since such actions can trigger an attack. Walk away slowly. If you have disturbed a nest and the insects swarm around you, lie face down and cover your head with your arms. Teach this technique to children.
- A severe allergic reaction to an insect sting is immediate and life-threatening. Therefore, an allergic child's emergency kit should be kept close at hand when the child is playing outdoors during insect season. An allergic child should also wear a medical alert necklace or bracelet to alert a rescuer who might find the child unresponsive.

■ INSECT STINGS ■
(Flying Insects)

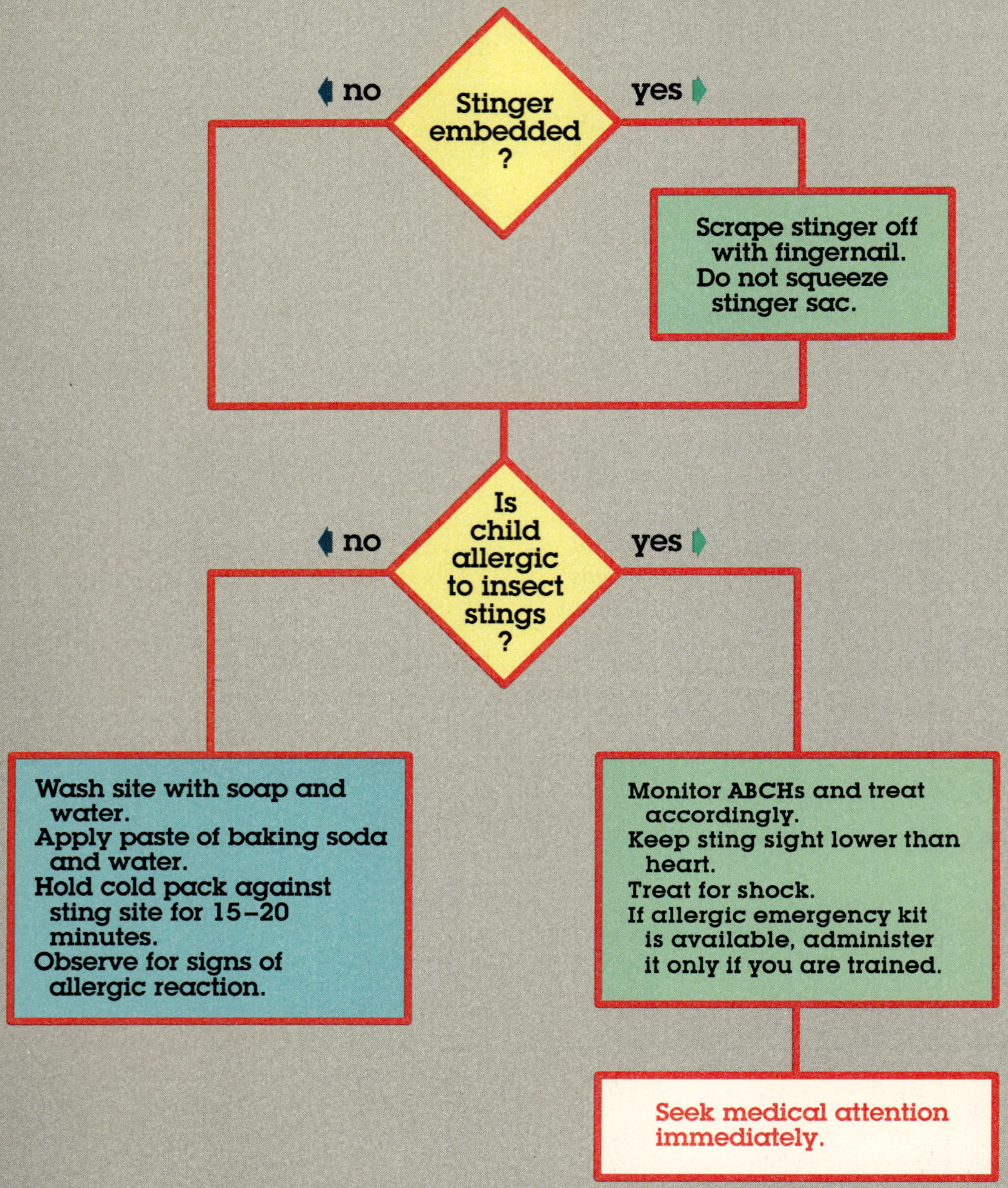

Lyme Disease

Lyme disease is a bacterial infection caused by the bite of an infected deer tick. In some areas of the United States, this tick is also known as a bear tick or sheep tick. The deer tick is smaller than the more common dog or wood tick and should not be confused with it.

Lyme disease has been found in nearly all of the American states, although it tends to concentrate in the Northeast, northern Midwest, Pacific Northwest, and California. The incidence in the Southeast is on the rise. The range of the disease is expanding as the ticks are carried farther inland by animals and birds.

Humans can contract the disease when they are out in the fields and woods where the deer tick lives. The months for greatest risk are May through August. In warmer regions of the United States, the risk of Lyme disease can exist year-round. Deer ticks are not found on sandy beaches. They can be as small as the head of a pin, and when engorged, are somewhat larger.

The deer tick picks up the Lyme disease bacteria by feeding on an infected animal. It then attaches itself to the clothing or exposed skin of a child who is walking in the woods or tall grasses. The tick bite is often not felt. If not removed, the tick can hang on for 2 to 4 days or longer, drawing blood for food, and becoming engorged, before letting go. The bacteria can be transmitted to the child while the tick is drawing blood. A deer tick bite does not always result in Lyme disease because not all deer ticks are infected. It is estimated that the number of deer ticks infected with Lyme disease ranges from 10 percent to 65 percent depending on the region of the country.

Signs and Symptoms

Early signs and symptoms of Lyme disease can appear from 1 to 3 weeks after the deer tick bite. Treatment at this stage is very effective.

- In approximately 60 percent to 75 percent of Lyme disease cases, a red rash develops at the site of the bite. This important early finding helps to diagnose the disease promptly. The rash can take more than one form but usually it appears as a flat or raised circle that expands over a period of several days. It sometimes resembles the shape of a doughnut as the red color of the center begins to fade. If left untreated, the rash will disappear in several weeks. Sometimes the Lyme disease rash does not follow this usual pattern. Show any suspicious rash to a health care provider.
- Additional early symptoms of Lyme disease, which can be mistaken for a flu-like illness, are headache, stiff neck, and aching muscles or joints, fever, swollen glands, and chills.

Later signs and symptoms of Lyme disease are more serious and can develop weeks and often months after

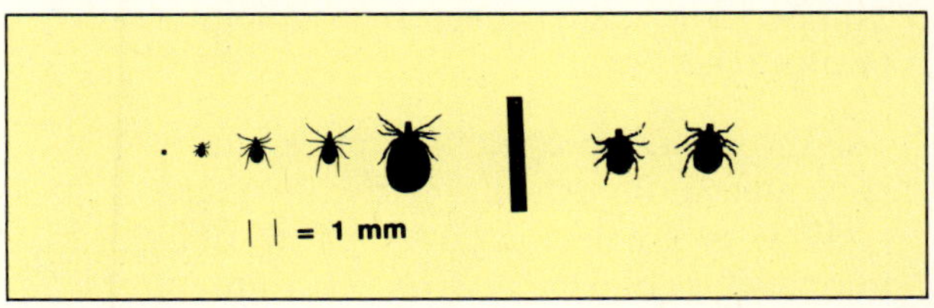

Near actual size, left to right, of larva, nymph, adult male, adult female, and engorged deer tick as compared to adult male and female dog tick
Source: Pfizer Central Research, Groton, Ct.

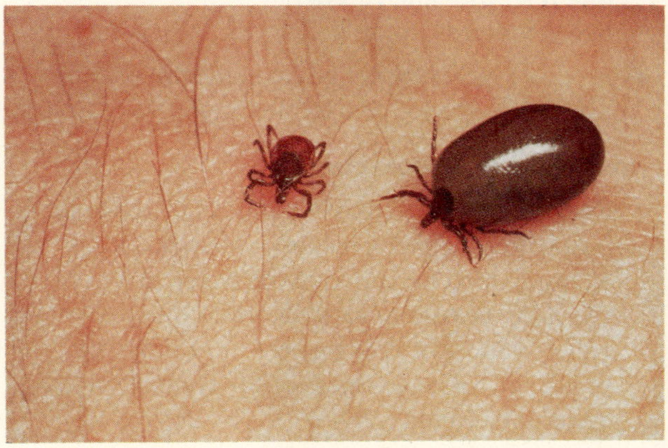

Unengorged and blood engorged deer ticks (seven times actual size)
Source: Courtesy of Dr. Michael Fergione, Pfizer Central Research

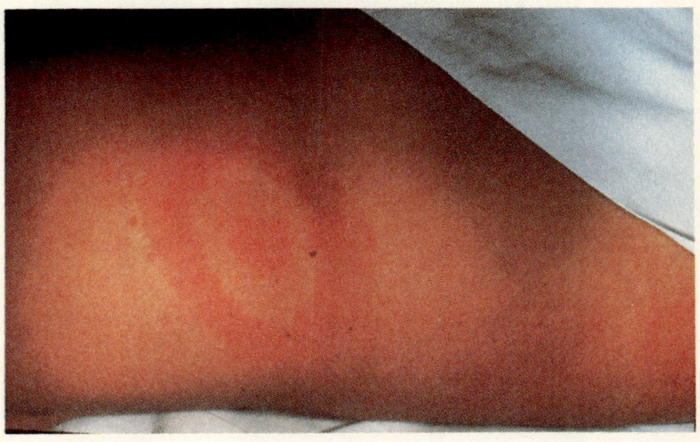

Lyme disease rash
Source: Courtesy of Dr. Alan MacDonald, Covenant Medical Center, Urbana, Il.

the tick bite. Recovery from this stage of the disease occurs more slowly.

- Painful swelling of joints, often the knees
- Heart problems causing an irregular heartbeat, dizziness, and weakness
- Nervous system problems causing headaches, neck stiffness, difficulty concentrating, and poor coordination.

Treatment

Lyme disease is usually diagnosed based on symptoms that the child and parents report. A blood test can help to confirm it, but not always. Lyme disease is not contagious.

- Treatment with antibiotics is started immediately.
- The child should rest until feeling well again. The rash will fade within days, while other flu-like symptoms might linger.
- A complete recovery can be expected if the disease is diagnosed and treated in the early stages.

Prevention and Detection

- Reduce exposure to infected ticks by covering legs with long pants tucked into socks, long-sleeved shirts tucked in at the waist, and sneakers instead of sandals when walking in tall grass, woods, or fields where ticks might be prevalent. Ticks are most easily spotted on light-colored clothing.

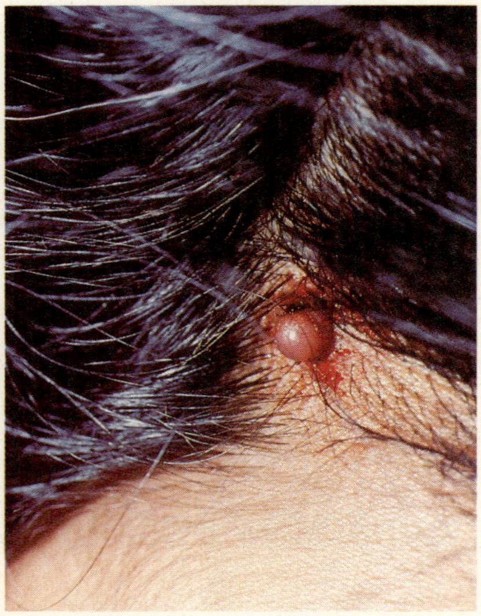

An embedded and engorged tick

Tick Removal

Most tick bites are harmless, although ticks occasionally carry diseases such as Rocky Mountain spotted fever and Lyme disease. Remove a tick as soon as it is discovered using the following method:

- Grasp the tick close to the skin surface where the mouth parts are attached. Use tweezers rather than fingertips because they are more accurate and reduce exposure to infection from the tick through breaks in the skin. Tug gently and firmly until it lets go. Do not twist or jerk because this might leave part of the tick in the skin.
- Wash the area with soap and water.
- Apply ice wrapped in a cloth to protect the skin.
- Calamine lotion can help to relieve itching. Know your center's policy about the use of this product.
- Do not attempt to remove a tick by using outdated methods such as coating it with petroleum jelly or fingernail polish, soaking it in alcohol, or holding a hot match against it. These methods are all ineffective and some are not safe.

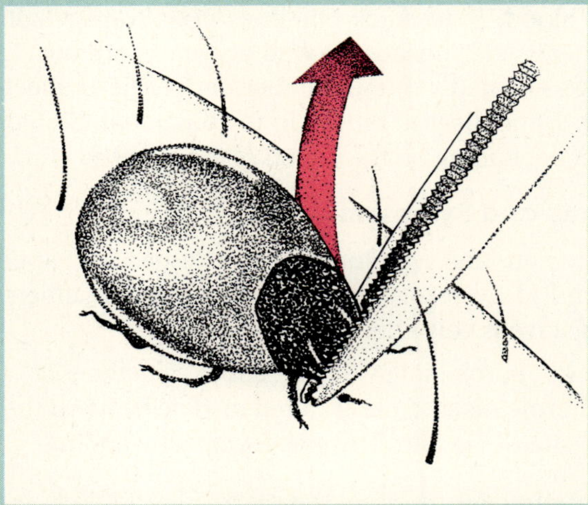

Remove a tick with tweezers. Tug gently and firmly until it lets go.

Tell the child's parent that a tick was removed. Both parents and child care providers should watch for a rash or signs of infection in the area of the tick bite, or for flu-like symptoms during the next several weeks. A health care provider should see any rash that develops up to 3 weeks after a tick bite.

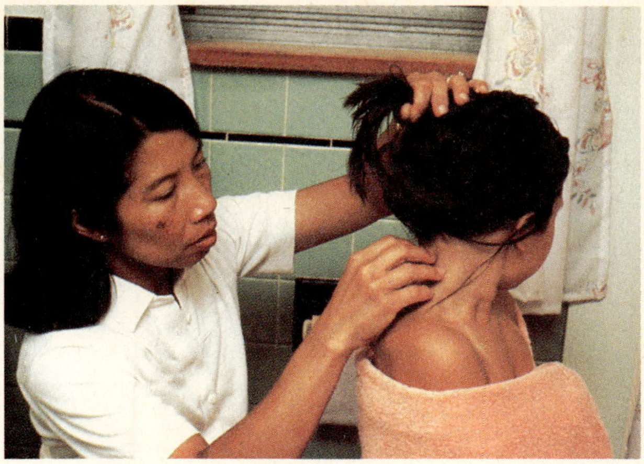

Checking for ticks
Source: Pfizer Central Research, Groton, Ct.

- Check children's skin daily for ticks. Pay special attention to the folds of the skin, the scalp, and the back of the neck. Use tweezers to remove the tick, and wash the skin with soap and warm water. Removing the tick within the first 24 hours greatly reduces the risk of infection.
- Observe the bite area daily for several weeks for a rash that might signal Lyme disease. Also watch for flu-like complaints for as long as 2 months. Early detection is important because Lyme disease is most easily treated in the early stages.
- Pregnant women should be especially observant for ticks. Although rare, it is possible for the Lyme disease bacteria to be passed to the unborn baby. A pregnant woman with symptoms should notify her health care provider immediately.
- Contact your local health department to find out where deer ticks are prevalent.
- Check pets for ticks. They can carry ticks on their fur and are also susceptible to Lyme disease. Use tick control products recommended by your veterinarian.

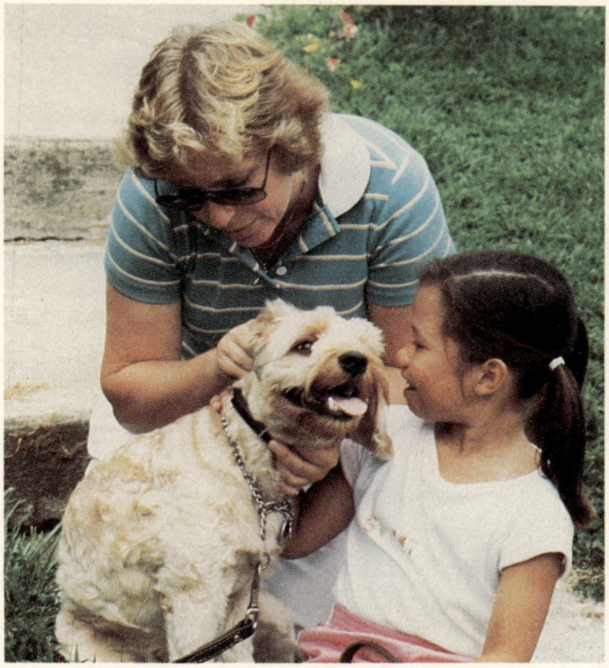

Source: Pfizer Central Research, Groton, Ct.

- Parents may use over-the-counter insect repellents. Products that contain 25 percent to 35 percent DEET are effective against ticks. Higher concentrations of DEET are available but can cause side effects and are not recommended. Permethrin is another repellent effective against ticks, but it is not approved for use in all states. Permethrin should only be applied to clothing, never directly to the skin.
- Insect repellents contain potent insecticides. Apply spray repellents only when out-of-doors, use sparingly, and wash hands after applying. Avoid breathing the repellent spray. Never apply it to an open wound or cut. Child care providers should never use insect repellents on children in their care.

■ TICK REMOVAL ■

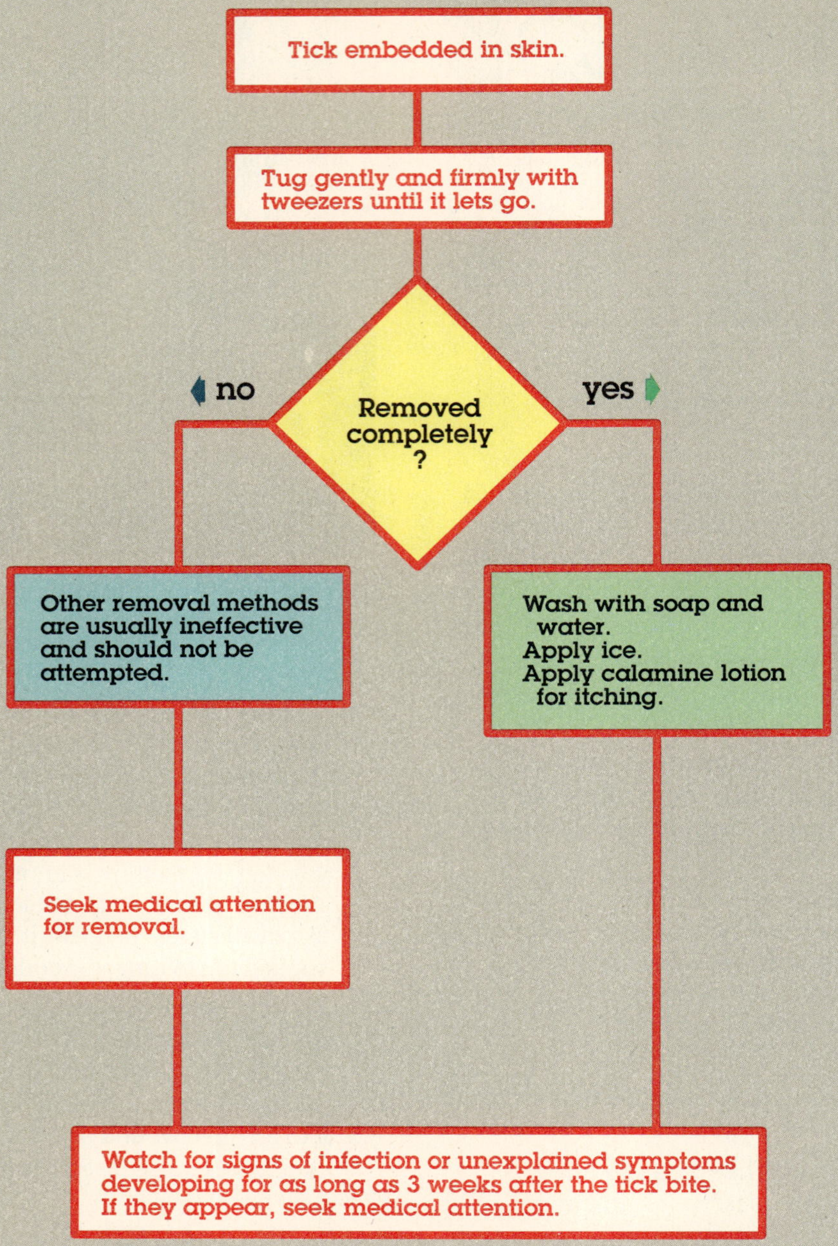

Swallowed Poisons

Check the correct response(s).

You suspect that a 3-year-old boy has swallowed children's flavored acetaminophen from an opened bottle. What information will you want to know when you speak to the poison control center?

1. ____ Did the child swallow any of the pills?
2. ____ About how many pills?
3. ____ How long ago did the child swallow them?

Mark the following statements true (T) or false (F).

1. ____ Always induce vomiting with syrup of ipecac in a conscious child who has swallowed a poison.
2. ____ Read the label of the poison container to find out the best treatment for a swallowed poison.
3. ____ Give the child a glass of water or milk before calling the poison control center.
4. ____ Corrosive chemicals cannot be vomited because the tissue of the throat and mouth will be damaged further.
5. ____ Everyone can reach a regional poison control center by using a toll-free telephone number for your area.
6. ____ As long as you keep medicines safely stored, it is OK to call medicine "candy" to convince a sick child to swallow it.
7. ____ There is no reliable way to tell a poisonous plant from a nonpoisonous plant.

Poison Ivy, Oak, and Sumac

Mark each action yes (Y) or no (N).

Which of the following might be useful after exposure to poison ivy, oak, and sumac?

1. ____ Wash the area immediately with soap and lots of running water.
2. ____ Apply calamine lotion to a rash that develops.
3. ____ Scrub the area frequently with pretreated towelettes.
4. ____ Use baking soda in a bath or as a paste if a rash develops.
5. ____ Use a moisturizing lotion to keep the skin soft if a rash develops.
6. ____ Avoid contact with other children because the rash will spread as the blisters weep.

Insect Stings

Mark each action yes (Y) or no (N).

Which are appropriate first aid measures for insect stings?

1. ____ Remove a stinger with tweezers or fingers.
2. ____ Wash the sting site with soap and water.
3. ____ Place a warm pack over the sting site.
4. ____ Arrange for a child with mild allergic reaction symptoms to be examined by a health care provider.
5. ____ A trained adult can treat an allergic child with the injection from the child's allergic emergency treatment kit.

8

Burns

■ Assessing a Burn ■ Heat Burns ■
■ Chemical Burns ■ Electrical Burns ■

A serious burn injury is a terrible incident that can leave a child with long-term physical and emotional scars. Curious children climb and grab; they do not have a clear understanding of what is dangerous, and they are fascinated by fire. The National Institute of Burn Medicine estimates that between 50 percent and 90 percent of all burns that occur in children under the age of 4 years can be prevented! Most burns of toddlers and preschoolers are scald injuries caused by hot liquids and grease. Flame burns are more commonly seen in children ages 5 to 12 years. Many burn injuries can be prevented if you make burn-proofing a part of child-proofing. Do you always place hot coffee out of a child's reach? Are your matches always returned to a safe, high, and hidden location? Are you teaching children that fire is a tool, not a toy?

The skin is sensitive to heat. Skin damage usually does not occur below 111°F. Temperatures between 111°F and 123°F cause significant tissue damage. Temperatures above 123°F destroy skin within seconds. Some states have a policy on water temperature limits in a child care setting. Know your state's policy.

Assessing a Burn

The severity of a burn is determined by three major factors: size, location, and depth. The age of the child and any preexisting medical problems also influence the seriousness of the injury as well as the course of the recovery.

More than 27,000 children are hospitalized each year with burn injuries. An estimated 400,000 more are treated in emergency rooms, physician's offices, and clinics. More than half of all childhood burns are seen in children under the age of 4 years.
Source: National Institute of Burn Medicine, Ann Arbor, Michigan

Preventing Burn Injuries

KITCHEN

Cooking

- Keep an eye on young children when you are cooking.
- Cook on back burners whenever possible to prevent children from touching hot burners. When cooking on front burners turn pan handles in to prevent them from being knocked over or pulled down.
- Supervise children when they are ready to learn to cook.
- Do not reach across a hot electric or lighted gas burner.
- Avoid storing foods, especially cereal, over the stove. Children might climb onto the stove to reach them.
- Do not place any hot liquids near the edge of a table or counter.

Electrical Appliances

- Use only UL-approved electrical appliances.
- Place all electrical appliances at the back of the counter.
- Do not allow electrical cords to dangle. Loosely coil electrical appliance cords so children cannot pull them down.
- Unplug electrical appliances when not in use.
- Keep electrical appliances away from water.
- Never leave a hot iron unattended. Unplug and remove it before you walk away.
- Cover electrical outlets to prevent children from sticking things into them.
- Do not overload extension cords. It is best not to use extension cords around infants and toddlers.

Barbecues

- Use only charcoal lighter fluid to light a barbecue. Never use gasoline or any other flammable liquid.

continued

- Never squirt charcoal lighter fluid on a burning fire.
- Keep the grill away from flammable walls and fences.
- Teach children to stay away from a barbecue in use.
- Do not throw hot embers on the ground because a barefooted child might step on them.

BATHROOM

- Set the temperature of the hot water heater at 110°F.
- Test the temperature of bath water before bathing babies and young children. Run cold water first, then hot to the desired temperature. Do not put a child in the tub until all water is turned off.
- Supervise toddlers and young children in the bathtub. If left unattended, they could scald themselves with hot water.
- Mark the hot water faucet with red fingernail polish or red tape.

BEDROOM

- Keep the child's crib a safe distance from radiators, heaters, and electrical outlets.
- Do not let cords dangle. Keep them away from children's reach.
- Avoid the use of space heaters in a child care center.

IN GENERAL

- Install smoke detectors and keep them operating properly. Change the batteries once a year and as needed.
- Smoke detectors should be located on each floor of a child care center or home. In the home, at least one detector should be located within 15 feet of each bedroom. Do not put a detector in the kitchen because even a small amount of smoke from the toaster can trigger the alarm. It is better to install the smoke detector a few feet away from the kitchen.
- Have a fire escape plan with a designated place to meet outside the building. Practice it.
- Keep emergency telephone numbers by the telephone.
- Open a window or door for fresh air if you smell gas or suspect a gas leak. Call the fire department or gas company for help. Do not light a match or turn on an electric light.
- Store corrosive chemicals only in a safe place. Safer still, don't store them; buy only a one-time-use quantity.
- Keep the fireplace screened and place barriers around wood stoves.

MATCHES

- Keep matches and lighters out of the reach of toddlers and preschoolers. Be firm about children not touching matches and lighters. Children can learn about fire safety at an early age. Parents should teach older children how to use matches and lighters safely.

These tips are adapted with permission from the National Institute for Burn Medicine, Ann Arbor, Michigan.

Size

Estimating the size of the burn will help you determine whether the burn is considered to be minor, serious, or critical. It also gives guidelines for appropriate first aid. The palm of the hand equals 1 percent of the body. Descriptions such as "the size of a quarter," "one side of the leg," or "half of the back," also help to define the size.

Location

Burns can be especially serious when they are located on one of four critical areas of the body—face, hands, genitals, and feet. Unfortunately, children commonly burn these areas when they reach up to stove tops, touch appliances, or spill hot liquids on themselves. Flame burns can be particularly serious because, in addition to the destruction of the skin, the fumes from the burning objects irritate the lining of the airway. This causes swelling and narrowing of the breathing passages.

Depth

The most familiar way to describe a burn injury is by depth. In the past, burns were classified as third, second, or first degree. These degrees were thought to describe how deeply the skin and nerves were damaged. Now, it is more common to describe burns as full-thickness, partial-thickness, or superficial as these terms are more descriptive of the depth of damage or destruction.

- ***Full-thickness burns*** (third degree). These burns severely damage or destroy the full depth of the skin. The length of time that a burning substance is in contact with the skin, as well as

Cris, age 6, was helping his mother decorate the Christmas tree when he accidentally leaned back into a table decoration with candles and ignited his sweatshirt. Cris had watched the Firebusters program and remembered to Stop, Drop, and Roll when your clothes catch fire. He was not injured as a result of his actions.

Five-year-old Abby, asleep in the mobile home of the grandparents she and her cousin were visiting, awoke at 1:00 a.m. to find fire and smoke in her room. Frightened as she was, Abby remembered the Learn Not to Burn presentation at her school a few months earlier. Abby dropped to the floor and crawled the length of the 65-foot home to awaken her grandparents and cousin. All four escaped unharmed, though the home was completely destroyed.

Kate, age 8, responded successfully to an early morning fire in her home. The fire had cracked windows with its heat, setting off the burglar alarm. Hearing this, Kate woke up coughing to a home filled with smoke. Her bedroom door was closed. Kate reacted quickly. Crawling on her hands and knees, she moved over to the door and felt the knob. It was hot. Kate then crawled back to her sleeping sister and woke her up. After breaking the window with a rocking chair as her father had taught her in their home escape planning, Kate made sure her sister was safely outside before leaving the burning house herself.

Marcus, age 9, was in the bathtub when he heard his six-year-old brother yelling. Jumping from the tub, he discovered that the younger brother had set his clothing on fire while playing with a lighter. Marcus first threw his towel at him. Realizing that this was not extinguishing the flames, he ordered his brother to "Stop, Drop, and Roll." The local fire department had presented two fire safety programs at Marcus's school in the previous six months.

Celelana's family's three-story apartment house was the target of an incendiary fire. When a smoke detector alerted her mother to the danger, she instructed her daughter to get out quickly. Six-year-old Celelana located her four-year-old sister, crying in her bedroom from fear of the smoke, and pulled her to the floor. She told the younger girl, "We must crawl under smoke to get out." Their mother found them both sitting on the grass in front of the house, which was by then engulfed in flames. Celelana told her she had learned the steps she followed from "Fireman Friendly" at her school.

Source: National Fire Protection Association, Quincy, Mass.

What Children Should Know

Children should know where the fire extinguishers are located. Extinguishers should be used only by a trained adult if the fire is small and contained.

Children should know the fire escape plan of their child care center. It should be posted in every room, and practiced. There should be two ways of exiting each room and a place where everyone should meet outside. Do not go back inside for any reason.

Children should know to use stairways, not elevators, when leaving a burning building.

Children should know to tie long hair back and not to wear loose-fitting clothes while cooking or standing next to an open flame. Hair and clothing can easily catch on fire.

Children should know that neither they nor their friends should play with matches or lighters. Instruct children to tell a teacher or parent if they find any.

Children should know the phrase, "Stop, drop, and roll." This will remind them to smother flames on their clothing by dropping to the ground and rolling. Running when clothes catch on fire helps the fire burn and increases the chance of inhaling smoke and flames. Also, teach children to cover their faces with both hands when rolling.

Children should know that a fire needs air to burn. Grease fires in a kitchen should be smothered with a lid, not doused with water.

Children should know to crawl to avoid breathing smoke and poisonous fumes when leaving a burning building. The cleanest air is found low to the ground.

Children should know that if they are in a burning building and come to a closed door, they should feel it with their hands. If the door is hot, there is smoke or fire on the opposite side. Do not open it.

Children should know that if they cannot escape a burning building, they should crawl to a room that has a telephone or a window to the outside. Call the emergency rescue number in your area. Signal for help from the window if there is no fire below that window.

Children should know that they should never go into a closet or under a bed. Rescuers won't be able to find them.

Children should know that the fire safety information they know might save a life.

Children should share what they know with their friends and parents.

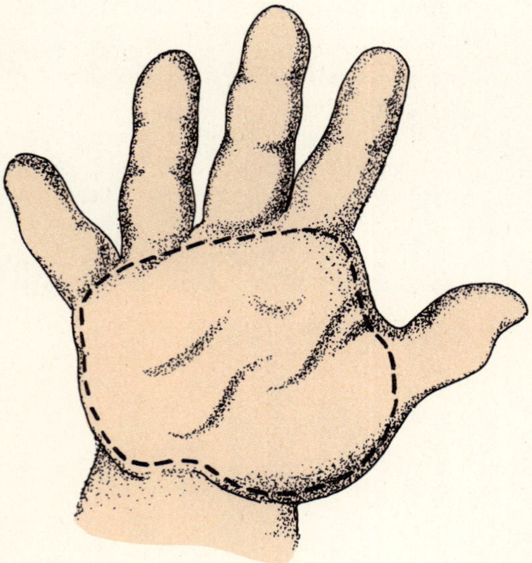

The palm of the hand equals 1% of the total surface area of the body.

the temperature, influence the depth of destruction. On the surface, full-thickness burns can appear red, raw, ash white, black, leathery, or charred. These deep burns also damage hair follicles, muscle, and other tissue. In addition, there is little or no pain in the area of full-thickness damage because the nerves are destroyed. The pain of a full-thickness burn results from the accompanying partial-thickness and superficial (second- and first-degree) burns that surround it. Burns caused by flames, very hot liquids, or electrical contact can cause full-thickness damage.

Full-thickness burns almost always require skin grafting. This is a surgical procedure that transplants healthy skin from another part of the body to the area where skin was destroyed. It is necessary because skin cannot regenerate after a full-thickness burn injury.

- ***Partial-thickness burns*** (second degree). These burns produce a painful and serious in-

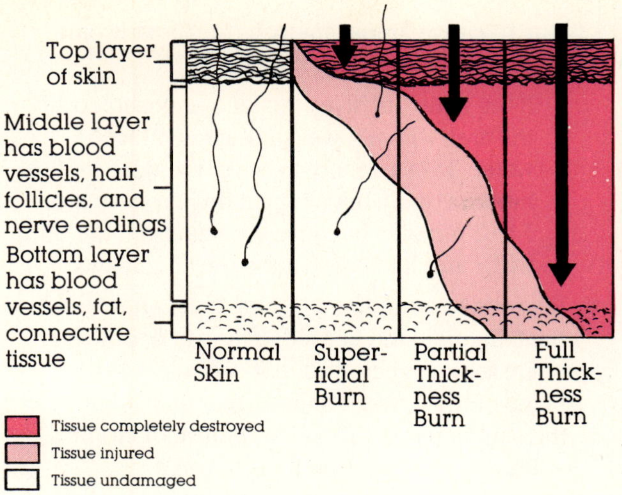

Depth of Burn.
Adapted with permission from the National Institute for Burn Medicine, Ann Arbor, Mi.

jury that damages, but does not completely destroy, the full depth of the skin. A partial-thickness burn appears dark red or mottled and develops blisters and swelling. Large blisters covering the entire burn area indicate a deep and more serious partial-thickness burn. Pain is severe, making medical care necessary for pain management as well as treatment of the burned skin. A large partial-thickness burn takes several weeks to heal and requires special dressings at home. Contact with a scalding-hot liquid and excessive exposure to the sun are examples of a partial-thickness burn.

- ***Superficial burns*** (first degree). These burns produce minor damage to the surface of the skin. A superficial burn causes redness, swelling, and pain that is mild in comparison to the deeper partial-thickness burn. The resulting color change of the skin varies from light pink to dark red depending on the child's skin tone. There is no blistering, as blistering is a sign of a deeper and more serious burn. A superficial burn heals completely within a few days. A simple sunburn that does not blister is an example of a superficial burn.

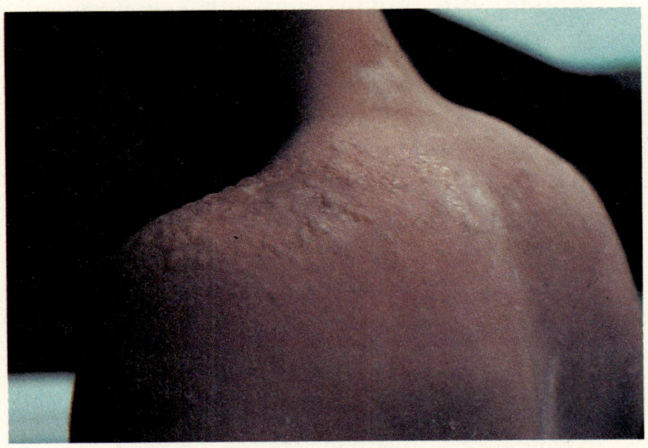

Partial-thickness burn-blistered shoulders

Flame-retardant Fabric

The most severe burns involve burning clothing. The type of fabric a child is wearing significantly contributes to the severity of a burn. New synthetic fibers are less flammable than the more natural fibers of cotton, nylon, and wool but create more damaging burns because the material actually melts onto the skin. In 1972, a federal law was passed requiring all children's sleepwear, sizes infant through 6X, to be flame retardant. This law has substantially reduced the burns caused by flames in younger children. The flame-retardant chemicals that are applied to clothing, however, can be removed if not laundered properly.

To protect the flame-retardant quality of children's clothing:

- Wash in warm water with a phosphate detergent only, not a laundry soap.
- Never use bleach or fabric softeners.
- Drip dry or dry on low settings.
- Do not iron.

Age

A burn is more serious on an infant and a young child than on an older child because the imbalance of body fluids caused by a serious burn injury is more difficult to correct in the younger child.

Preexisting medical problem

A chronic medical condition, such as heart or kidney disease, diabetes, asthma, or an immune system disorder, makes it difficult for the child with a serious burn injury to recover easily and fight off infection.

First Aid for Burns

In many burn injuries, swift first aid action can limit the extent of the damage and help speed the child's recovery. Delayed or improper first aid can allow a burn injury to become more serious, increase the risk of infection, and slow healing.

> **First aid for all burns includes:**
> - Stop the burning process.
> - Check and monitor the airway, breathing, and circulation and treat accordingly.
> - Cool the burn with water, regardless of the source of the burn.

Burns alone do not cause unconsciousness or bleeding. Other injuries should be suspected in a child with these additional problems.

The following first aid sections are organized according to the source of the burn. Each includes the three essential treatment steps listed above and specifics of first aid care that are particular to that burn.

Heat Burns

Heat burns are common among young children. They can be divided into burns caused by flames and burns caused by such other hot sources as liquids, grease, and appliances.

Flame Burns

The severity of a flame burn is influenced by the type of clothing the child is wearing and whether smoke and flames are inhaled.

- * **Stop the burning process.** Smother flame burns by using a blanket or rolling the child on the floor or grass. Prevent the child from running because this fans the flames and helps the fire burn.
- Check for consciousness by calling the child's name. Burn injuries do not cause unconsciousness. Other injuries should be suspected if the child is unconscious. **Check and monitor the airway, breathing, and circulation and treat accordingly.** Swelling of the airway can occur rapidly following a flame burn or it can take as long as 24 hours. Continue to monitor the child's breathing closely and watch for any signs of breathing difficulties.
- * **Cool the burn with water** to dull the pain. This treatment is most effective during the first couple of hours immediately following the injury.
  - Use a sink, tub, or other clean container. If outside, lake, stream, pool, or ocean water may be used. Avoid using *forceful* running water from a faucet or a hose because this can cause further injury to the already damaged skin.
  - If the injury involves the face or chest, cover the area with a towel saturated with cold water. Take care not to cover the nose and mouth completely. Repeat this process every 1 to 2 minutes because the heat from the burn will warm the water in the towel quickly.
- Remove surrounding clothing that can retain heat. Saturate the burned area with cool water while removing clothes that can retain heat. Many of the newer synthetic materials melt onto the skin and are difficult to remove. If clothing adheres to the skin, do not remove it.
- Send someone to call for emergency medical help, if necessary.
- Treat the child for shock by elevating the legs 8 to 12 inches and by keeping the child warm.
- Never place ice directly on a burn because ice, too, can burn the fragile skin that remains. Also avoid using ice water because it can cause rapid loss of body heat leading to hypothermia, a life-threatening condition in which the body temperature is reduced to a dangerously low level.
- Never apply ointments, including burn ointments, petroleum jelly, creams, butter, margarine, toothpaste, or other home remedies to a burn. These products trap the heat of the burn and cause further pain and damage. If the burn requires medical care, the product applied must be removed before appropriate medical treatment can be given.
- Never break blisters. Blisters protect the burn and prevent infection.
- Apply a dry, sterile dressing.

Nonflame Heat Burns

- **Stop the burning process.** Immerse these burns immediately in cool tap water.
- Check for consciousness by calling the child's name. Remember that burn injuries alone do not cause unconsciousness. **Check and monitor the airway, breathing, and circulation and treat accordingly.**
- **Cool the burn with water** to dull the pain. This treatment is most effective during the first couple of hours immediately following the injury.
  - Use a sink, tub, or other clean container. Avoid using *forceful* running water from a faucet or a hose because this can cause further injury to the already damaged skin.

- If the injury involves the face or chest, cover the area with a towel saturated with cold water. Take care not to cover the nose and mouth completely. Repeat this process every 1 to 2 minutes because the heat from the burn will warm the water in the towel quickly.

- Remove surrounding clothing that can retain heat and cause further pain and damage. If clothing adheres to the skin, do not remove it.
- Send someone to call for emergency medical help, if necessary.
- Treat the child for shock.
- Never place ice directly on a burn because ice, too, can burn the already damaged skin. Also avoid using ice water because it can cause rapid loss of body heat leading to hypothermia, a life-threatening condition in which the body temperature is reduced to a dangerously low level.
- Never apply ointments, including burn ointments, petroleum jelly, creams, butter, margarine, toothpaste, or other home remedies to a burn. These products trap the heat of the burn and cause further pain and damage. If the burn requires medical care, the product applied must be removed before further treatment can be given.
- Never break blisters. Blisters protect the burn and prevent infection.
- Apply a dry, sterile dressing.

Chemical Burns

Although not commonly seen in child care centers, chemical burns sometimes occur from industrial-strength cleaning products and many chemicals typically stored in garages and basements. A corrosive chemical begins to burn the skin on contact. By diluting and removing the chemical immediately, damage can be reduced.

- Brush off a dry or solid chemical substance, such as lime, before flushing with water. Small amounts of water can activate some dry chemicals and cause more damage to the skin than when dry.
- Stop the burning process by flooding the area with cool running water under low pressure from a faucet or a hose for 10 to 15 minutes. Do not use water under high pressure, such as from a garden hose attachment, because such pressure could drive the chemical deeper into the tissue.

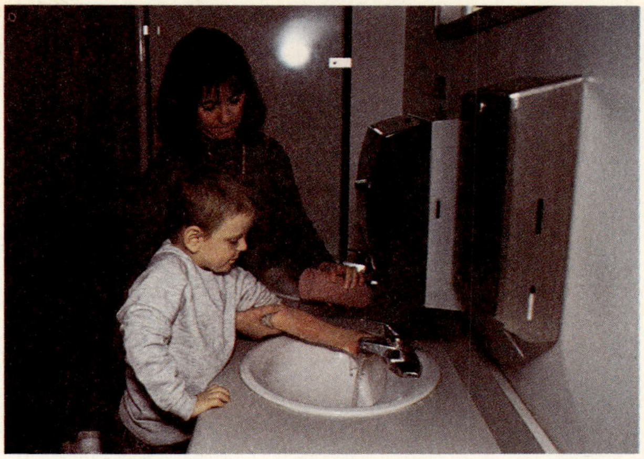

Washing/flooding a chemical burn

- Remove all clothing in the area of the spill because it might be contaminated with the chemical.
- Call the local poison control center for advice on further treatment.
- Do not break blisters on the skin if they develop. Treat as you would for heat burns of the same extent and depth.
- Apply a dry sterile dressing.

When to Seek Medical Treatment for a Burn Injury

If you are unsure of the severity of the burn and whether medical treatment is necessary, consult the following list of guidelines. The child should be seen immediately by a health care provider if:

- Pain is severe enough that the child is inconsolable and not able to be distracted.
- The child is under 5 years of age with a partial-thickness burn larger than the size of a quarter.
- The child has a full-thickness burn of any size.
- The child has a chronic medical problem.
- There are partial-thickness or full-thickness burns on the child's face, hands, feet, or genitals, or the burn encircles an arm, leg, or the chest.
- Another injury accompanies the burn.
- The child might have inhaled smoke or flames.
- Signs of abuse are present, such as cigarette burns, a clear mark of submersion on a burned extremity, or a burn injury with an explanation that does not seem plausible.

■ HEAT BURNS ■

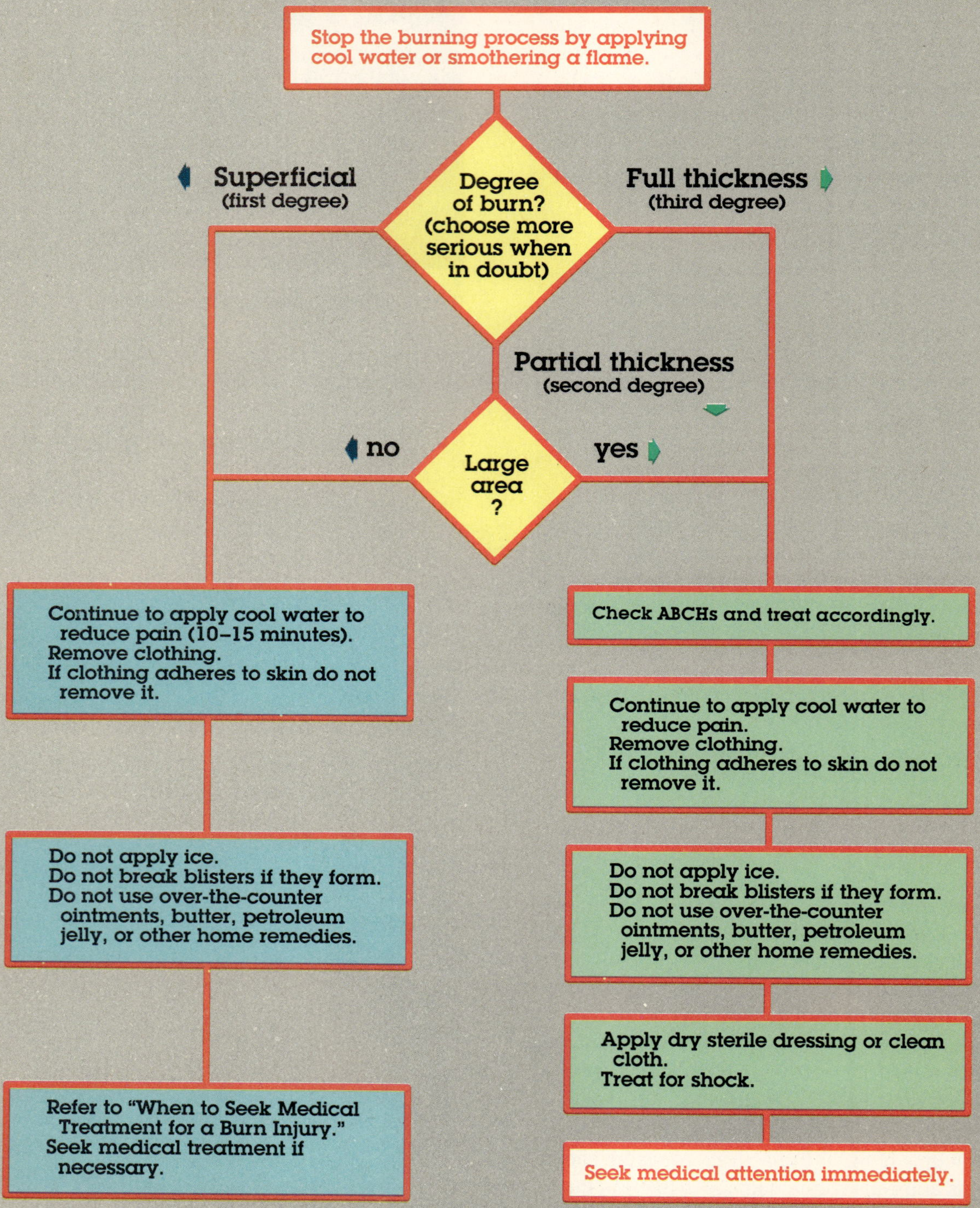
Stop the burning process by applying cool water or smothering a flame.
Degree of burn? (choose more serious when in doubt)
Superficial (first degree)
Full thickness (third degree)
Partial thickness (second degree)
Large area ?
no
yes
Continue to apply cool water to reduce pain (10–15 minutes). Remove clothing. If clothing adheres to skin do not remove it.
Do not apply ice. Do not break blisters if they form. Do not use over-the-counter ointments, butter, petroleum jelly, or other home remedies.
Refer to "When to Seek Medical Treatment for a Burn Injury." Seek medical treatment if necessary.
Check ABCHs and treat accordingly.
Continue to apply cool water to reduce pain. Remove clothing. If clothing adheres to skin do not remove it.
Do not apply ice. Do not break blisters if they form. Do not use over-the-counter ointments, butter, petroleum jelly, or other home remedies.
Apply dry sterile dressing or clean cloth. Treat for shock.
Seek medical attention immediately.

■ CHEMICAL BURNS ■

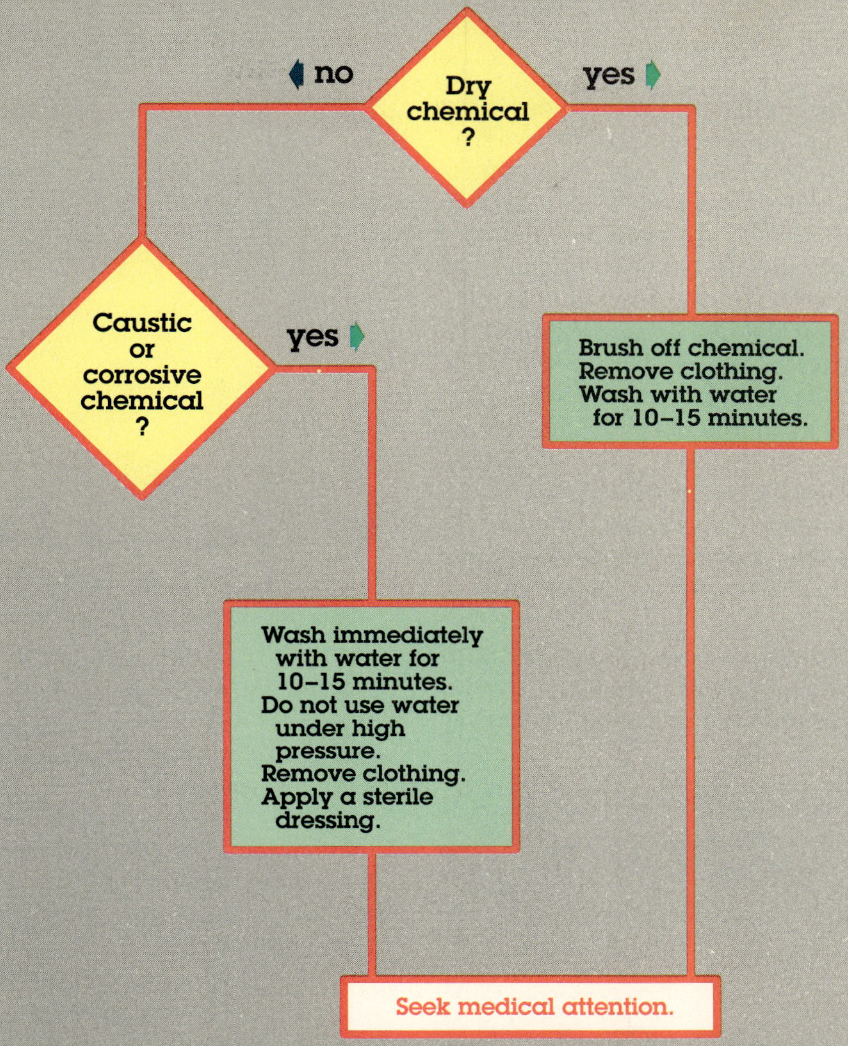

Chemical Burns of the Eye

See Eye Injuries, Chapter 6.

Electrical Burns

Electricity, when used properly, is one of our safest and cleanest sources of power. Because its use is so routine, we tend to forget the enormous energy potential behind the seemingly innocent household plug. Even household current of 110 volts can be deadly under certain conditions, such as using an appliance with wet hands or while standing on a wet floor.

Electricity follows the path of least resistance. In the body, this path is along the nerves and through the body fluids. Electrical current enters a child's body at the point of contact and travels rapidly through the body, generating heat and causing destruction. Usually the electricity exits where the child is touching a metal object or the ground. There might or might not be a burn on the skin. Although the damage to the skin might appear to be small, the internal damage can be extensive.

Electrical current that passes through the body can cause severe damage or life-threatening injuries such as full-thickness burns or respiratory and cardiac arrest.

> Electricity travels best in water—the body of a child is more than 75 percent water.
> *National Institute for Burn Medicine, Ann Arbor, Michigan*

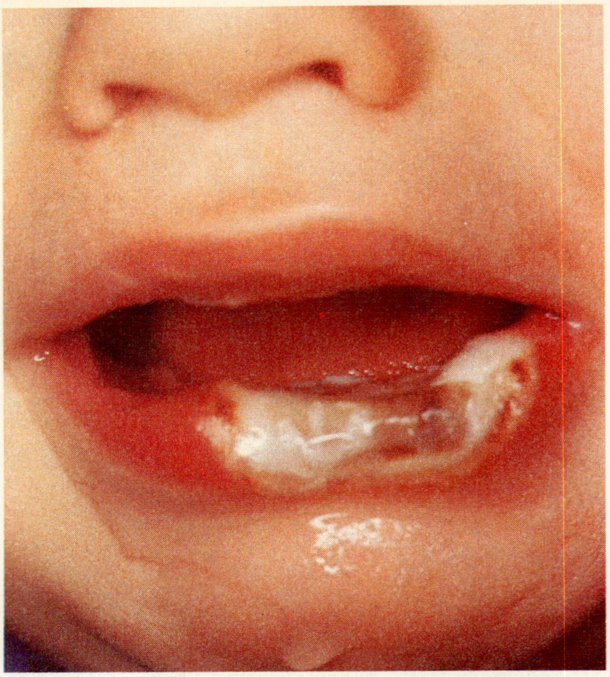

Full-thickness electrical burn after biting through an electrical cord

Outdoor Power Lines

Although a downed power line seldom occurs, adults should know how to proceed safely when dealing with this very dangerous situation. The power must be turned off before a first aider approaches a child who is in contact with the wire. *Never* attempt to move downed wires unless you are trained and equipped with tools capable of safely handling high voltage.

If the child is trapped in a car with a power line fallen across it, tell the child to stay in the car. To prevent electrocution, the power must be disconnected before the child gets out of the car. This can be done only by the electric company. Stand at least 15 feet from the car and prevent bystanders from entering the danger area.

Indoors

Most indoor electrical burns result from the use of faulty electrical appliances or from improper or careless use of electrical equipment. Typical electrical injuries of young children include biting through an electrical cord and sticking a metal paper clip or safety pin into a wall outlet.

Most children who receive an electrical shock will be knocked away from the electrical source by the force generated from the contact. Although the child will be upset and shaken, there are no lasting effects from this type of shock.

If the child remains in contact with the electrical source, it is a life-threatening emergency. The child is "hot" with electricity and will pass the electricity to whoever touches the child. Electricity causes strong muscle contractions that result in the child's holding on tightly to the damaged electrical cord or faulty appliance. The child is unable to let go until the electricity is turned off. The fastest and most effective way to stop the flow of electricity is to unplug the appliance if the plug is undamaged and you can reach it without coming in contact with the child. Otherwise, you must turn off the electricity by using the wall switch, circuit breaker, fuse box, or outside switch box.

Do not attempt to kick an appliance with your foot or to push it away with another object, even if the object is thought not to conduct electricity. Because the child is gripping the "hot" appliance or cord, your attempt is likely to be ineffective. Go directly to the power source to turn off the power. All child care providers should know where the main power source is located and how to turn it off.

First Aid

Once the danger to a rescuer is eliminated, first aid can begin.

- Check for consciousness by calling the child's name. Check and monitor the airway, breathing, and circulation and treat accordingly.
- Send someone to call for emergency medical help.
- Treat for shock by elevating the legs 8 to 12 inches and keeping the child warm.
- Check for burns. Most electrical burns are full-thickness burns. Electricity can also ignite clothing causing a flame injury. Treat as you would other burns of the same depth.

Any child who sustains a severe electrical shock needs immediate medical attention because of the possibility of respiratory or cardiac arrest. In this event, the burn injury, even if full thickness, becomes secondary.

A strong electrical shock can cause severe internal damage as well as burns. Recovery can take many months.

■ ELECTRICAL INJURIES ■

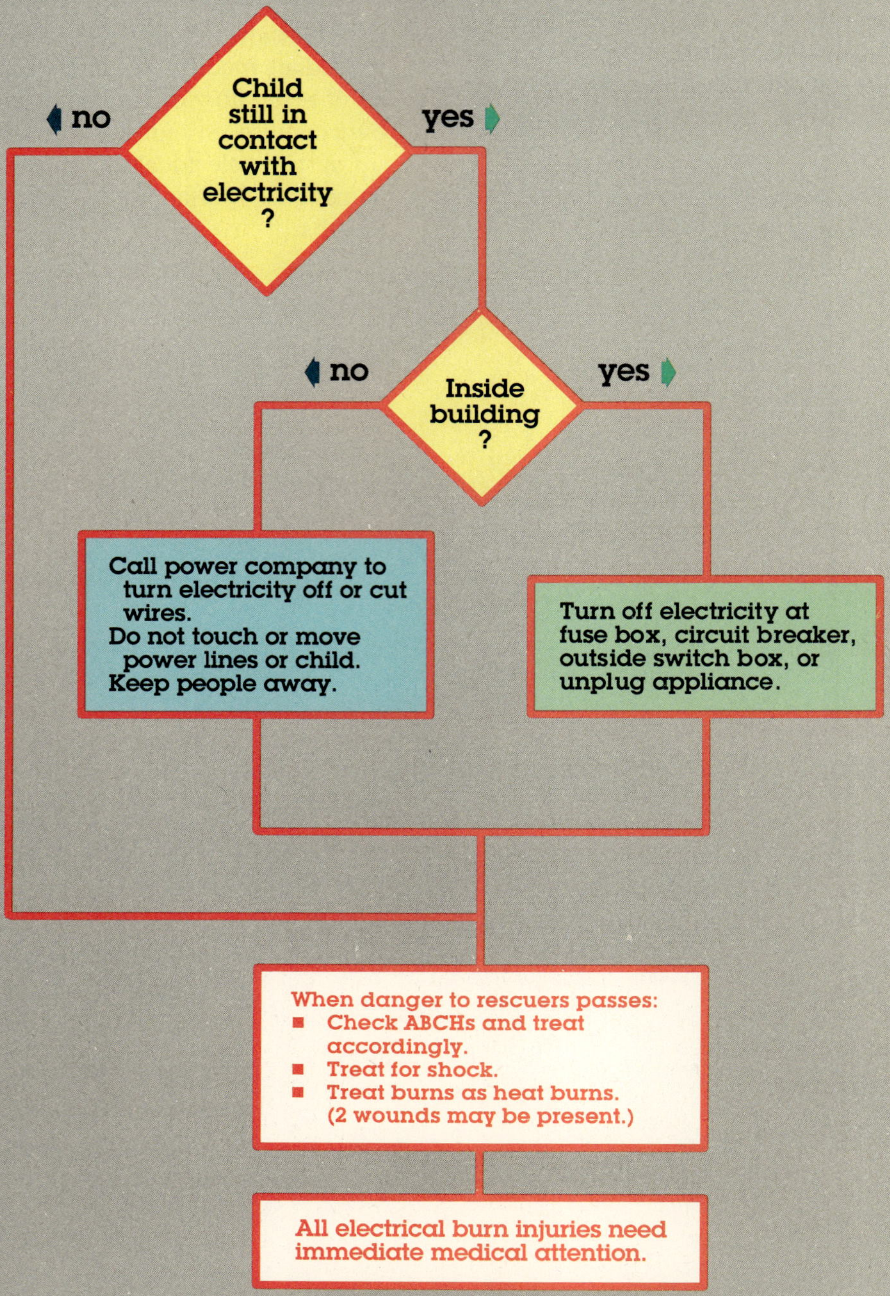

Heat Burns

Choose the best answer.

1. ____ What is the first step in caring for a child with a burn?
   - **A.** Check the ABCs and treat accordingly.
   - **B.** Stop the burning process by smothering the flame or dousing the burn with water.
   - **C.** Treat for shock.
   - **D.** Cover the burn with a clean dressing.
2. ____ What should you do to ease the pain of a burn?
   - **A.** Cover the burn with petroleum jelly or any over-the-counter burn ointment.
   - **B.** Cover the burned area with a clean dressing.
   - **C.** Place the injured part in a sink filled with warm water.
   - **D.** Place the injured part in a sink filled with cool water.
3. ____ The type of burn characterized by reddening, blisters, and deep intense pain is called a:
   - **A.** Superficial burn (first degree)
   - **B.** Partial-thickness burn (second degree)
   - **C.** Full-thickness burn (third degree)
4. ____ Which type of burn is characterized by little or no pain and skin that can be ash white, black, leathery, or charred?
   - **A.** Superficial burn (first degree)
   - **B.** Partial-thickness burn (second degree)
   - **C.** Full-thickness burn (third degree)
5. ____ Which body areas are especially sensitive to being burned?
   - **A.** Face
   - **B.** Hands
   - **C.** Feet
   - **D.** All of the above
6. ____ A child's hand size represents what percentage of the body?
   - **A.** 1%
   - **B.** 5%
   - **C.** 10%

Mark each action yes (Y) or no (N).

When giving first aid for a burn, you should:

1. ____ Apply petroleum jelly to the burn.
2. ____ Apply butter to the burn.
3. ____ Apply cool water to the burn.
4. ____ Apply ice to the burn.
5. ____ Apply a dry, sterile dressing and secure it in place.
6. ____ Open blisters before applying a burn ointment.

Chemical Burns

Choose the best answer.

1. ____ When washing chemicals from the body, it is best if the water is:
   - **A.** Applied to the area under high pressure.
   - **B.** Applied to the area under low pressure.
   - **C.** Kept in a large basin into which the affected body part is submerged.
2. ____ What is the first step in caring for a child who has spilled a dry chemical on his skin?
   - **A.** Read the chemical container's label as to proper procedures.
   - **B.** Flush with water.
   - **C.** Brush off the dry chemical before flushing with water.
   - **D.** Cover the area with a dry, sterile bandage.

Electrical Burns

Choose the best answer.

1. ____ If a child is stranded in a car with a power line fallen across it, the child should be instructed to:
   A. Stay in the car.
   B. Jump from a car window.
   C. Exit through the door.
2. ____ If you are near a child who is in contact with downed high-power electrical lines, you should:
   A. Try to move any wires with wood poles or handles.
   B. Try to pull the wires away from the child.
   C. Use wood poles or handles to try to pull the child away from any wires.
   D. Wait until the power company can cut the wires or disconnect them.
3. ____ Where does electricity produce the most damaging burns?
   A. On the skin
   B. Deep under the skin
4. ____ First aid for a child who has received an electric shock can include:
   A. CPR
   B. Burn first aid
   C. Shock first aid
   D. All of the above
5. ____ The first step in caring for a child receiving an electrical shock is to:
   A. Pull the appliance away from the child.
   B. Pull the child away from the appliance.
   C. Unplug the appliance from the wall socket.

9

Cold- and Heat-Related Injuries

■ Frostbite ■ Frostnip ■ Heat Stroke ■
■ Heat Exhaustion ■ Heat Syncope ■ Sunburn ■

Outdoor play is a healthy activity enjoyed by most young children. It should be encouraged year-round. Some seasonal weather conditions have the potential to harm a child's health if the length of time and conditions of exposure exceed safe limits.

Cold-Related Injuries

Frostbite

Frostbite is the freezing of body tissue. Both air temperature and length of time that the child is exposed determine the extent of the damage. Children are more susceptible to frostbite than adults because they have a smaller amount of body fat to insulate them against the damaging cold. Frostbite is seen frequently on hands, fingers, cheeks, ears, nose, and toes. In severe cases, body tissue dies from the lack of circulating blood and oxygen caused by the cold temperature.

Signs and Symptoms

Initially, exposed or underprotected skin is cold and mildly painful, but the pain subsides as the exposed skin becomes numb in the freezing process. The signs and symptoms become apparent when the child comes indoors.

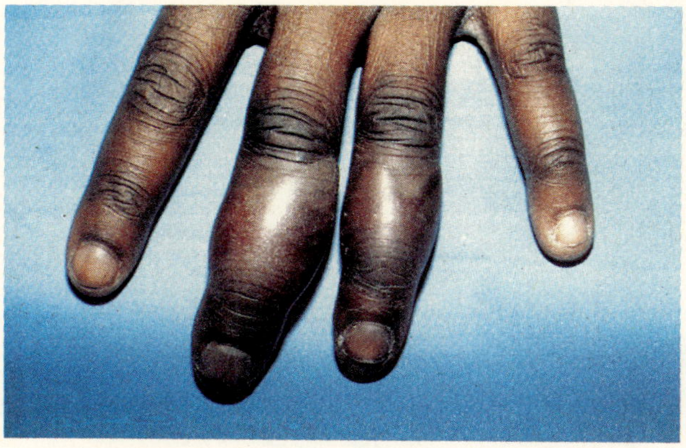

Swollen frostbitten fingers

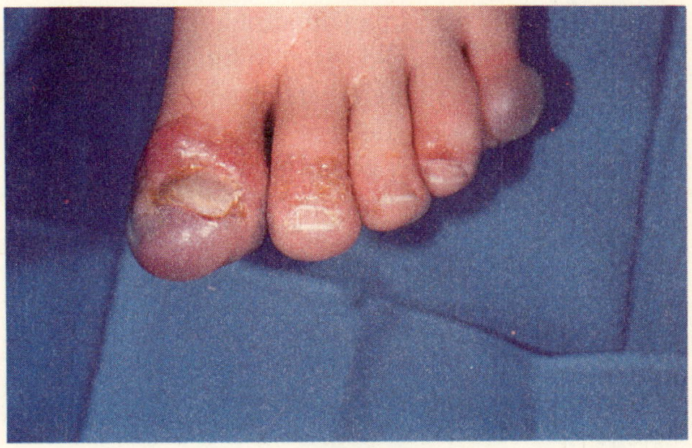

Blistered frostbitten toes

- Tingling and burning of the frostbitten area
- Aching or throbbing pain, which can be severe
- Difficulty moving the body part
- Skin color change to milky white, grayish yellow, or pale blue that might change to red, purple, or blue-black once thawing begins
- Swelling of the frostbitten area as it starts to thaw
- Waxy-looking skin
- Skin feels hard, but tissue underneath feels soft
- Blistered skin, indicating a more serious degree of frostbite

First Aid

- Remove clothing from affected area.
- Examine the area for frostbite if the child complains of pain and has difficulty using the body part.
- Do not break any blisters that form.
- Slightly elevate the area to decrease pain and swelling.
- Place gauze pads between fingers or toes to prevent them from sticking together and to absorb moisture.
- Cover any blisters that rupture with a sterile gauze pad.
- Keep the child warm.

- Offer a warm drink, but never an alcoholic beverage.
- Have the child seen by a health care provider immediately.

Cautions

- Do not attempt to rewarm the area yourself by using a hot water bottle, warm water, heating pad, radiator, blow dryer, fireplace or other poorly measurable heat sources. Leave this care to medical professionals who will warm the area rapidly using a carefully controlled technique.
- Never rub the area in an attempt to stimulate circulation. This could result in further damage to fragile skin and underlying tissue.
- Never rub snow on the area.
- Handle the area very gently to avoid rupturing the ice crystals that form under the skin.
- Do not allow a child to walk on feet that might be frostbitten.

Preventing Frostbite

Frostbite is seen when children are inadequately dressed and are outdoors sledding, skiing, and playing for long periods of time. The relatively short exposure and the close supervision of outdoor winter play at a child care center reduce the risk of frostbite occurring to a child in your care. Nonetheless, take these precautions when outdoors with children during the freezing weather:

- Always dress appropriately for cold-weather play including mittens, snow pants, boots, and hats that cover ears.
- Be sure that mittens and hats stay on.
- Observe for white spots forming on cheeks that might indicate mild frostbite.
- Bring a child indoors immediately who complains of a cold, numb, tingly, or painful area on the body.
- Check the temperature and limit outdoor play time accordingly during the cold-weather months. See How Cold Is it?
- Teach others about the importance of frostbite prevention. Once frostbitten, the injured body area will be more susceptible to future episodes of frostbite. In addition, a child who has had frostbite will continue to be very sensitive to the cold and can experience tingling, loss of feeling, and pain during cold weather for many years.

Winter Wardrobe

	Advantages	Disadvantages	Wear In
WOOL	Stretches without damage; insulates well even when wet	Heavy weight; absorbs moisture; may irritate skin	Layer 1, 2 or 3
COTTON	Comfortable and lightweight	Absorbs moisture	Layer 1 (for inactive people) or 2
SILK	Extremely lightweight and durable; very good insulator; washes well	More expensive; does not transfer moisture quickly	Layer 1
POLYPROPYLENE	Lightweight; transfers moisture quickly and dries quickly	Does not insulate well; low melting point; surface may pill up	Layer 1 or 2 (for active people)
DOWN	Durable, lightweight; most effective insulator by weight	Expensive; loses insulative quality when wet; difficult to dry	Layer 2 or 3 (especially in dry, extreme cold)
NYLON	Lightweight; wind- and water-resistant; durable	May not allow perspiration to evaporate; low melting point; flammable	Layer 3
SYNTHETIC POLYESTER INSULATION	Does not absorb moisture, therefore insulates even when wet	Heavier than down; does not compress as well	Layer 2 or 3 (especially in wet weather)

Source: National Safety Council, Family Safety & Health.

How Cold Is It?

Wind can make the temperature feel lower than the thermometer registers. If the thermometer reads 20° F and the wind speed is 20 mph, the exposure is comparable to −10° F. This is called the wind-chill factor. A rough measure of wind speed is: If you feel the wind on your face, the speed is about 10 mph; if small branches move or dust or snow is raised, 20 mph; if large branches are moving, 30 mph; and if a whole tree bends, about 40 mph.

Determine the wind-chill factor by:

1. Estimating the wind speed by checking for the signs described above.
2. Looking at a thermometer reading outdoors.
3. Matching the estimated wind speed with the thermometer reading in the "Wind-Chill Factor" table below.

Frostnip

Frostnip is also caused by exposure to the cold but is less serious than frostbite. It is seen on the same body areas as frostbite—hands, fingers, cheeks, ears, nose, and toes.

Signs and Symptoms

- Tingling and awareness of cold, indicating that circulation is slowed and unable to warm the area.
- A white spot or patch on the nose or a cheek.
- Pain and numbness.

First Aid

- Cover the area with a scarf, glove, or mitten. This should promote the return of a healthy skin color quickly.
- Come indoors to prevent the area from becoming frostbitten.
- Do not rub the area hoping to promote circulation.
- Warm the frostnipped area by blowing warm breath on it, and by holding the part between warm hands.
- A child can warm his hands and fingers by placing them in his armpits.

Frostnip should be resolved within 10 to 15 minutes after coming inside. If it is not, reexamine the area for signs of frostbite.

Heat-Related Injuries

Most children love the summer and the seemingly endless hours of outdoor play. Adults enjoy having them there for all the healthy reasons that being outside implies. Yet it is important for child care providers

Wind-Chill Factor

Estimated Wind Speed (in MPH)	Actual Thermometer Reading (°F)											
	50	40	30	20	10	0	−10	−20	−30	−40	−50	−60
	Equivalent Temperature (°F)											
calm	50	40	30	20	10	0	−10	−20	−30	−40	−50	−60
5	40	37	27	16	6	−5	−15	−26	−36	−47	−57	−68
10	40	28	16	4	−9	−24	−33	−46	−58	−70	−83	−95
15	36	22	9	−5	−18	−32	−45	−58	−72	−85	−99	−112
20	32	18	4	−10	−25	−39	−53	−67	−82	−96	−110	−124
25	30	16	0	−15	−29	−44	−59	−74	−88	−104	−118	−133
30	25	13	−2	−18	−33	−48	−63	−79	−94	−109	−125	−140
35	27	11	−4	−20	−35	−51	−67	−82	−98	−113	−129	−145
40	26	10	−6	−21	−37	−53	−69	−85	−100	−116	−132	−148
(Wind speeds greater than 40 mph have little additional effect.)	Little danger (for properly clothed person). Maximum danger of false sense of security.				Increasing danger. (Flesh may freeze within 1 minute.)			Great danger. (Flesh may freeze within 30 seconds.)				

■ FROSTBITE ■

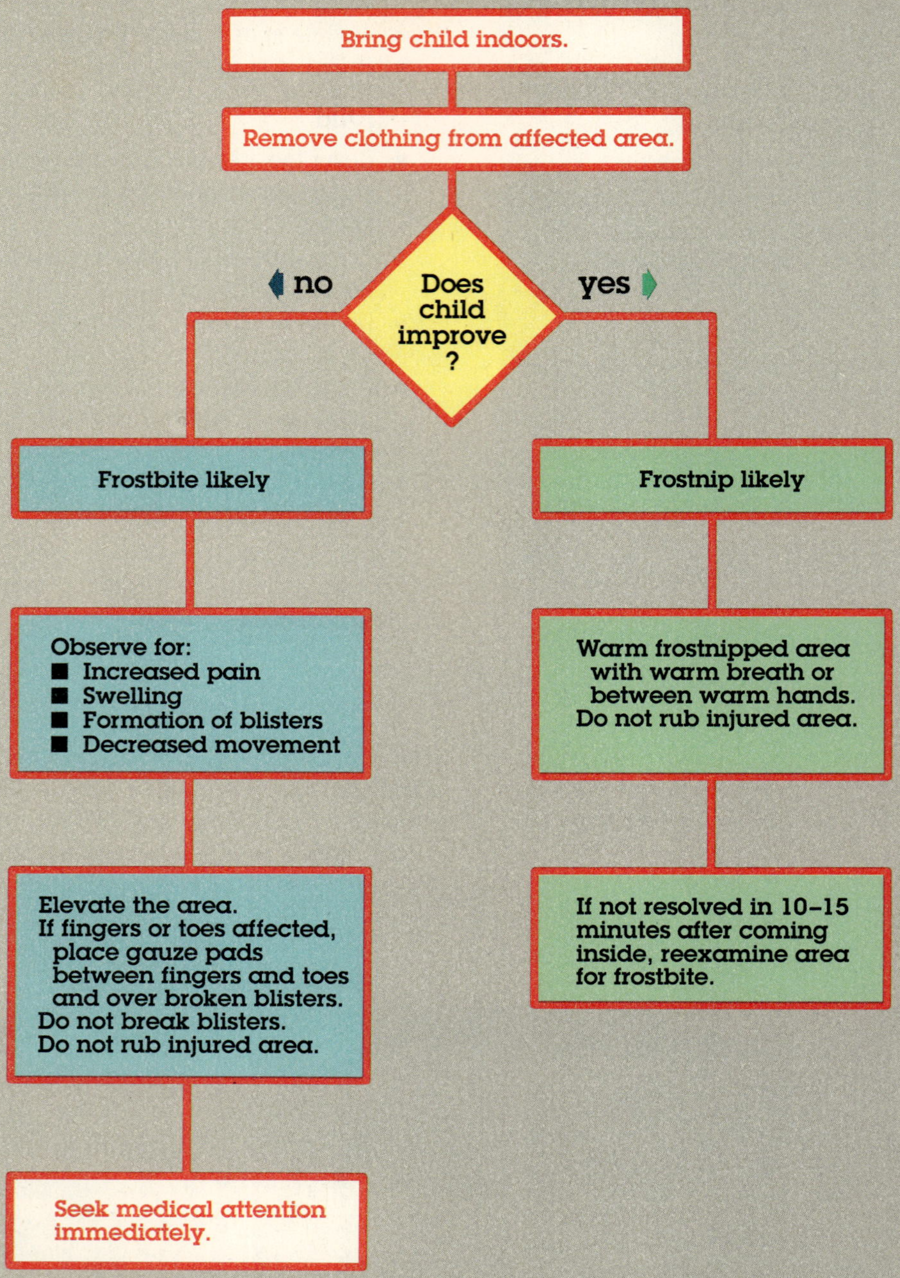
Bring child indoors.
Remove clothing from affected area.
Does child improve ?
no
yes
Frostbite likely
Frostnip likely
Observe for:
■ Increased pain
■ Swelling
■ Formation of blisters
■ Decreased movement
Warm frostnipped area with warm breath or between warm hands. Do not rub injured area.
Elevate the area.
If fingers or toes affected, place gauze pads between fingers and toes and over broken blisters.
Do not break blisters.
Do not rub injured area.
If not resolved in 10–15 minutes after coming inside, reexamine area for frostbite.
Seek medical attention immediately.

to know that the sun and the heat can be dangerous and occasionally deadly. Use common sense and the recommendations in this section to avoid heat-related injuries.

Heat-related injuries are caused by overexposure to high temperatures. These injuries can be mild or life threatening depending on the degree of heat and the length of time that the child is exposed.

Heat Stroke

Heat stroke is a life-threatening medical emergency in which the body becomes unable to regulate its temperature. It can develop suddenly and is the least common and most dangerous heat-related emergency.

Sweating is how the body cools itself in warmer weather. When exposed to excessively high temperatures, the mechanism that regulates the body's cooling system and triggers sweating ceases to function; without that process, the result is a life-threatening rise in body temperature. A child who is left in a closed car on a hot day, where temperatures can rise far above 100° F, is at risk for developing heat stroke.

Signs and Symptoms

Mild signs and symptoms are headache, dizziness, nausea, and vomiting. Severe signs and symptoms can rapidly follow the mild signs and symptoms or they can appear abruptly without warning.

- Body temperature can approach 106° F, or higher
- Skin is hot and dry because the sweat glands are not functioning
- Rapid breathing and pulse
- Face flushed
- Confusion and lethargy
- Collapse and loss of consciousness
- Seizures

Brain, liver, and kidney damage and death can result if the body is not cooled quickly

First Aid

Rapid treatment of heat stroke is essential because every minute of delay increases the likelihood of serious complications or death.

- Check the airway, breathing, and circulation and treat accordingly.
- Send someone to call for emergency medical help.
- Move the child to a cool place.
- Remove clothing such as shirt and pants.
- Apply cool, wet towels to the child's head, trunk, and limbs. Take care not to cover the nose and mouth. Continually fan the child to speed the evaporation of water.
- Place ice packs on the body in areas with abundant blood supply such as the neck, armpits, and groin. Wrap the ice in a cloth to protect the skin.
- Care for seizures, if they occur. See Seizures, Chapter 11.
- Do not give aspirin or acetaminophen in an attempt to reduce the fever because they will have no effect.

Hospitalization is always necessary for a child with heat stroke.

Heat Exhaustion

Heat exhaustion occurs when the body loses too much water and salt through sweating. In children, it is often

Heat Stroke–	Heat exhaustion–
–Dry, flushed, hot skin	–Moist, pale, cool skin
–Very high body temperature	–Normal or subnormal temperature
–No sweating	–Heavy sweating
–Life threatening	–Serious, not life-threatening

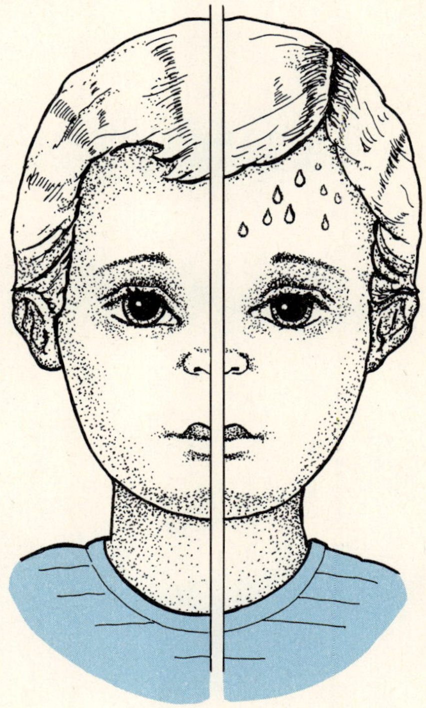

Comparison of heat stroke and heat exhaustion

■ HEAT-RELATED EMERGENCIES ■

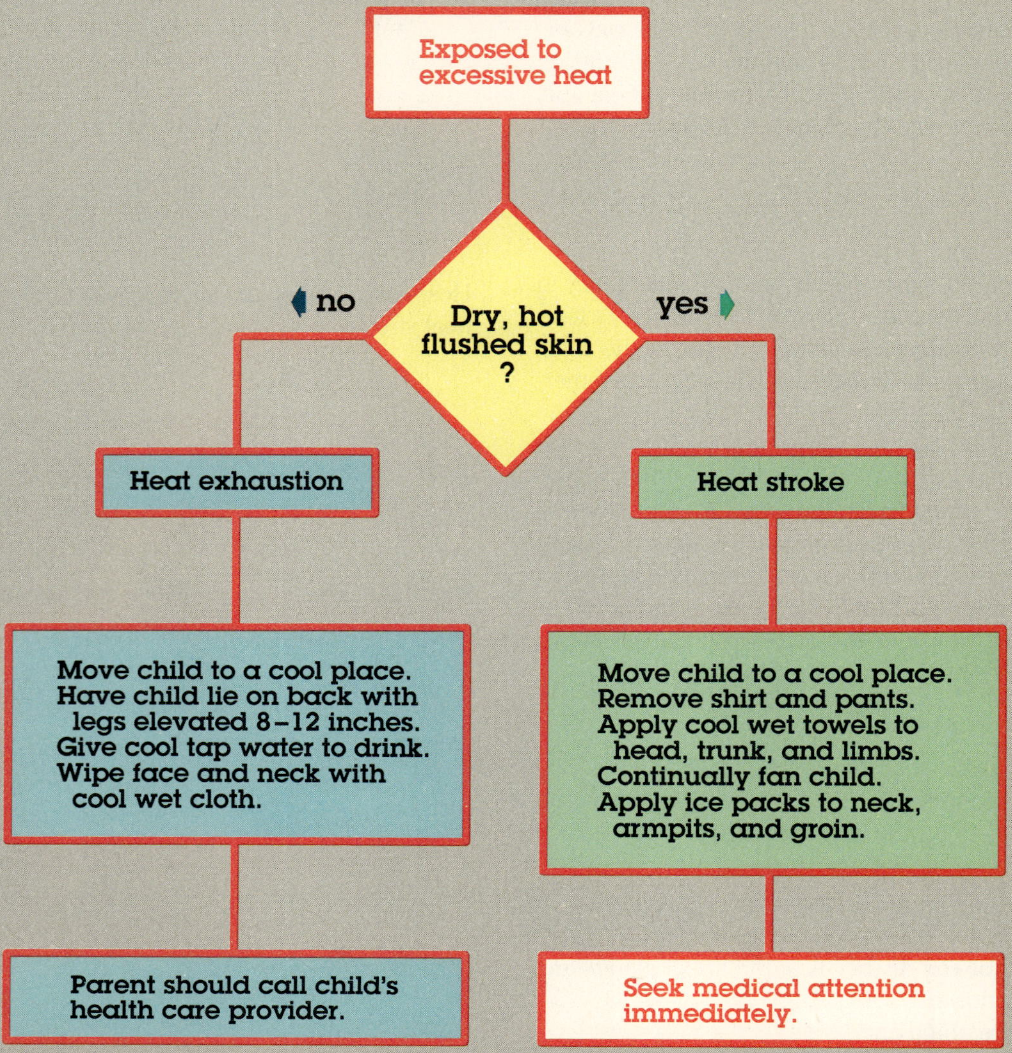

the result of prolonged physical activity in high temperatures. This condition differs from heat stroke in that the body is sweating and the temperature remains normal. Heat exhaustion is less critical than heat stroke, but it requires prompt attention to correct it.

Signs and Symptoms

- Skin pale and cool with heavy sweating
- Fast and weak pulse
- Tiredness and weakness
- Dizziness and feeling faint
- Pounding headache
- Nausea and vomiting
- Muscle cramps
- Body temperature remains normal

First Aid

- Move the child to a cool place. Have the child lie down with feet elevated 8 to 12 inches.
- Give cool water to drink.
- Wipe the child's face and neck with a cool, wet cloth.
- Ask the child's parent to come and take the child. Suggest that the parent call the child's health care provider.

Heat Syncope

A child can easily develop heat syncope from overexposure to the sun, and it can occur easily in a child who is sensitive to the sun. This condition resembles fainting in that the child feels light-headed but does not usually faint. Minor first aid measures are very effective in treating heat syncope.

Signs and Symptoms

- Lightheadedness
- Headache
- Nausea

First Aid

- Have the child lie down in a cool place to rest.
- If not nauseated, give cool water to drink.

The child should begin to feel better within 15 minutes but should not participate in strenuous outdoor activity for the remainder of the day.

Preventing Heat-Related Injuries

1. Encourage children to drink cool tap water frequently on hot days, as often as every 2 hours. Fruit juices and popsicles are fine as treats, but they contain sugar which can make it difficult for the body to absorb fluid. It is possible for a child to become dehydrated before feeling thirsty.
2. Provide cooling entertainment, such as a sprinkler or a wading pool.
3. Avoid vigorous physical activities between 11 A.M. and 2 P.M. when the sun's rays are the most intense.
4. Read a story in the shade of a tree to enjoy the outdoors on very hot days.
5. Never leave a child in a closed vehicle.

Heat Cramps

See Muscle Cramps, Chapter 10.

Sunburn

Unprotected skin is exposed to the harmful ultraviolet rays of the sun whether the day is sunny or cloudy. Repeated exposure to the sun causes early aging of the skin and changes that can allow skin cancers to occur later in life. Skin can be damaged by ultraviolet rays without burning, and the harm from repeated unprotected and under-protected exposures resulting in a tan are cumulative.

Signs and Symptoms

A mild sunburn is usually a superficial burn and has the following signs and symptoms:

- Redness
- Pain and tenderness, especially when trying to move the burned area
- Can worsen as the day progresses, even hours after coming inside

A more serious sunburn is a partial-thickness burn and has these additional signs and symptoms:

- Blisters on the burned area
- Fever and chills
- Pain that can be so intense the child will not tolerate clothing on the area
- Nausea
- Dehydration

First Aid

- Give the child cool baths or apply cool compresses to the sunburn several times per day.
- Do not apply greasy ointments or home remedies such as butter, toothpaste, or shortening to the sunburn.
- Parents may apply over-the-counter sunburn remedies to nonblistered skin, if desired. These

products do not speed healing, but they do reduce pain and soothe the skin. Child care providers should know their center's policy about the use of these products.

- Parents may give a mild analgesic such as acetaminophen for pain. Child care providers should know their center's policy concerning the use of acetaminophen.
- Parents should consult the child's health care provider concerning a sunburn that blisters, or if the child has any of the symptoms that accompany a more serious sunburn.

Sunburn Precautions

We now know that the summer sun is not as friendly as the warm rays make us feel it is. Protecting skin from the sun is essential to reduce sunburn and to protect against the long-term damage that years of exposure to ultraviolet rays can produce.

1. Limit children's exposure to the direct sun between the hours of 11:00 A.M. and 2:00 P.M. when the sun's rays are the most intense.
2. Parents should provide a sunscreen along with written permission to use it. All children should wear a sunscreen with a sun protection factor (SPF) of at least 15, regardless of the skin's tanning ability. This number indicates the amount of protection the product provides. For instance, a child wearing a sunscreen with an SPF of 4 can remain in the sun four times longer than without skin protection before skin damage occurs.
3. Choose sunscreens that block both UVA and UVB rays because they provide protection against the widest range of ultraviolet rays.
4. Apply sunscreen liberally to frequently exposed areas, such as the face, the back of the neck, the shoulders, behind the knees, and the tops of the feet. There are sunscreen products made exclusively for children that do not sting sensitive skin. However, do not apply any sunscreen products to an open cut or rash.
5. Apply sunscreen 20 to 30 minutes before going outside because this allows the protective ingredients time to be absorbed below the surface of the skin. Reapply sunscreen frequently while out-of-doors as even a sunscreen with an SPF of 15 can be washed away by playing in water or sweating.
6. The reflection of ultraviolet rays off the water at a pool, lake, or ocean, as well as off the sand at the beach increases the intensity of the sun's rays. When in these locations, cover-ups such as shirts and hats are essential additions to sunscreen protection. Use an umbrella to provide children with a shaded area.
7. Children under the age of 1 year require special protection. They should have minimal exposure to direct sun and are safest if not taken to a beach where they risk dehydration in addition to sunburn. When exposed to direct sun they should have all skin covered and wear a hat. Manufacturers of sunscreens recommend that their products not be used on infants under the age of 6 months.
8. Some antibiotics can increase a child's sensitivity to the sun's rays. Check all medication containers for warning labels.
9. Do not tell a child that a tan is a sign of good health. It is important to educate even young children about the risks of sun exposure to prevent unnecessary sunburns now and sun-related health problems later.

Frostbite

Mark each action yes (Y) or no (N).

1. ____ Rewarm a frostbitten part by wrapping a heating pad around it.
2. ____ Rub the frostbitten area to restore circulation.
3. ____ A child with frostbitten toes should not walk.
4. ____ Wrap frostbitten fingers snugly together to speed rewarming.
5. ____ Break any blisters that might form.
6. ____ Suspected frostbite should be seen in an emergency medical facility immediately.

Heat-Related Injuries

Mark each description HE (heat exhaustion) or HS (heat stroke).

1. ____ Skin sweating
2. ____ Related to inability to sweat
3. ____ Skin dry
4. ____ Normal body temperature
5. ____ Body temperature extremely high
6. ____ Requires prompt attention but is seldom life threatening
7. ____ Can be sudden and life threatening
8. ____ Related to extreme loss of water and salt

Check (√) the correct first aid steps to take when a child collapses and has very hot, dry and red skin:

1. ____ Send someone to call for emergency medical help.
2. ____ Wrap the child in wet towels.
3. ____ Continually fan the child.
4. ____ Apply ice wrapped in a towel to neck, armpits, and groin.

10

Bone, Joint, and Muscle Injuries

■ Fractures ■ Sprains ■ Dislocations ■ Spinal Injuries ■ Muscle Cramps ■ Sports-Related Injuries ■

Fractures

A fracture is a partial or complete break in a bone caused by a twist or a direct blow. Fractures are common in children, even though the bones and ligaments of healthy children are more flexible than those of adults. These injuries are especially worrisome in children because any damage to the growth plate of a bone (the area of the bone where growth takes place) can cause shortening of the bone and irregular growth. Fractures often involve damage to the surrounding muscles, nerves, and blood vessels, causing bleeding, swelling, and pain.

a. Closed fracture

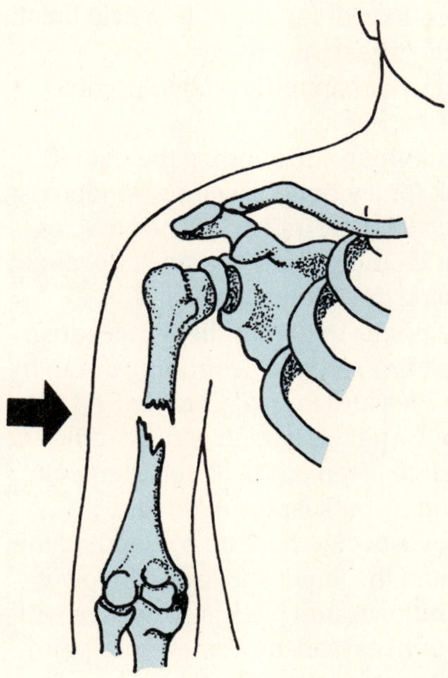

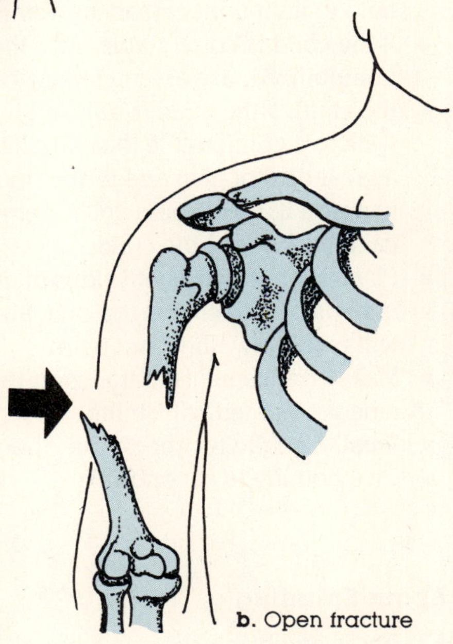

b. Open fracture

Types of Fractures

- ***Closed (simple) fracture.*** The skin is not broken and there is no wound at the site of the fracture.
- ***Open (compound) fracture.*** The skin over the fracture is open and torn. The wound is caused either by the bone breaking through the skin or by a direct blow that breaks the skin at the time of the fracture. The bone is not always visible. Open fractures are more serious than closed fractures because there is greater blood loss and greater chance of infection.

Signs and Symptoms

- ***Pain and tenderness.*** The child will complain of a sharp pain at the site of the injury.
- ***Swelling.*** This is caused by bleeding and can occur immediately after a fracture.
- ***Deformity.*** The break in the bone permits it to take an unnatural shape or bend. This is not always obvious. Compare the injured body part with the uninjured side of the body when checking for deformity.
- ***Loss of use.*** The child might be able to move the injured part slightly but will not have full range of motion.

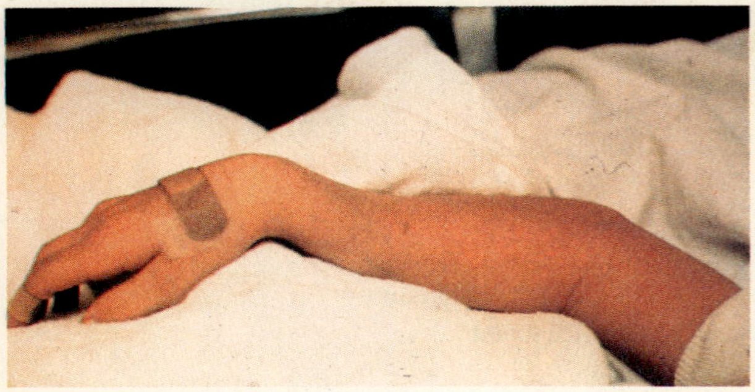

Forearm fracture

First Aid

- Always check for life-threatening injuries first. Broken bones, except for spinal or pelvic breaks, are seldom life threatening.
- Ask the child what happened and to point to where it hurts.
- Remove the clothing surrounding the injured area to check for a wound, swelling, tenderness, or deformity. Move the injured part as little as possible. Cut clothing at the seams, if necessary to avoid moving the injured area.
- Use pressure points to control heavy bleeding that can result from a bone protruding through the skin. See Pressure Points, Chapter 5.
- Cover the bone and the wound with a sterile dressing or large clean cloth. Never attempt to clean a wound if you suspect a fracture.
- Immobilize a suspected fracture by padding the injured area and the joints above and below it with towels, pillows, and jackets. This care will help to limit unnecessary movement and pain.
- If the child is comfortable once the fracture is immobilized, use an emergency carry to move the child. If the child is able, allow the child to walk to a comfortable location. If the child is in a great deal of pain and further movement will increase it, you should call for emergency medical help to move the child.
- Place ice packs on both sides of the injured area rather than directly on top of it, and elevate. This will reduce swelling and pain.
- Make arrangements to transport the child to an emergency medical facility.
- Treat the child for shock. See Shock, Chapter 4.
- Give nothing to eat or drink.

About Splinting

A splint is an object, such as a board, that is secured to an injured body part where a fracture is suspected. It supports the injured area and prevents further movement.

A splint should be applied only by a trained emergency medical technician. Emergency medical technicians routinely apply them and use specialized equipment best suited to the injury. Their knowledge and expertise allow them to apply a splint with minimal risk of further damage.

Some knowledge of splinting can be useful for older children and adults, especially in remote areas, but if emergency medical care is nearby, splinting is not recommended for several reasons:

- A young child in pain cannot be relied on to be cooperative.
- Splints can be applied incorrectly due to inexperience. A splint that is applied too tightly or positions a limb incorrectly can restrict circulation to the limb and cause further pain and damage.
- Unnecessary movement of the injury during splinting can cause additional pain and damage to the bone, soft tissue, blood vessels, and nerves.

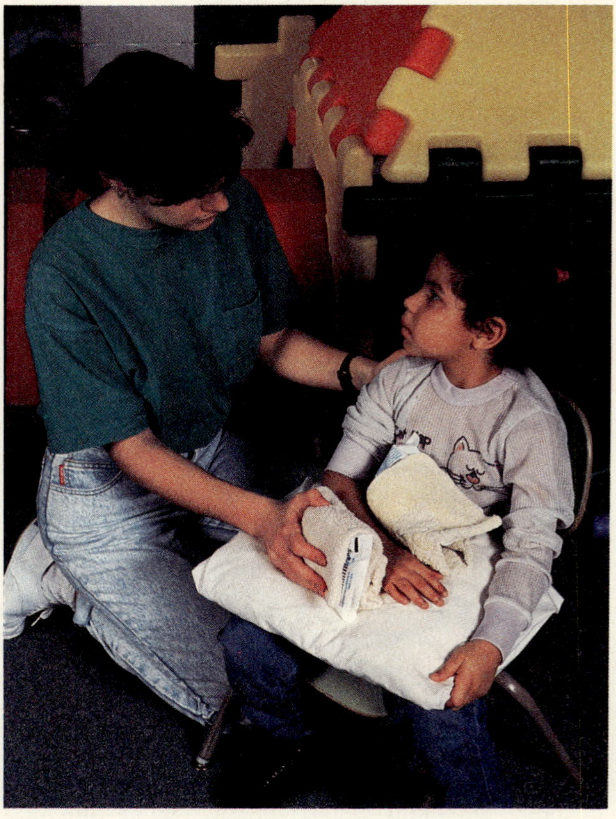

First aid for a suspected fracture

In a child care setting, the immobilization of a suspected fracture by padding the injury with towels and pillows is preferred to splinting. Immobilization provides substantial stability and minimizes movement with less chance of causing additional harm.

Sprains

A sprain is a twisting of a joint, along with tearing of the supportive muscles and ligaments. It is sometimes difficult to distinguish between a fracture and a sprain because the symptoms are often similar. Any child with a suspected fracture or sprain needs to have an X-ray.

First Aid

The following first aid measures of rest, ice, and elevation are effective when treating sprains, strains, bruises, and other injuries where there is damage to the soft-tissue areas of the body. For best results, begin first aid immediately after the injury occurs.

REST. Do not allow the child to continue using the injured body part. Have the child sit or lie down while you continue first aid treatment.

ICE. Apply a cold pack to the injured area for periods of 10 to 15 minutes. Wrap the cold pack in a cloth to protect the skin. The application of a cold pack reduces the pain, bleeding, and swelling that accompanies a soft-tissue injury. Continuous use of a cold pack is not recommended because it can result in frostbite.

ELEVATION. Elevate the injured body part. This with the application of ice helps to control the local internal bleeding, swelling, and pain.

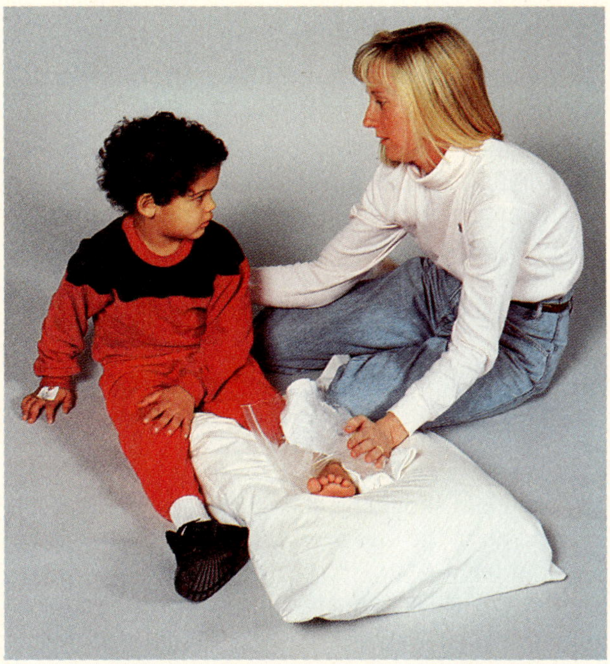

Rest, ice, and elevation for soft tissue injuries

Dislocations

A dislocation is the separation of a bone from a joint. In children, it is commonly seen in fingers and elbows. It takes only a small amount of force for the bone of a child to be dislocated, because children's bones and ligaments are very flexible. This is why adults are cautioned against roughly pulling the forearm or hand of a child. A simple, quick tug on a child's hand to prevent him from stepping from a curb or to protect against a stumble can be enough to dislocate an elbow. Babies and children should never be lifted by their hands. Always lift them by placing your hands underneath their armpits.

Signs and Symptoms

- Pain and tenderness. A dislocated bone can be very painful if the nerves and ligaments are torn.
- Swelling. This is caused by bleeding within the tissues.
- Deformity. This is caused by the unnatural shape of the bone outside of the joint socket. Sometimes the bone will naturally relocate itself immediately, but often it needs to be returned to its proper position by a health care provider.
- Loss of use. Any movement will cause pain if the bone remains dislocated. If the dislocation corrects itself naturally but the child continues to have reduced movement and discomfort, the child's parent should call the health care provider.

First Aid

Dislocations, although often very painful, are not life threatening.

- Ask the child what happened and to point to where it hurts.
- Remove clothing surrounding the injured area to check for swelling, tenderness, or a deformity. Avoid moving the injured part.
- Immobilize the injured area by having the child hold it firmly against the body or by padding it with a towel or pillow to prevent further movement and discomfort.
- Apply a cold pack to the injured area to decrease pain and swelling. Wrap the cold pack in a cloth to protect the skin.

- Do not try to reposition a dislocated bone because blood vessels and nerves can become trapped between the bones, causing further injury. Repositioning of a dislocation should be done by trained medical personnel only.
- Give nothing to eat or drink.
- Ask the parent to have the child seen in an emergency care facility for an X-ray.

Spinal Injuries

A spinal injury damages the bony spinal column that surrounds and protects the nerves of the spine. These nerves allow us to feel sensation and to move our bodies. Serious injury to the spinal column and nerves causes paralysis, or permanent loss of feeling and movement below the area of the injury.

Spinal fractures are becoming increasingly common in children. They most often result from the bending, twisting, or jolting involved in a violent car or bicycle accident or in a sports-related injury. Motor vehicle accidents are the leading cause of spinal cord injury in children under the age of 16 followed by sports-related injuries, acts of violence (mostly all from gunshot wounds), and falls. Any child who is found unconscious after a violent injury must be treated as if suffering from a spinal injury.

It is important to know there might not be any immediate damage to the nerves of the spine following a spinal fracture. However, if the child is allowed to sit up after such an injury or is otherwise improperly handled, the spinal nerves can be damaged. This is why immobilizing the neck and spine of a child with a suspected spinal injury is so important.

Signs and Symptoms

- Painful movement of the arms and/or legs. Pain can be sharp or radiate down the legs.
- Numbness, tingling, weakness, or burning sensation in the arms or legs.
- Paralysis of the arms or legs. Loss of movement in the arms and hands might indicate nerve damage to the neck or upper spine. Loss of movement of the legs and feet might indicate nerve damage in the lower spine. The child's hand should be able to grasp your hand firmly, and the child should be able to push the toes firmly against your hand.
- Deformity, or unnatural angle of the child's head and neck.

First Aid

- Check for consciousness by calling the child's name. Check and monitor the airway, breathing, and circulation and treat accordingly. If CPR is necessary, and you are training in CPR, the child must be positioned on the back, move the child by rolling the head, neck, and spine as one unit. See Skill Scan: Rolling an Unconscious Child.
- NEVER MOVE AN UNCONSCIOUS CHILD EXCEPT TO SAVE A LIFE. If the child is in a life-threatening situation such as near a burning car and must be moved, use an emergency move found in Skill Scan: Emergency Moves for an Unconscious Child.
- Send someone to call for emergency medical help.
- Wait for trained medical personnel to move the child. A child with a suspected spinal injury requires a cervical collar and immobilization on a spine board. Splinting a spinal injury should be done only by emergency medical personnel. A child care provider can immobilize a suspected spinal injury without causing further harm, but should not attempt to splint it.
- Immobilize, or support to keep from moving, the head, neck, and spine by padding them with towels, blankets, or jackets. Do not change the child's position. Tell the child not to move, if consciousness regained.
- A child who has been injured in the water and might have a spinal injury should be floated carefully to shore. Before removing the child from the water, the child should be secured to a backboard by trained emergency medical personnel.

If the child is conscious, continue with the following first aid steps:

- Ask the child what happened and where it hurts.
- Carefully remove the child's shoes and observe for any reluctance or inability to move the toes or fingers.
- Ask the child to wiggle the toes and fingers. If the child is unable to move, or if movement causes additional pain along the spine, this might indicate damage to the spinal column or spinal nerves.
- Ask if the child can feel you give the foot or hand a gentle scratch.
- The child should be able to grip your hand firmly and point the toes against gentle pressure from your hand.

Even if the child can move his extremities and is painfree, do not hesitate to call for emergency medical help if the injury was exceptionally traumatic or you are unsure of the child's condition.

■ FRACTURE/DISLOCATION ■

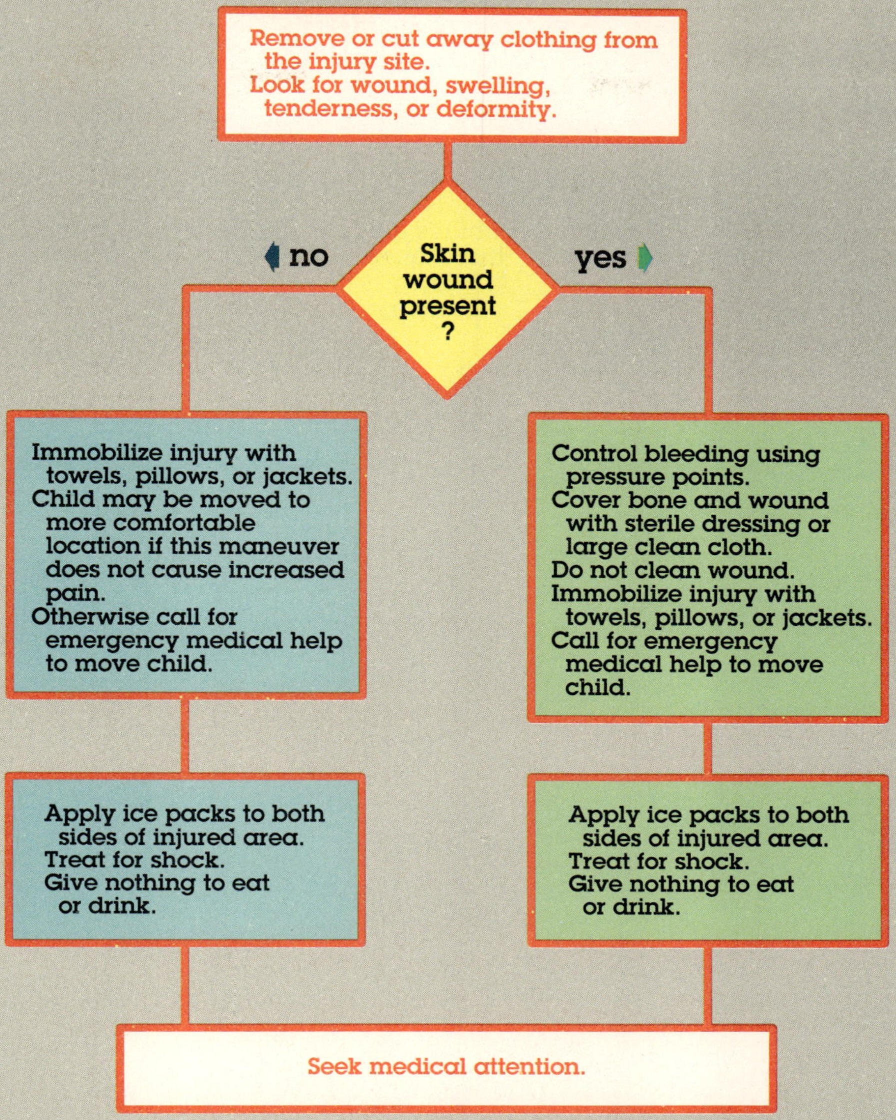

■ SPINAL INJURY ■

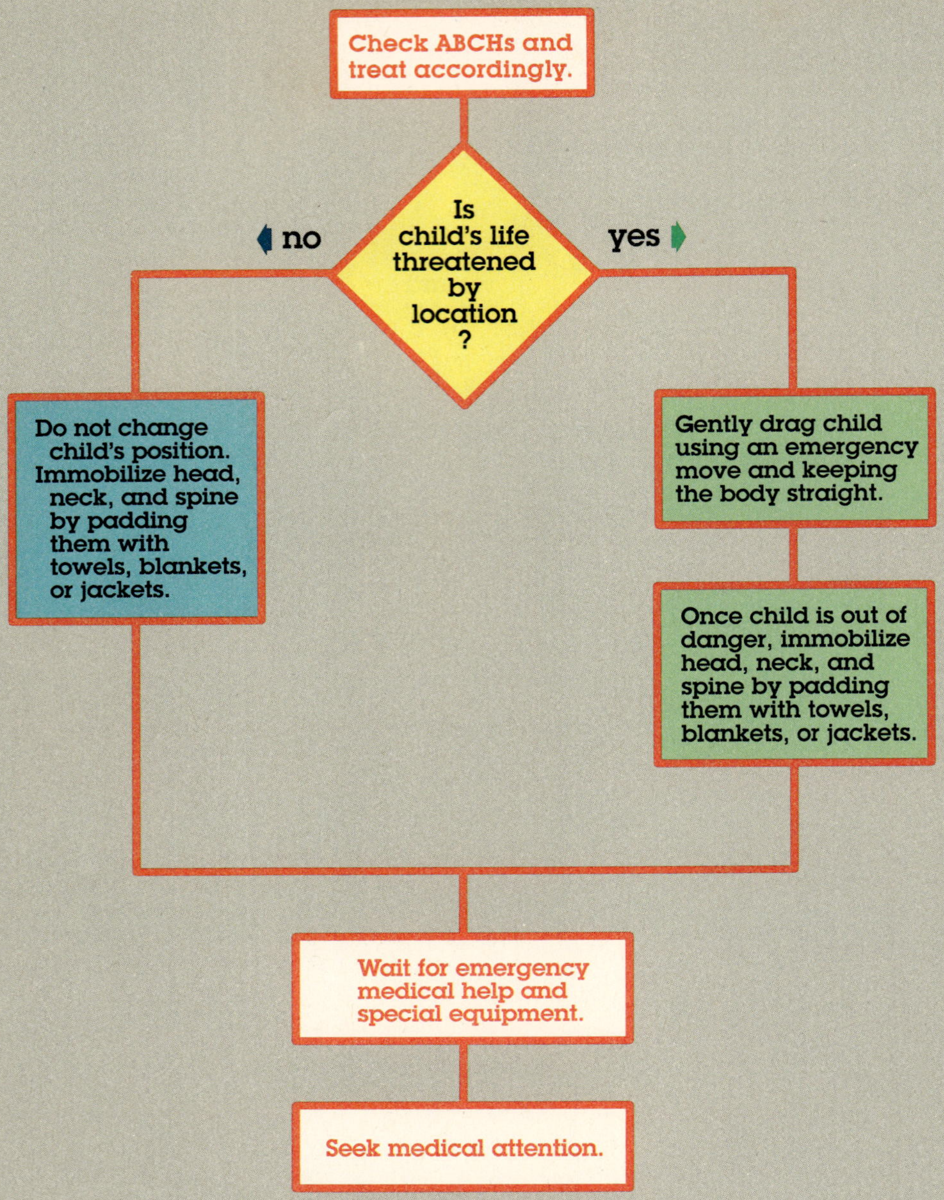

Muscle Cramps

A muscle cramp is an uncontrolled spasm of a muscle that causes pain and temporary loss of movement. Usually the cramp strikes a leg muscle and can last from a few minutes to a few hours. There are several causes of muscle cramping. Among those commonly seen in children are the overuse of a muscle and the loss of water and salts through heavy sweating.

First Aid

- Attempt to relieve a cramp by gently stretching the affected muscle. A gradual stretching of the muscle can help to lengthen spasmed muscle fibers and relieve the cramp. Let the child control the progress of the stretching because too rapid stretching can cause additional spasm and pain.
- Apply an icepack wrapped in a towel to help the muscle to relax.
- Apply pressure to relax the affected muscle, but do not massage it.
- Replace lost fluid by drinking cool water. Sports, or electrolyte drinks can also be helpful but not in large amounts. The high sugar content makes it difficult for the body to absorb fluid.
- Do not give salt tablets. They can irritate the stomach and further upset the body's balance of fluid. Salt is best replaced in combination with other electrolytes.

Sports-Related Injuries*

Children as young as ages 5 and 6 participate in organized sports. The pressure from coaches to win, not just to play, can be enormous. Most injuries can be attributed to repetitive overuse or overtraining which results in stress fractures, sprains, tendonitis, torn cartilage, bursitis, and shin splints.

The U.S. Consumer Product Safety Commission reports that four million children seek treatment in hospital emergency rooms every year because of sports-related injuries, and it estimates that another eight million are treated by family physicians for these injuries.

Be aware of the following guidelines when children participate in organized sports activities. They can help to prevent a sports injury.

- An individual who is responsible for coaching an organized sport should have experience, training, and education in the health risks of training children too vigorously.
- All coaches (paid as well as volunteer) should be trained in first aid or CPR.
- Children should have a complete physical exam before participating in sports activities.
- Children should know what safety equipment is necessary and have it available to them. Equipment should fit properly.
- Playing areas should be free of hazardous debris.
- Time should be included for warm-up and cool-down activity.
- Pain is an indication that something is wrong. Do not attempt to work through it. Seek medical attention.

**Adapted from* Sports and Injuries, *The National Youth Sports Foundation For the Prevention of Athletic Injuries, Inc.*

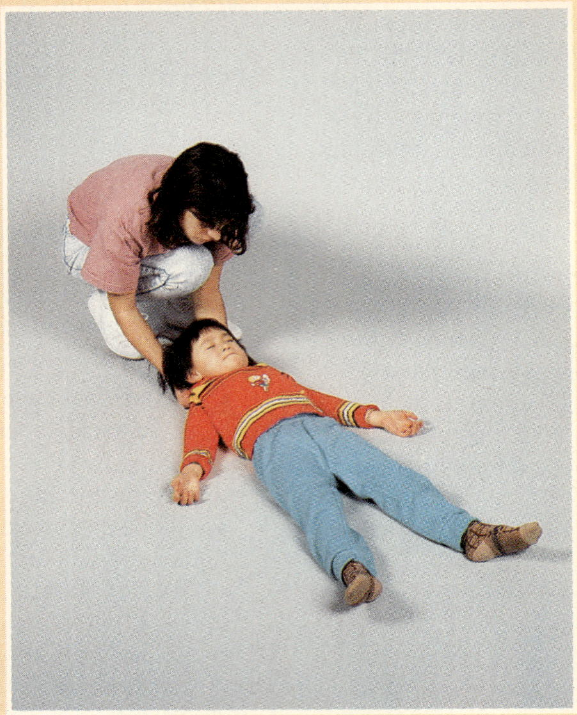

Clothing drag. Firmly grasp clothing around the collar and support the child's head on your wrists while pulling the child away from danger.

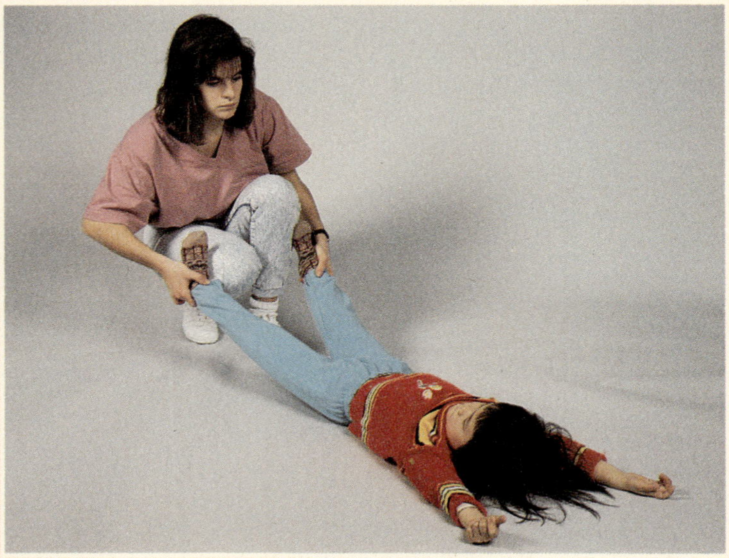

Ankle drag. Firmly grasp the child's ankles and pull the child away from danger. Use only on smooth surfaces.

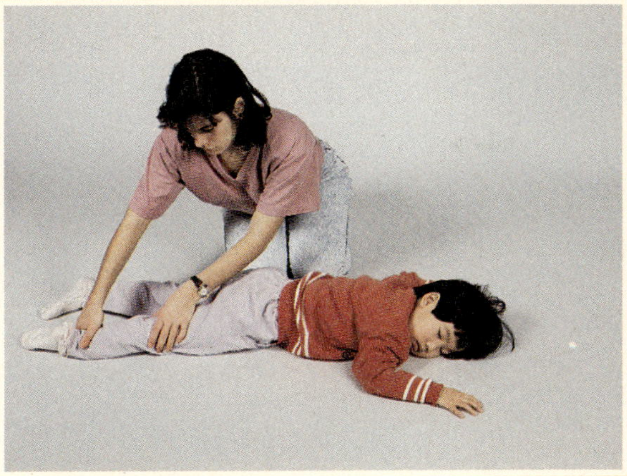

1. Straighten child's legs.

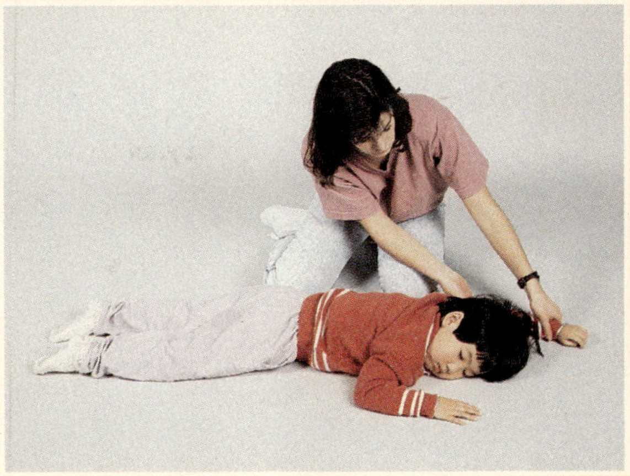

2. Move child's arm closest to you above child's head.

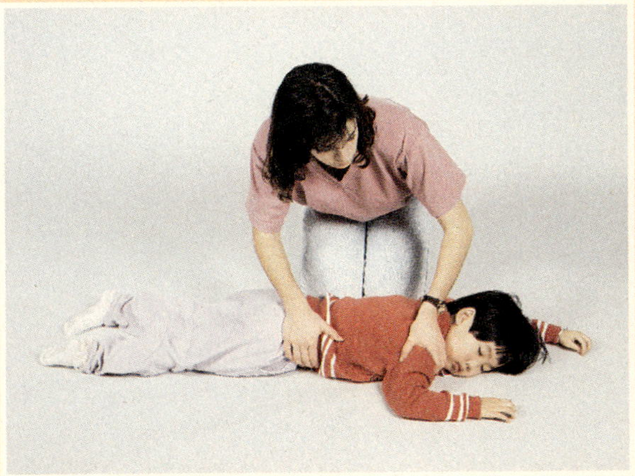

3. Place one hand on child's shoulder and other hand on child's hip.

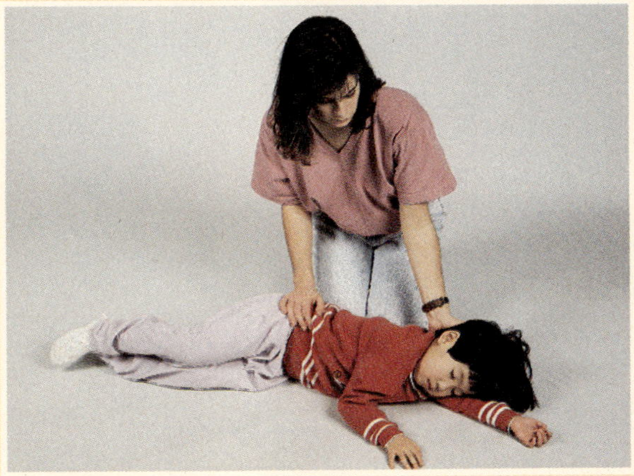

4. Roll child onto side and move hand from shoulder to support back of neck.

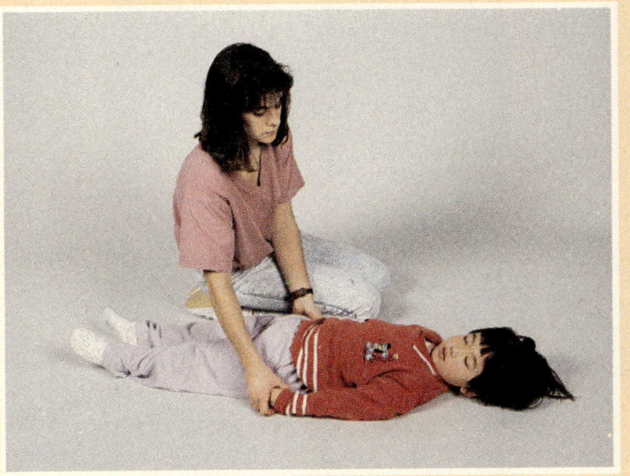

5. Place child's arms alongside body.

SKILL SCAN: Checking for Spinal Injury

CHECKING FOR SPINAL INJURY IN THE UPPER PART OF THE BODY:

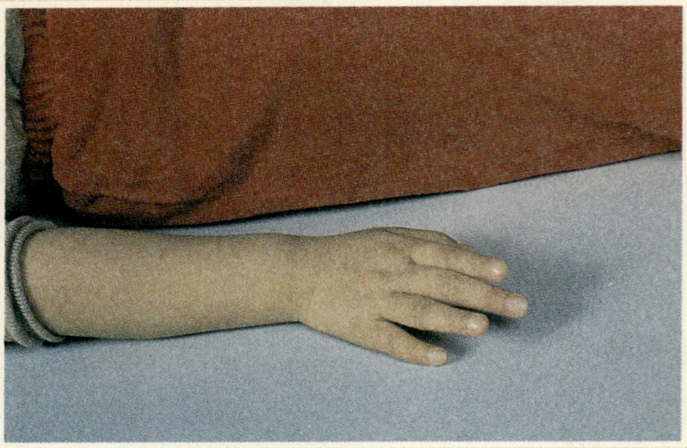

Ask child to move fingers.

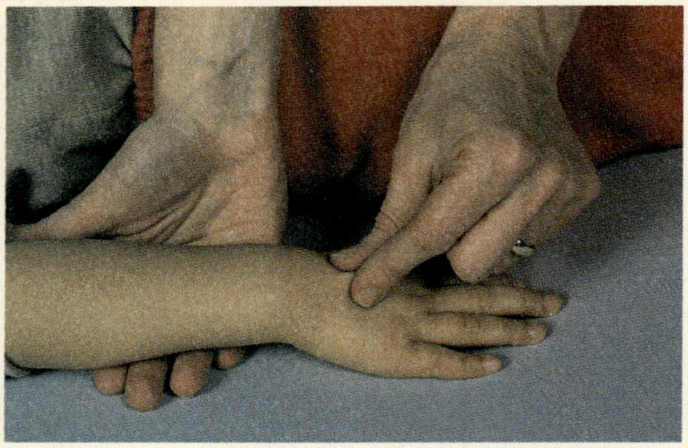

Ask if child can feel a gentle pinch on the hand.

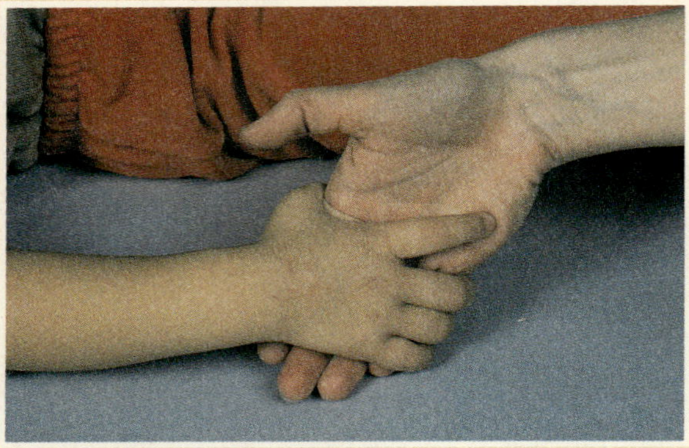

Ask child to grip your hand firmly.

CHECKING FOR SPINAL INJURY IN THE LOWER PART OF THE BODY

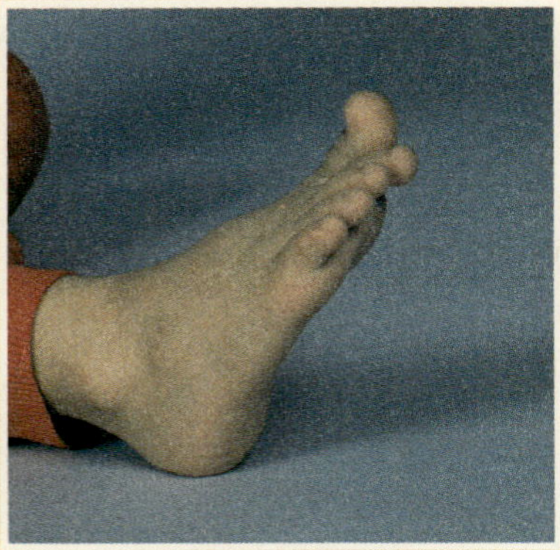

Ask child to move toes.

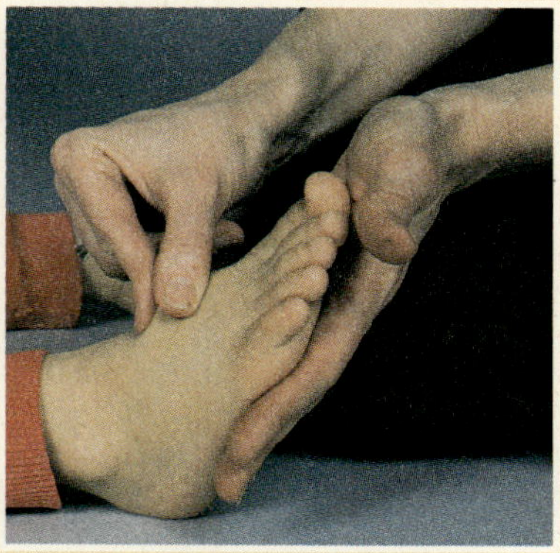

Ask if child can feel a gentle pinch on the foot.

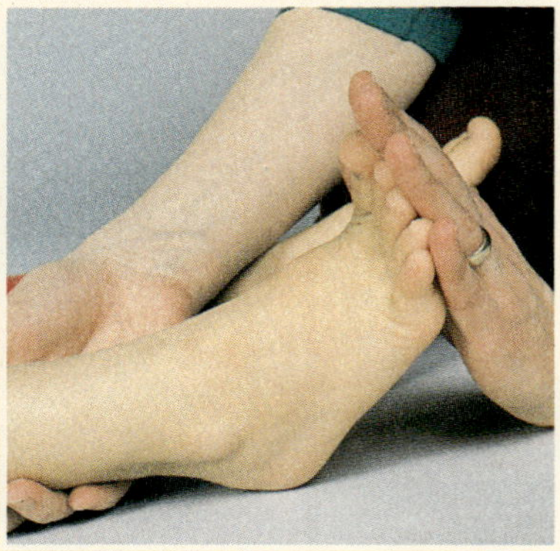

Ask child to point toes against gentle pressure from your hand.

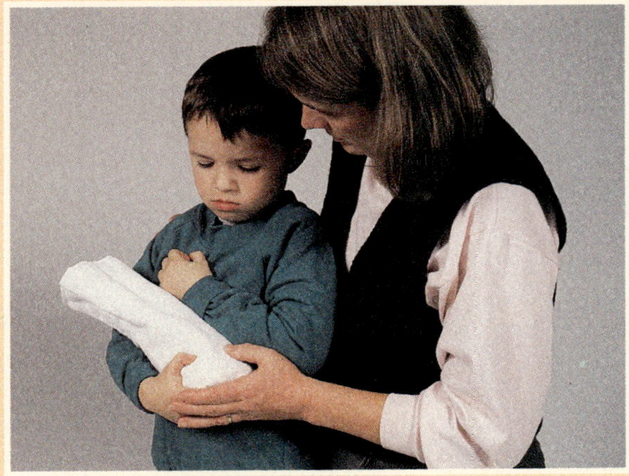

Upper arm/elbow

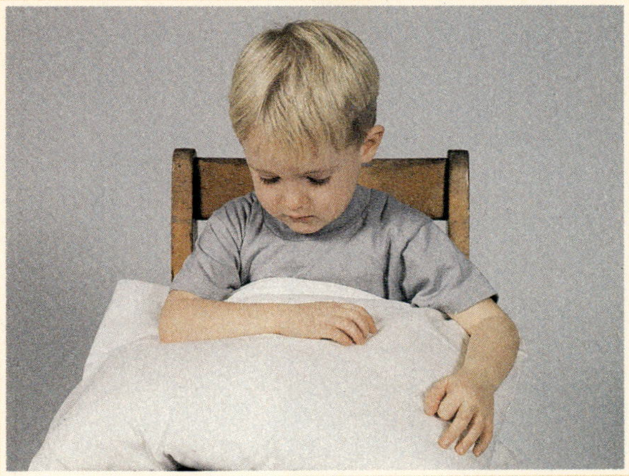

Lower arm/wrist

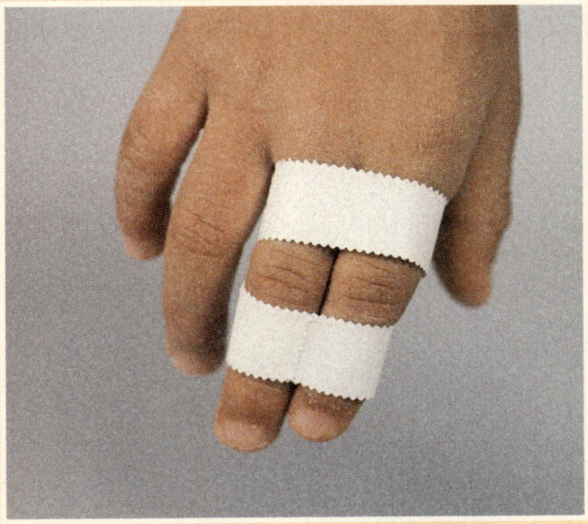

Finger

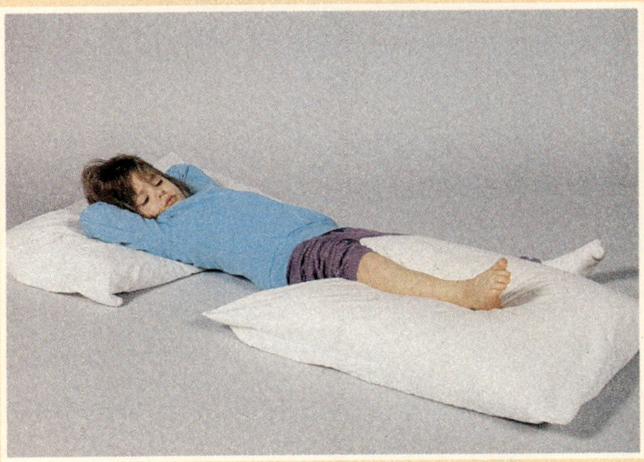

Leg/ankle

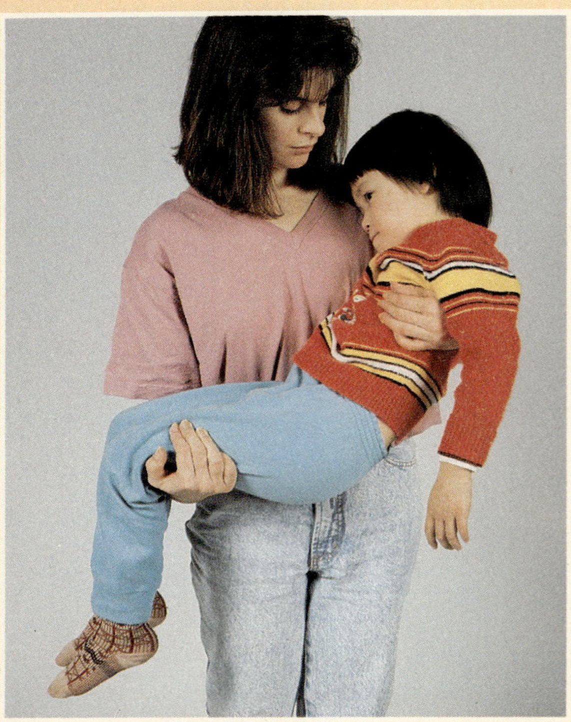

Cradle carry

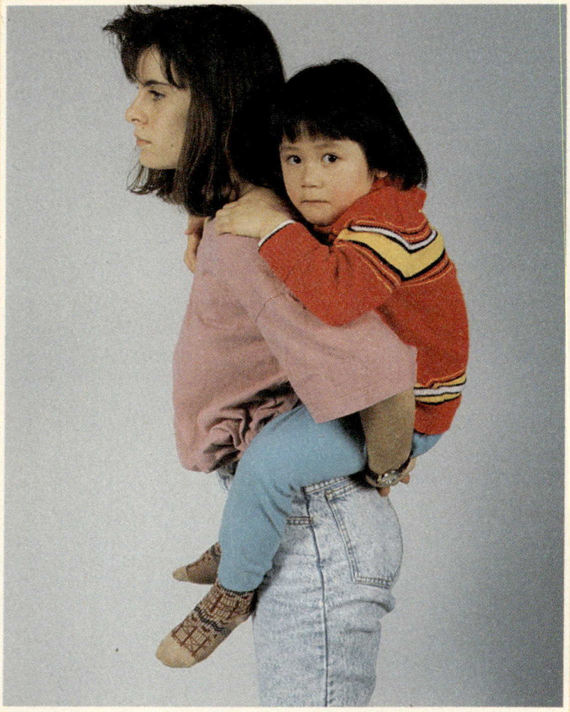

Piggyback carry

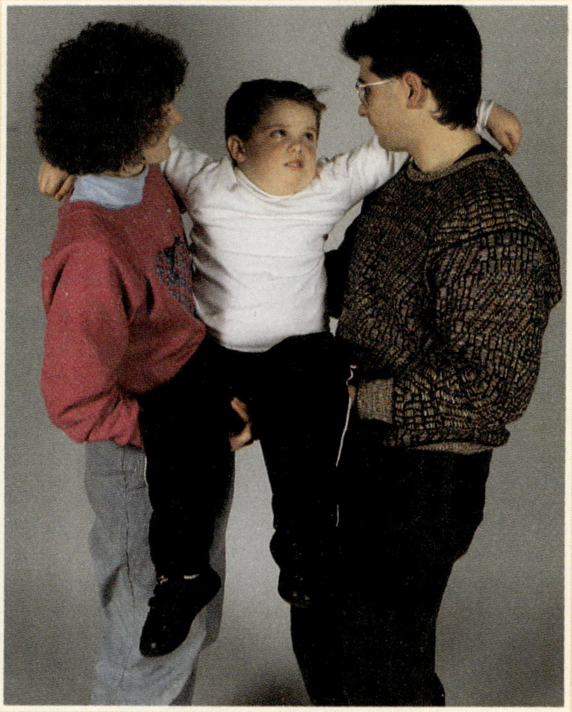

Two-handed seat carry

Fractures

Mark the following either true (T) or false (F).

1. ____ Fractures in children are worrisome because damage to the growth plate can cause shortening of the bone.
2. ____ Fractures only damage bones.
3. ____ A closed fracture breaks the skin.
4. ____ The bone is not always visible in an open fracture.

Check (√) the correct sign or symptom of a fractured bone:

1. ____ Pain and tenderness
2. ____ Swelling
3. ____ Deformity
4. ____ Limited movement
5. ____ Fever
6. ____ Vomiting

Check (√) the correct first aid measures for a fractured bone:

1. ____ Remove the clothing surrounding the injury.
2. ____ Apply gentle, firm pressure to reinsert a bone if the fracture is open.
3. ____ Realign a fracture before immobilizing and applying ice.
4. ____ Cover an open fracture with a sterile dressing or large clean cloth.

Sprains

Check (√) the correct first aid measure for a child with a sprained ankle.

1. ____ Apply ice or a cold pack to the injured area and elevate it.
2. ____ Apply a warm pack to the injured area.
3. ____ Have the child rest.
4. ____ Keep the injured part lower than the heart.
5. ____ Keep the injured ankle below the level of the heart.

Dislocations

Check (√) the correct first aid measure for a child with a dislocated elbow:

1. ____ Apply ice or a cold pack to the injured area and elevate it.
2. ____ Apply a warm pack.
3. ____ Have child bend elbow to reposition a dislocated elbow.
4. ____ A dislocation injury will improve with time and the child does not need to be seen by a health care provider.

Spinal Injury

Mark true (T) or false (F):

1. ____ Serious injury to the spinal nerves causes paralysis.
2. ____ Movement of the injured child following a spinal fracture poses little risk to the spinal nerves.
3. ____ Loss of movement in the arms and hands might indicate nerve damage to the neck or upper spine.
4. ____ A child who is found unconscious after a violent injury must be treated as if a spinal injury has occurred.
5. ____ There might not be any immediate damage to the nerves of the spine following a spinal fracture.
6. ____ Motor vehicle accidents are the leading cause of spinal cord injury in children.
7. ____ Never move an unconscious child except to save a life.

11

Medical Emergencies

■ Asthma ■ Croup ■ Epiglottitis ■ Sudden Infant Death Syndrome and Infant Apnea ■ Dehydration ■ Diabetes ■ Fevers ■ Febrile Seizures ■ Seizures ■ Meningitis ■ Reye's Syndrome ■ Near-Drowning ■

Asthma

Asthma is one of the most common chronic diseases of childhood today. The U.S. Public Health Service estimates that there are more than 2.5 million children who suffer from asthma. According to the American Lung Association, asthma is on the increase in both children and adults, due primarily to increased exposure to environmental pollutants and irritants.

A child with asthma experiences sporadic breathing difficulties that are often called "attacks." During these attacks, the lining of the airways throughout the lungs swell, narrowing and therefore partially obstructing these passages. The lungs increase their normal production of mucous secretions which can further narrow the airways. Additionally, the muscles surounding the chest tighten making breathing difficult. During a severe episode of asthma, exhaling is more difficult than inhaling and a child might have a feeling of suffocation.

Signs and Symptoms

Asthma attacks can vary in length and intensity. Some children might experience an annoying cough lasting for several days, weeks, or even months, while other children might have such difficulty breathing that they cannot even complete a sentence.

A child experiencing an asthma attack can have one or all of the following signs and symptoms:

- Coughing. The lungs normally secrete mucus to act as a lubricant in the lungs and to help remove foreign particles from the airway. During an asthma attack, the lungs secrete large amounts of the mucus which narrows and blocks the airway. Coughing is the body's response to try to clear the airway. A child with asthma eventually learns how to cough up this mucus to clear the airway. Coughing is often more frequent at night.
- Wheezing. The wheezing breath sound is heard not only when a child inhales, but also when exhaling, and is caused by the narrowing of the airway.
- Chest tightness and shortness of breath. This is especially common following vigorous exercise. During a severe attack, a child must concentrate much energy on breathing. If you look closely, you will see the child's nostrils flaring and see the child using abdominal and neck muscles to help pull air into the lungs.
- Increased pulse and respiratory rate. These increase in response to an increased need for oxygen.

In some children, asthma is so mild that it is termed "hidden" asthma. These children have a persistent mild case of asthma. The signs and symptoms are not pronounced and the disease can go unnoticed. Commonly, these children have more frequent upper respiratory infections and mild coughs. These children are not able to take long deep breaths. The airway of a child with hidden asthma is only mildly obstructed but this can affect the child's level of activity, especially during vigorous exercise.

First Aid

- Help the child to sit straight up in a quiet area.
- Give asthma medication as prescribed by the child's health care provider. Asthma medication can be in the form of a prescription capsule, tablet, liquid, or aerosol which must be supplied by the child's parent. Some oral asthma medications have a very unpleasant taste. Do not administer the medication more frequently than prescribed. A medication release form, signed by the child's health care provider, must be kept as part of the child's medical record.
- Give the child plenty of clear fluids. This will help to thin the mucus in the lungs and make it easier for the child to cough up the secretions.
- Check the child's pulse and respirations.
- Keep the child at rest until there is improvement.

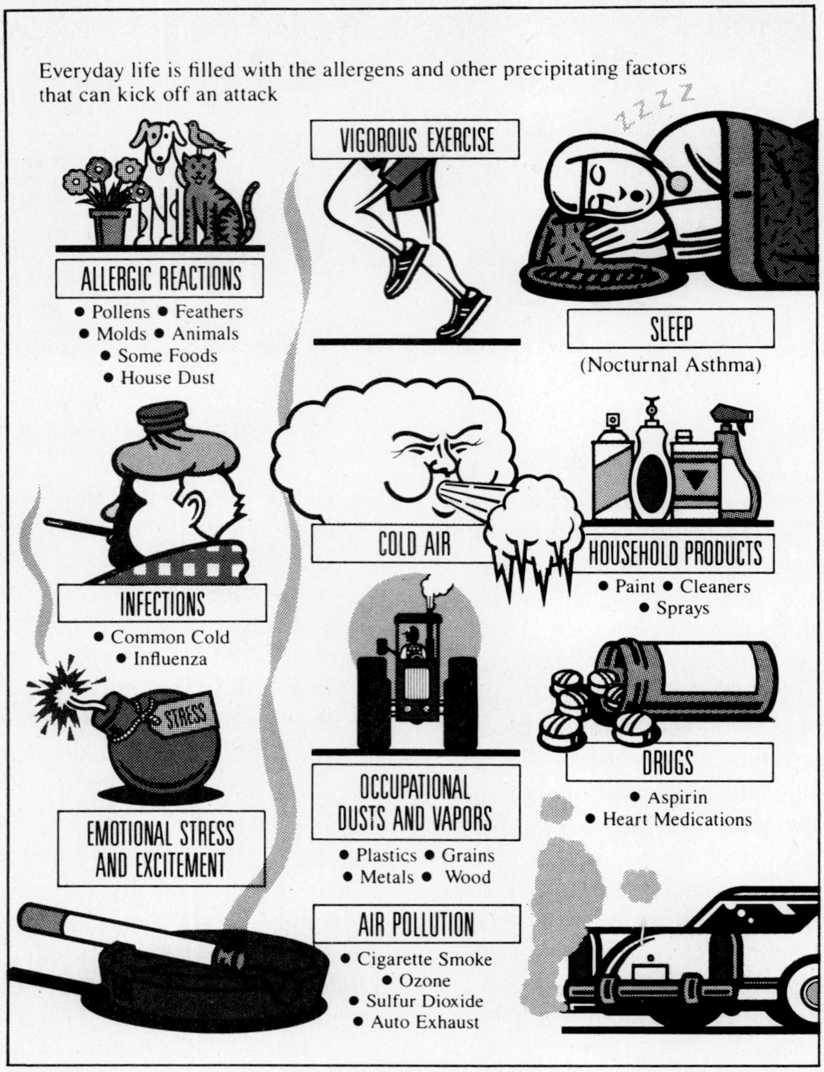
Everyday life is filled with the allergens and other precipitating factors that can kick off an attack
ALLERGIC REACTIONS
• Pollens • Feathers
• Molds • Animals
• Some Foods
• House Dust
VIGOROUS EXERCISE
SLEEP
(Nocturnal Asthma)
INFECTIONS
• Common Cold
• Influenza
COLD AIR
HOUSEHOLD PRODUCTS
• Paint • Cleaners
• Sprays
STRESS
EMOTIONAL STRESS AND EXCITEMENT
OCCUPATIONAL DUSTS AND VAPORS
• Plastics • Grains
• Metals • Wood
DRUGS
• Aspirin
• Heart Medications
AIR POLLUTION
• Cigarette Smoke
• Ozone
• Sulfur Dioxide
• Auto Exhaust

Chart and Source: American Lung Association®—The "Christmas Seal" People®

Call the child's parent to have the child seen by a health care provider if:

- The child is unable to speak easily.
- The child has flaring nostrils and is working very hard to breathe, using the muscles of the neck and abdomen.
- The child's lips have a blue discoloration.
- The child does not improve within 30 to 45 minutes after taking medication.

Children with asthma must be taught as early in life as possible about their disease. Although children in a child care setting will always need supervision in taking medication, they need to know what their medicine does and how and when to take it. Routine physical activity should be encouraged. Vigorous physical activity may also be encouraged if the child's asthma is well controlled. Children and their providers need to know which allergic substances and irritants trigger the asthma attacks and how to avoid these triggers. Even though asthma cannot be cured, most asthma can be controlled.

Asthma Triggers

Children with asthma, because of an increased sensitivity of the lung tissue, have a heightened reaction when exposed to various allergic substances and nonallergic irritants. These substances are called asthma triggers. Some common asthma triggers are:

- ***INFECTIONS.*** Upper respiratory infections can trigger an episode of asthma. These infections are usually viral and are not helped by antibiotics.
- ***ALLERGIES.*** Common substances that trigger allergic responses are dust, mold, pollen, feathers, and animal fur. Additionally, certain medications and, infrequently, foods such as eggs,

milk, grains, and chocolate can cause an asthma attack. It is important to know that a child must be exposed to a substance, at least once, to be sensitized. After the initial contact, repeated exposures can cause the child to have an asthmatic reaction. Therefore, the first time a child comes in contact with a dog, or is exposed to a pollen, there will be no reaction, even though the child might later develop an allergy to these substances.

- ***IRRITANTS.*** These substances irritate the lining of the airway causing coughing, runny nose, watery eyes, and tightness in the muscles of the chest. Air pollution and the breathing of secondhand cigarette smoke are major irritants to a child with asthma.
- ***EXERCISE.*** According to the American Lung Association vigorous exercise such as running can trigger an episode of asthma in more than 80 percent of the children with the disease. The exercise that is least likely to stimulate an episode of asthma is swimming. Asthma attacks resulting from exercise are often controlled with medication taken prior to the activity.
- ***WEATHER.*** Changes in the weather can stimulate an asthma attack in a child with the disease. Windy days in the spring and fall stir up pollens and dust in the air, and the dry cold air of winter can irritate the lining of the airways.
- ***EMOTION.*** Although psychological factors are not a cause of asthma, they can influence the course of an attack. Emotional stress or the extreme excitement of laughing or crying, in a child who has asthma, can result in rapid breathing and an episode of wheezing. Additionally, a child who is experiencing tightness in the chest and breathing difficulties will feel anxious. This anxiety is worsened if the adult care giver appears anxious, as well. Try to remain calm so as to reassure the child.

Croup

Croup is an acute, spasmodic swelling of the vocal cords. It is caused by a viral infection, although the same symptoms can appear as a result of an allergic reaction. Croup is not a disease itself, but a group of respiratory symptoms. It is most common in infants and young children, with episodes lasting from 3 to 5 days. The symptoms are more pronounced in children than in adults because their airways are smaller. In an adult, croup appears as a mild form of laryngitis.

Signs and Symptoms of Mild Croup

- Barklike cough
- Hoarseness

Signs and Symptoms of Severe Croup

- The above symptoms of mild croup
- Difficulty breathing
- Flaring nostrils and use of abdominal muscles to pull air into the lungs
- Blue discoloration around the nose and lips

An attack of croup typically occurs at night when the child wakes with a hoarse, barking cough and difficulty breathing. There is usually no fever.

First Aid

- Immediately take the child, along with a favorite book or stuffed animal into the bathroom and close the door. Hold the child on your lap outside the shower and turn on the hot shower to produce misting. This misting helps to decrease the swelling of air passages. Holding the child close to a cool mist vaporizer produces the same effect.
- The child's breathing should improve significantly within 10 to 15 minutes. If the child's breathing does not improve after 20 to 30 minutes of treatment, contact the child's health care provider. If you need to take a child with croup to an emergency facility, it is best to open the car windows fully to allow the child to breathe cold air. This helps to decrease some of the swelling and make it easier for the child to breathe.

Epiglottitis

Epiglottitis is a bacterial, upper respiratory infection that is experienced by children under the age of 5 years. The epiglottis is a flap of skin that closes over the opening to the airway during swallowing to prevent food and fluid from entering the airway An infection of this tissue, although uncommon, represents a life-threatening emergency.

Signs and Symptoms

- Difficulty breathing and flaring nostrils. The child must use the accessory muscles of the neck and chest to pull air into the lungs.
- The child assumes a position of sitting upright with neck and nose outstretched.
- Drooling. The child is unable to swallow saliva due to swelling of the epiglottis.
- High fever.

■ ASTHMA ■

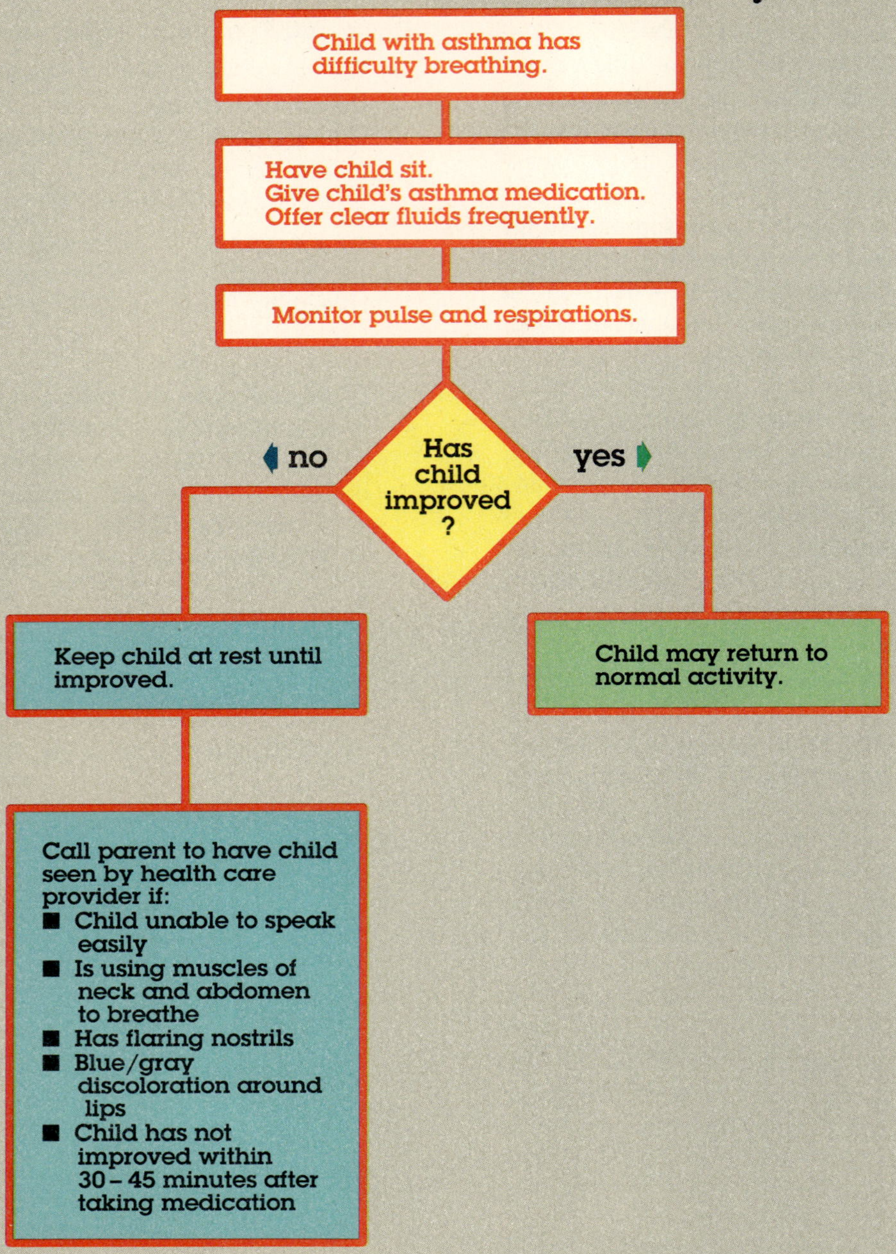
Child with asthma has difficulty breathing.
Have child sit.
Give child's asthma medication.
Offer clear fluids frequently.
Monitor pulse and respirations.
Has child improved ?
no
yes
Keep child at rest until improved.
Child may return to normal activity.
Call parent to have child seen by health care provider if:
■ Child unable to speak easily
■ Is using muscles of neck and abdomen to breathe
■ Has flaring nostrils
■ Blue/gray discoloration around lips
■ Child has not improved within 30 – 45 minutes after taking medication

Treatment

- A child who experiences signs and symptoms of epiglottitis needs to be seen in an emergency medical facility immediately.
- Keep the child as calm as possible because crying makes it more difficult for the child to breathe.
- Monitor the airway, breathing, and circulation. Begin CPR, if necessary.

A vaccine is now available, known as the HIB vaccine, that protects infants and young children from such serious bacterial illnesses as epiglottitis and certain types of meningitis. All children should receive this vaccine as part of their early childhood immunization program.

Sudden Infant Death Syndrome (SIDS) and Infant Apnea*

Sudden Infant Death Syndrome (SIDS) is the sudden and unexpected death of an apparently healthy infant which cannot be explained by autopsy or by the child's health history. It is a leading cause of death in babies under the age of 1 year, with most infant victims being between the ages of 2 and 4 months. SIDS crosses all racial and socioeconomic boundaries. Most SIDS deaths occur during the night or at nap time, and the greatest number of cases occur in the winter months. Often the infant had a viral respiratory illness 1 to 2 weeks before the death.

The exact causes of SIDS are not yet understood. SIDS researchers are working to discover a means of early detection and prevention as well as to search for the underlying causes. This involves learning more about how a healthy infant develops and functions. No association has ever been found between SIDS and childhood immunizations.

When a baby dies of SIDS, parents or child care providers often blame themselves, but it is no one's fault. It could not have been prevented. In fact, in the few observed cases of deaths attributed to SIDS, CPR techniques were unsuccessful in resuscitating the infants. Support groups are available for families who have suffered the loss of an infant to SIDS. Health care providers can help parents find a SIDS support group.

Another condition of infancy that can be confused with SIDS is infant apnea. Apnea is a temporary stoppage of breathing. Only a tiny percentage of SIDS victims experience episodes of apnea before death.

Adapted from "Facts on Sudden Infant Death Syndrome," courtesy of the Sudden Infant Death Syndrome Alliance.

Short periods of apnea—less than 15 seconds—are normal and safe. Many infants pause in their breathing in this manner. Apnea becomes life threatening when it is prolonged. Prolonged apnea can cause the infant to choke or gag and to become limp. The skin color can become pale and blue or gray. Many children with prolonged infant apnea respond successfully to CPR. Most infants outgrow apnea by the age of 6 months.

Dehydration

Dehydration is a dangerous loss of fluids from the body. It occurs when the total amount of water a child loses (through sweating, urination, diarrhea, and vomiting) is greater than what is taken in. Water accounts for over half of a child's body weight. A young child with a fever loses water quickly. You need to watch closely for signs of dehydration if a child is ill with any of the following:

- Vomiting
- Diarrhea
- Fever
- Heat exhaustion
- Refusal or inability to drink fluids—for instance, if there is pain from chicken pox blisters in the throat

Dehydration is of special concerns in infants and young children because water accounts for up to three-quarters of their body weight and dehydration can occur within even a few hours.

Signs and Symptoms

- A decreased amount of urine that is deep gold in color and has a strong odor because it is more concentrated.
- No tears when crying.
- Dry cracked lips with little or no salivation.
- Unusually thirsty
- Irritable or fussy
- Dry skin; no sweating.
- Sunken eyes.
- Listlessness, sleepiness.
- Poor skin turgor. To determine this, lightly pull up a pinch fold of skin and release it. Skin with poor turgor returns slowly to normal position or remains "tented."
- A sunken fontanel (soft spot) in infants under the approximate age of 1 year.

First Aid

A child with severe dehydration must be hospitalized to receive intravenous fluids. Most dehydration is mild, and early treatment can prevent a life-threatening emergency. Follow these guidelines:

- Offer small but frequent sips of water or an oral electrolyte solution available in many grocery and drug stores.
- Do not give sweetened drinks such as apple juice, soft drinks and gelatin.
- Call a parent if a child shows signs of dehydration. A parent should contact the child's health care provider if unsure of how to correct the problem.

Diabetes

Childhood diabetes is a chronic disease in which the body cannot produce insulin. Insulin is a hormone produced by the pancreas and is needed by the body to transport food, in the form of a sugar called glucose, into the cells. Normally, the cells use glucose for energy. Without insulin, glucose is present in the bloodstream but it is unable to enter the cells. The cells receive no nourishment, no matter how much food the child eats. This is known as type I, or insulin-dependent diabetes and affects about one million people, almost all of them children.

Diabetes is not yet a curable disease. It is controllable through a balance of these three components:

1. Administer daily injections of insulin to ensure that insulin is always present in the blood to transport glucose to the cells.
2. Eat foods at regular times to keep the correct balance between insulin and glucose in the blood.
3. Regulate exercise to promote good health and to maintain balanced insulin and glucose levels.

Diabetes can produce two separate medical crises, each with its own distinct signs and symptoms.

Hyperglycemia (High blood glucose)

Hyperglycemia is an abnormally high level of glucose in the blood. Persistent high levels are thought to cause damage to blood vessels throughout the body. They can also eventually damage organs such as the heart and kidneys, and can impair the child's general circulation. Children with hyperglycemia are particularly susceptible to infections. Children with diabetes are always fighting hyperglycemia because they cannot produce insulin.

Diabetes Explained

During normal digestion, much of the food we eat is broken down into a sugar called glucose which the body uses as fuel for the cells. Glucose enters the bloodstream where it is transported from the blood into the cells with the help of insulin. The pancreas, an organ of digestion, normally produces insulin whenever food is eaten and releases that insulin into the blood. The insulin then attaches to the glucose and transports it from the blood into the cells to nourish them. Without insulin, the glucose is available in the bloodstream but is unable to get to those cells. The cells do not get nourished, and the body begins to starve. This leads to weakness and fatigue. In addition, the high level of glucose in the blood makes the body particularly susceptible to infection.

The accumulating glucose is filtered out of the blood by the kidneys and spills into the urine. This process requires extra water which produces thirst. The glucose in the urine is lost, leaving the body unnourished, and producing insatiable hunger. The body turns to its supply of stored fat to make energy, which produces significant weight loss. These are three telling signs of the development of diabetes–weight loss, thirst, and hunger.

Unlike glucose, fat does not require insulin to transport it into the cells. However, in using fats for energy, the body produces unhealthy wastes called ketones. A buildup of ketones in the blood results in a condition known as ketoacidosis. If ketoacidosis is left untreated, it can lead to coma and death. The buildup of ketones in the blood produces a fruity odor to the breath, which is another indicator of developing diabetes.

Signs and Symptoms

The following signs and symptoms of hyperglycemia can occur in a child with an undiagnosed case of diabetes. They might also occur in a child who is known to have diabetes, indicating illness or that the insulin dose or food intake needs to be readjusted. Recognition of these signs might take several days or even weeks.

- Excessive thirst
- Excessive hunger
- Excessive urination
- Fruity breath odor
- Sudden unexplained weight loss
- Weakness
- Overly tired and irritable
- Bed-wetting
- Drowsiness in advanced cases

A child without diabetes can show one or two of these symptoms occasionally. But a child with developing or poorly controlled diabetes will show several of these signs persistently. Often it is the sudden onset of bed-wetting and unexplained weight loss that causes the parent to take the child to a health care provider. Child care providers should report any of these recurring signs and symptoms to the parent.

First Aid

Hyperglycemia is not an immediate medical emergency in terms of first aid. However, it will require prompt attention once diagnosed. A child who consistantly demonstrates one or more of these signs and symptoms should be seen by his/her health care provider. Untreated, hyperglycemia will result in further deterioration of the child's health.

- Call the parent's attention to the child's persistent signs and symptoms.
- Urge the parent to have the child examined by a health care provider as soon as possible. A child who is known to have diabetes also needs to be examined in order to have the insulin dose adjusted and diet reviewed.

Hypoglycemia (Low blood glucose)

Hypoglycemia is an abnormally low level of glucose in the blood. It is the most frequent medical emergency for the child with diabetes and can be life threatening. It comes on quickly and must be treated immediately.

Normally, insulin levels rise and fall in response to meals and snacks eaten. In childhood or type I diabetes, insulin is given by injection before breakfast and later toward the end of the day. It circulates in the blood all day long. As long as there is sufficient glucose in the bloodstream, a balance is maintained. If the blood glucose level falls below a critical point, hypoglycemia occurs.

In childhood diabetes, hypoglycemia is also known as *insulin shock.* The most common causes of insulin shock are: receiving too much insulin, not eating enough food, and being unusually physically active. Hypoglycemia is most likely to occur when a snack or meal is served late or skipped.

Sign and Symptoms

Symptoms of hypoglycemia can vary among children. Be observant for sudden changes in the child's personality and behavior that might indicate hypoglycemia. Some children are not able to recognize an oncoming reaction.

Initial signs and symptoms:

- Trembling
- Weakness
- Sweating
- Dizziness
- Irritability
- Hunger

If left untreated, these additional signs will occur:

- Confusion
- Impaired thinking and coordination
- Drowsiness
- Loss of consciousness or seizure

First Aid

Hypoglycemia can be life threatening if ignored. Correcting the condition requires sugar. The child's parent should supply you with a suitable sugar source such as sugar cubes, sugar packets, honey, candies, frosting, or orange juice to be kept on hand. The parent will also instruct you on the amount to give to the child. A school-aged child with diabetes should carry a sugar source at all times.

A child care provider should be alert for the signs and symptoms of hypoglycemia, or insulin shock in a child with diabetes.

- Give the child a fast-acting sugar. This sugar should raise the blood glucose level in 10 to 15 minutes and make the child feel better once again.
- Observe the child and expect to see an improvement in 10 to 15 minutes.
- If there is no improvement in 15 minutes, give the same amount of the sugar again and notify the parent.
- If there is still no improvement in another 15 minutes, send someone to call for emergency medical help.
- If a child with diabetes is found unconscious, place a small amount of table sugar under the child's tongue. Do not attempt to give sugar in a liquid form. Monitor airway, breathing, and circulation and treat accordingly. Position the child on the side. Send someone to call for emergency medical help.

Special Considerations for the Child with Diabetes

Diabetes is a lifelong illness that affects every aspect of the child's life. Constant daily insulin injections and testing blood for glucose, as well as following lifelong diet restrictions make diabetes a demanding disease.

The delicate balance between glucose and insulin levels in the blood is affected by the child's diet, physical activity, illness, and stress. Controlling the disease successfully in a child requires a team effort from the child, parents, health care provider, and child care provider.

Diet

A child with diabetes needs a diet of foods that are high in nutritional value and low in concentrated sugar. It is essential for meals and snacks to be eaten at regular intervals to maintain the balance between glucose and insulin. Most children with diabetes need a morning and afternoon snack. Parents will give child care providers specific instructions about their child's diet. A child care provider is responsible for making snacks and mealtimes pleasant.

Parties and holiday celebrations present special problems when restricted foods are plentiful in the classroom. Food exchanges and substitutions that allow a child to eat special treats are occasionally permitted but should be discussed with the child's parent.

Physical Activity

Most children with diabetes should be encouraged to participate fully in all activities of the child care center or school. Parents should provide information on any necessary restrictions. Strenuous activity can upset the balance between insulin and glucose in the blood and cause insulin shock. Do not restrict the child's activities for fear of insulin shock; instead, understand that the child's diet can be adjusted to ensure that the child has the additional energy necessary for energetic play or a special activity.

Illness and Stress

Illnesses and stress increase the demands on the body because they upset the balance between glucose and insulin. A child care provider must be especially watchful of a child with diabetes who is ill or stressed.

Diabetic Emergency Summary Chart

	Hyperglycemia	**Hypoglycemia (insulin reaction)**
Cause	Too much sugar and too little insulin	Too little sugar and too much insulin
Develops	Slowly, over a period of days or weeks	Suddenly, within seconds or minutes
Signs	Persistent hunger Persistent thirst Frequent urination Dry mouth and skin Unexplained weight loss Stomachache	Trembling Dizziness Weakness Sweating Irritability Hunger Headache
Advanced Signs	Flushed skin Vomiting Abdominal pain Fruity breath Difficulty breathing Loss of consciousness	Anger Confusion Blurred vision Impaired thinking and confusion Loss of consciousness
Treatment	Insulin	Give sugar in form of table sugar, honey, regular soft drinks, frosting
Correctable	Over a period of days or weeks in a hospital	Usually at home or child care center within 15 minutes of eating sugar

■ HYPOGLYCEMIA ■

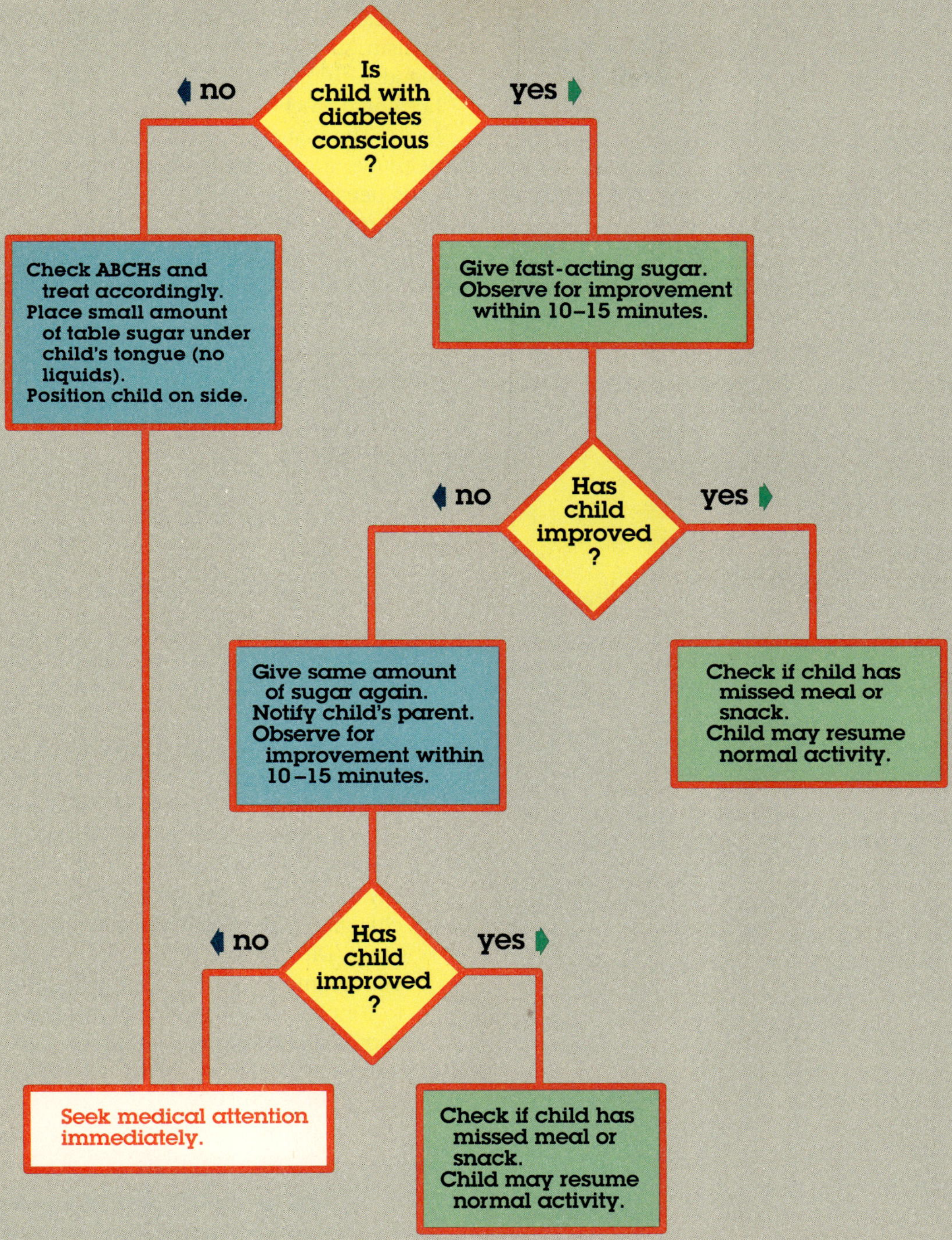

A Few More Answers about Diabetes

Where does diabetes come from?
Childhood diabetes has no clearly evident source. All people can inherit genes that make them more susceptible to the risk of developing type I diabetes. A gene is a tiny part of a chromosome that determines the characteristics for that child from sex and eye color to some health problems. However, genes might need to be stimulated by a viral illness and an immune system problem for diabetes to develop.

Could the child's diabetes have been prevented?
No. There are some stresses, such as illness or infection, that might cause the diaetes to show its presence earlier in life, but diabetes cannot be prevented.

Does eating a lot of sweets cause diabetes?
No. Despite what people think, there is no evidence to suggest that this is true. You will not use up your body's supply of insulin eating too many sweet foods. Eating a diet high in sweets can contribute to dental cavities, childhood obesity, and poor nutrition. None of these are desirable, but they are not causes of diabetes.

Will diabetes go away after insulin treatment and leave the child cured?
No. At present, there is no cure for diabetes. It is a lifelong, controllable health condition. Once controlled and then well managed, the child will develop physically, emotionally, and socially.

Is diabetes contagious?
No. You cannot catch diabetes from another individual. Activities such as sharing a drinking cup or a piece of food, or touching blood or saliva, are not ways of developing diabetes.

Fevers

Fevers are very common in young children. The appearance of a fever triggers a period of discomfort for the child and concern from parents and child care providers. A fever is not harmful, and in fact, it is beneficial. However, a prolonged fever can be of concern when the illness responsible for the fever is not diagnosed. A fever is not an illness; it is a symptom of an illness.

Why does a child get a fever? When the body's immune, or defense system detects an invading organism, such as a bacteria or virus, certain cells in the blood surround the invader. This triggers a series of hormonal reactions that tells the body to "turn up the heat." The higher temperature created by the fever is helpful to the cells that are destroying the bacteria or virus because they can work more effectively at temperatures above normal.

The normal body temperature is 98.6°F, but it is not unusual for a young child's fever to run as high as 104°F or 105°F during an illness. A temperature can be measured orally, rectally, or under the arm (axillary). Readings can vary depending on where the temperature is taken. A rectal temperature reading can be as much as a degree higher than an oral temperature reading, and an axillary temperature reading can be as much as a degree lower. The method you use depends on the age of the child.

Measuring a Rectal Temperature

A rectal temperature gives the most accurate temperature reading. However, it is unnecessarily intrusive to children over 1 year of age. To take a rectal temperature:

- Use a rectal thermometer which has a wider bulb than the oral thermometer, making it less likely to break, and a disposable cover. Shake a glass thermometer firmly several times until reading is below normal.
- Lay the infant on the back or stomach on a changing table. Use the belt to hold the child in place. Dip the bulb of the rectal thermometer in petroleum jelly, gently insert it into the rectum ½ to 1 inch in depth and hold it in place by putting your hand firmly on the buttocks, with the thermometer sticking out between your fingers.

Recommended Methods for Taking Temperatures in Children

	Rectal	Axillary	Oral
under 1 year	•	•	
2 years		•	
3 years		•	
4 years		•	•
5 years and older			•

- A digital thermometer must be left in place for 30 to 60 seconds or until it registers with a beeping sound or a light; a glass thermometer must be left in place for 60 to 90 seconds.

Measuring an Axillary Temperature

To take an axillary temperature:

- Use either an oral or rectal thermometer with a disposable cover. Shake a glass thermometer firmly several times until the reading is below normal.
- Place the bulb of the thermometer against the child's underarm skin and hold it in place by gently pressing the child's arm against the side.
- A digital thermometer must be left in place for 30 to 60 seconds: a glass thermometer must be left in place for 10 minutes.

Measuring an Oral Temperature

This method is not recommended for children age 4 and under because it is beyond their understanding and skill.

- Use an oral thermometer with a disposable cover. Shake a glass thermometer firmly several times until the reading is below normal.
- Place the bulb of the thermometer under the child's tongue, close the lips, and have the child hold the thermometer in place with the fingers.
- A digital thermometer must be left in place for 30 to 60 seconds; a glass thermometer must be left in place for 3 minutes.

If the child drinks a cold beverage several minutes before the temperature is taken, the reading could be inaccurate.

Forehead and Oral Strips

The forehead strips must be held against the skin until a reading appears on the strip. The oral plastic strips are held under the tongue for several minutes until a reading appears on the strip. The accuracy of these strips varies depending on the length of time and the conditions under which they are stored.

Caring for a Child with a Fever

A child's temperature remains elevated while the immune system fights the invading bacteria or virus. It is not possible to speed up the process or "cure" a fever. It is possible, however, to reduce a high fever. A moderate fever (99°F to 102°F) can promote the body's infection-fighting system without the discomfort and concern that a fever above 102°F can generate.

- Separate the child from the group. A fever is often associated with a contagious illness. The child should remain at home until he is fever-free for 24 hours or, if necessary, examined by a health care provider.

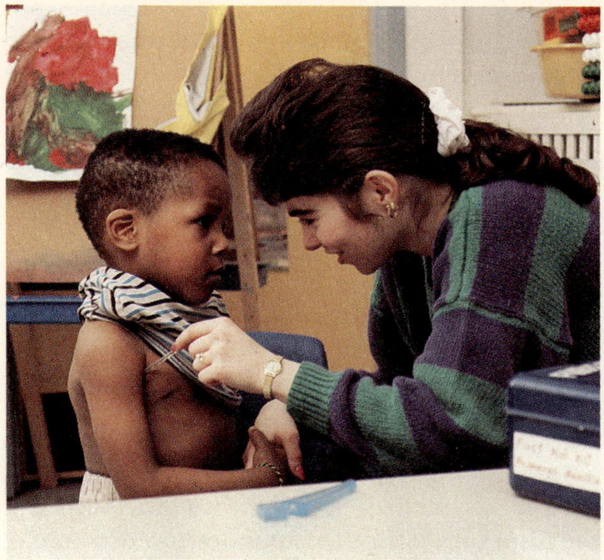

Taking an axillary temperature

- Encourage sips of clear fluids, such as water, tea, flat ginger ale and cola, finely crushed ice, popsicles, and gelatin. A fluid is considered clear if you can see through it when it is held up to the light. Apple juice is also a clear fluid, but it can cause diarrhea in some children. Milk and orange juice are not clear fluids.
- Dress the child as lightly as possible, but do not allow the child to shiver. Shivering can increase the body's temperature.
- Sponge bathe a child if the fever is over 103°F. Rub the skin briskly using tepid water (75°F to 90°F) and a face cloth. Also dampen the head, because a large percentage of body heat is lost through the head. The resulting drop in body temperature is caused by the evaporation of the water from the skin and the release of heat from dilating surface blood vessels. The inside temperature is reduced by the circulation of cooled blood from the surface down into the organs and tissue while the warm blood travels to the surface and is cooled.
- Do not use rubbing alcohol as it can be absorbed through the skin.
- Give acetaminophen if you have written permission from the child's parent and physician. Know your center's policies about administering medication.
- Ask the child's parent to come for the child as soon as possible.

Fevers in children under the age of 6 months (and especially under 3 months) are most worrisome because infants cannot fight infections as easily as older children and can more easily become dehydrated. The following are guidelines for notifying a child's parent:

Age	Temperature
0 to 6 months	over 100°F rectally
6 to 12 months	over 101°F rectally or 100°F axillary
1 year and older	over 101°F orally or 100°F axillary

Cleaning a Thermometer

Thermometers should be washed in tepid water (75 to 90°F), rinsed in a bleach solution made of 10 parts water to one part bleach, and then allowed to air dry. The use of disposable thermometer covers is recommended.

Febrile Seizures

In a small percentage of children, a rapid rise in fever can cause a seizure. A febrile seizure is not related to a chronic seizure disorder and has no effect on the child's neurologic or brain function.

A child who has experienced a febrile seizure is more likely to have a future episode. A child care provider should begin fever reducing measures promptly when a fever develops. A febrile seizure rarely occurs in children under the age of 6 months and is most common between the ages of 18 months and 3 years. It seldom occurs in children over the age of 6 years.

Care of a Child Having a Febrile Seizure

- Treat as you would for grand mal seizure.
- Any child who experiences a seizure for the first time should be seen in an emergency medical facility. If the child has had a previous febrile seizure, call the parent to take the child to his health care provider.

Seizures

A seizure or a convulsion is an indication of a disturbance of electrical impulses of the brain. These disturbances cause a variety of body responses ranging from a few seconds of staring, to longer pauses and loss of attention, to collapse on the floor with loss of consciousness and the strong shaking of large voluntary muscles.

Causes of Seizures

- High fever
- Head injury
- Drug overdose
- Drug reaction
- Serious illness
- Poisoning
- Brain abnormalities
- Genetic factors

Sometimes a specific cause of the seizure can be identified but, more commonly, the cause remains unknown. Even without knowing the exact cause, a health care provider can usually treat the child with medication to control the seizures or reduce their frequency.

Aura

Some children experience an aura immediately before having a seizure. This is an internal warning system that can be a noise, visual change, funny taste, feeling in the stomach, numbness, or other sensation that causes the child to know a seizure is about to happen. Recognizing this warning sign, the child can lie down before the seizure occurs. Other children experience no aura or cannot recognize it as such, and will not know that a seizure is about to occur.

Grand Mal Seizure

A grand mal seizure involves the entire body. A child who experiences a grand mal seizure loses consciousness and temporarily stops breathing. The child resumes breathing as the seizure progresses and regains consciousness when the seizure ends. During the seizure, the body becomes rigid, the eyes roll back, and the neck and back arch slightly. The entire body has jerky or shaking movements. There is increased saliva production causing drooling or foaming at the mouth. The child might be incontinent of urine and stool.

First Aid

The uncontrolled movements of a child experiencing a seizure can be frightening to watch. A seizure must run its course. There is nothing you can do to interrupt it or alter it. The child care provider must remain calm in order to observe the seizure and protect the child from injury.

- Move toys and furniture out of the way so that the child is not injured during the seizure.
- Roll the child onto one side to allow saliva to drain and to keep the tongue from blocking the airway.
- Do not restrain the child's movements.

■ SEIZURE ■

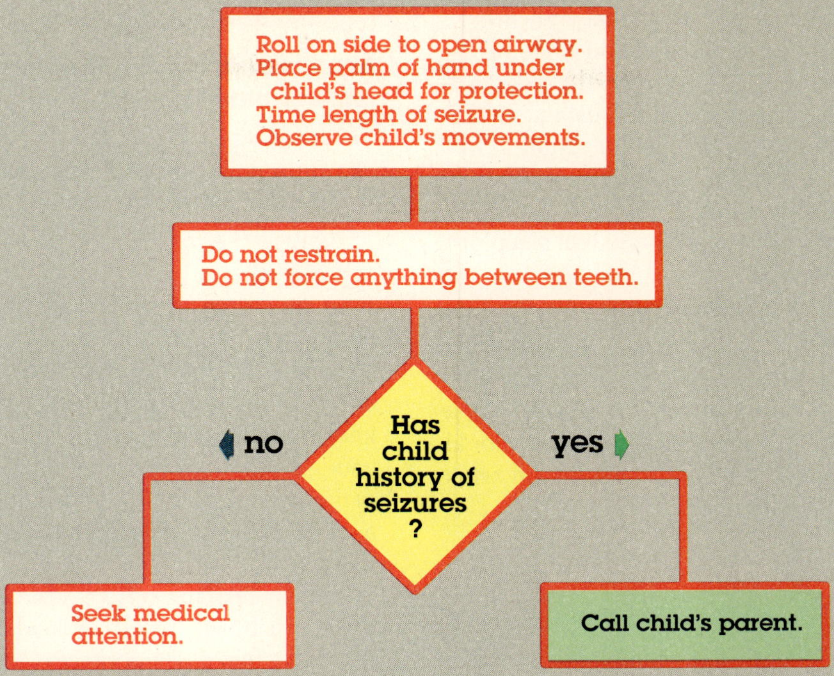
Roll on side to open airway.
Place palm of hand under child's head for protection.
Time length of seizure.
Observe child's movements.
Do not restrain.
Do not force anything between teeth.
Has child history of seizures ?
no
yes
Seek medical attention.
Call child's parent.

- Slide the open palm of your hand under the child's head, allowing the head to bump against the padding of your hand rather than the floor.
- Do not force anything between the child's teeth.
- Observe and time the seizure so that you can describe the body parts affected and estimate the length of the seizure. A seizure might seem to last longer than it actually does, especially if you are frightened. Your detailed description will be important to the child's health care provider.
- Let the child rest following the seizure. A child recovers from a seizure slowly and will sleep or be drowsy for a while.
- Do not give anything to eat or drink until the child is fully alert.

A child who is experiencing a seizure for the first time will need immediate medical care. If a child has a known seizure disorder, your child care center should have instructions from the child's doctor on what measures to take following the seizure.

Meningitis

Meningitis is an infection and inflammation of the meninges, the protective membranes that cover the brain. It also affects the spinal fluid, a watery cushion surrounding the brain and spinal cord.

The disease is transmitted from person to person by contact with contaminated saliva, nasal discharge, or droplets from a sneeze. The infecting organisms initially enter the body through the throat and lungs and make their way into the blood. In the blood, they travel to the brain where they infect the meninges. Meningitis can be caused by both viruses and bacteria.

Although meningitis can strike at any age, it usually occurs in infants and young children under the age of 5 years. The disease can spread easily through a child care center where children are in close contact with one another. Young children share mouthed toys and have not yet learned the importance of washing their hands after coughing, sneezing, or wiping their noses. In addition, their immature immune systems do not fight infection well.

Signs and Symptoms

The signs and symptoms of meningitis differ slightly, depending on the age of the child.

In infants:

- Fever
- Irritability or lethargy
- High-pitched cry
- Unusual swelling of an infant's soft spot, or fontanel located on the top of the head.
- Vomiting.
- Poor feeding
- Rash that appears as either fine red spots that look like broken blood vessels or larger purple blotches that can cover the body.

In older children, in addition to the above signs and symptoms:

- Headache
- Neck pain (Any movement of the neck stretches the meninges and causes pain.)
- Sensitivity to light
- Seizures

Most children who suffer from meningitis will recover completely, but some forms of meningitis can cause blindness, deafness, muscle weakness, brain damage, and in some cases, death. A vaccine is now available, known as the HIB vaccine, that protects infants and young children from some of the more serious forms of meningitis. All children should receive this vaccine as part of their early childhood immunization program.

Because of the seriousness of the disease and the long-term health risks involved, parents of children who have had close contact with a child with meningitis should contact their health care provider to find out about preventive treatment.

Reye's Syndrome

Reye's Syndrome is an uncommon disease that affects all organs of the body, especially the liver and brain. The incidence of Reye's Syndrome is reported to be 1 to 2 cases per 100,000 people. The National Reye's Syndrome Foundation believes that the true number might actually be higher because reporting the disease is not required. Reye's Syndrome primarily affects children from infants through teenagers, and is occasionally seen in adults. The disease is not contagious.

Reye's Syndrome strikes quickly and is most likely to occur following a viral infection such as influenza, an upper respiratory infection, or chicken pox. Usually it begins during the recovery period of the illness, but it can strike as late as two weeks after the initial illness. A child with Reye's Syndrome requires hospitalization for treatment.

Signs and Symptoms

Initial signs and symptoms include:

- Unexpected and continuous vomiting following a recent viral infection
- Listlessness and wanting to be left alone
- Drowsiness

Later signs and symptoms which can follow the above in as little as 12 hours:

- Confusion and delirium
- Moaning or screaming
- Combativeness and other irrational behavior
- Convulsions
- Coma

Signs and symptoms in infants do not follow the same pattern as in older children. For example, continuous vomiting, which is a significant sign in older children, might not occur in infants.

Signs and symptoms include:

- Rapid or irregular breathing
- Listlessness
- Diarrhea

Fever is not usually present. Fortunately, the sudden and severe beginning of Reye's Syndrome almost guarantees that the child's health care provider will be called promptly.

First Aid

Left untreated, Reye's Syndrome can be fatal. Children stand the best chance of recovery when treatment is started promptly. Recognizing the signs and symptoms of Reye's Syndrome is the most important intervention a child care provider can perform.

- Notify the child's parent of the signs and symptoms and ask the parent to come for the child immediately.
- Encourage the parent to call the child's health care provider.
- Treat for vomiting. (See Vomiting, Appendix B.)

Reye's Syndrome and Aspirin

Although there is no known cause of the disease, some studies suggest that there is a link between the development of Reye's Syndrome and the use of aspirin for viral illnesses such as influenza, upper respiratory infections, and chicken pox. The U.S. Surgeon General, the Food and Drug Administration, and the Centers for Disease Control now recommend that children not be given aspirin (also called salicylate) and products that contain aspirin for fever unless specifically recommended by a health care provider. Many manufacturers of aspirin now voluntarily label their products with this warning. Many pharmacies are placing warnings beside their aspirin products. Do not, however, attempt to rule out Reye's Syndrome in a very ill child who did not take aspirin; Reye's Syndrome can develop without the use of aspirin as well.

Near-Drowning

Drowning is the fourth leading cause of injury resulting in death among children. More than one third of all drownings happen to children ages 4 and under. Drowning can be a silent killer and it can happen quickly. Equally sad are the near-drowning victims who survive but suffer brain damage and a reduced quality of life. Near-drowning refers to surviving a prolonged period of time under water without oxygen.

A drowning or a near-drowning can occur in any body of water in which the nose and mouth of a child can be submerged. Besides the obvious large bodies of deep water, drownings can also occur in toilets, bathtubs, sinks, water buckets, fish tanks, and wading pools with only inches of water.

As a child care provider, you must diligently supervise the children in your care in and around water.

The following situations are true water emergencies and require you to take immediate life-saving action:

- Child panicking or struggling in water of any depth
- Child floating face down or submerged below the water surface
- Child limp with face in shallow water

First Aid

- Yell for help to alert others to the emergency.
- Rescue the child from the water. If the child is unconscious or injured following a dive, suspect that a spinal injury has occurred. Keep the head, neck, and spine straight. To do this, float the child onto a large full-body board and lift the child out of the water gently, supporting the head and neck.
- Determine consciousness, check airway, breathing and circulation, and treat accordingly. If you cannot give rescue breaths to the child, you must assume that the airway is obstructed and you must begin airway obstruction techniques. See Unconscious Choking Child and Infant sections in Chapter 3.
- If the child vomits, which is likely following a near-drowning, roll the child onto the side as a unit. Clear the vomitus from the mouth with your finger.

- Send someone to call for emergency medical help. Any child who survives a near-drowning incident, even if revived immediately with basic life-support techniques, must be taken to an emergency medical facility.

Numerous successful rescues have occurred after prolonged submersions in cold water. This is because the body's oxygen requirement is reduced in cold water, making it possible for the brain to survive longer without oxygen than the accepted 4 to 6 minutes.

Rescues

If a child is in trouble in the water, the adult rescuer should only attempt a rescue for which the rescuer has been trained or is otherwise capable of performing. Rescuers should never jeopardize themselves and risk becoming additional victims. The following are rescue methods that can be used in attempting to reach a child in the water:

- Reach a conscious, struggling child from the shore with a branch, pole, rope, or towel. If the child is beyond this reach, throw anything that floats, such as a styrofoam kickboard, a life jacket, a large, empty, airtight plastic container, or wood.
- Use a boat if one is available to rescue a child if the child is far off shore. Pull the child into the boat over one of the ends, not over the side of the boat.
- Swim to a child only if you are trained. Take a towel or object that floats for the child to grasp. For the safety of each of you, do not let the child grab you.
- Extend a light-weight pole or branch or throw a rope to a child who has fallen through the ice. Have someone grab your waist to stabilize you. Tell the child to spread the arms over the ice to distribute weight evenly. If you have nothing to extend and there are enough people present, try to reach the child by forming a human chain. Lie flat on the ice and grab the ankles of the person ahead of you.

Prevention

- All children should learn to swim at a young age.
- All pools should be surrounded with a locked fence.
- Rescue flotation devices should be kept near pools.
- Supervising children in and around water means that adults cannot take their eyes off the children even to glance at a magazine.
- Teach children respect for the water. Safe play and fun play go together in the water.
- Never leave a child alone for even a few seconds in or near any body of water including the bathtub.
- Empty bathtubs, wading pools, and water buckets immediately after use.
- Keep the toilet lid down.
- Teach children never to walk on ice on a pond or other body of water without adult permission and supervision.

Asthma

Mark each statement yes (Y) or no (N).

1. Which of the following signs and symptoms might a child having an asthma attack experience.

   A. ____ Coughing
   B. ____ Wheezing
   C. ____ Tightness in the chest
   D. ____ Fever
   E. ____ Increased pulse
   F. ____ Increased respiratory rate

2. Common asthma triggers include:

   A. ____ Upper respiratory infection
   B. ____ Dust
   C. ____ Animal fur
   D. ____ Vigorous exercise
   E. ____ Dry, cold air

Diabetes

Check (√) the correct signs and symptoms of hypoglycemia.

1. ____ Trembling
2. ____ Weight loss
3. ____ Dizziness
4. ____ Hunger
5. ____ Skin rash
6. ____ Sweating

Mark each statement true (T) or false (F).

1. ____ Hyperglycemia is easily corrected in the home or child care center.
2. ____ It might take several days or weeks until symptoms of hyperglycemia are recognized.
3. ____ Hypoglycemia is most likely to occur when a snack or meal is served late or skipped.
4. ____ Repeat sugar treatment for hypoglycemia if child has not improved in 1 hour.

Croup/Epiglottitis

Mark the following statements true (T) or false (F).

1. ____ Croup is a viral illness.
2. ____ Epiglottitis is a bacterial illness.
3. ____ Croup usually occurs in the morning.
4. ____ Cold air and humidity help a child with croup to breathe more easily.
5. ____ A child with epiglottitis has difficulty swallowing and might drool.

Fevers

Mark the following statements true (T) or false (F).

1. ____ A fever is a symptom of an illness.
2. ____ A fever helps to fight infection.
3. ____ A normal body temperature is 99.6°F.
4. ____ Axillary (under the arm) temperatures are recommended for children under the age of 5.

Mark the following yes (Y) or no (N).

If a child in your care has a temperature of 103°F you should do the following:

1. ____ Separate the child from the group and have the child lie down in a quiet area.
2. ____ Offer sips of clear fluids.
3. ____ Remove outer layer of clothing.
4. ____ Administer acetaminophen or aspirin appropriate for the child's age and weight.
5. ____ Place a cool cloth on child's forehead.

Seizures

Answer true (T) or false (F).

1. ____ All children who have seizures experience an aura.
2. ____ A grand mal seizure involves the entire body.
3. ____ A child who experiences a grand mal seizure remains conscious but cannot speak.
4. ____ A febrile seizure can occur in a child if a very high fever is allowed to continue for several hours.

Mark the following yes (Y) or no (N).

Correct first aid for a grand mal seizure includes:

1. ____ Give the child small sips of clear fluids.
2. ____ Protect the child from injury by restraining the arms.
3. ____ Position the child on the back to maintain an open airway.
4. ____ Gently slide a spoon or pencil between the teeth of a child having a grand mal seizure.
5. ____ Move toys and furniture out of the way so that the child is not injured during a grand mal seizure.

Meningitis

Mark the following true (T) or false (F).

1. ____ Meningitis can spread easily when children are in close contact with one another.
2. ____ Meningitis can be spread by children sharing mouthed toys.
3. ____ Meningitis can be spread by poor handwashing after changing the diaper of a child with infected stool.
4. ____ The cause of meningitis is unknown.

Dehydration

Mark the following true (T) or false (F).

Which of the following are signs of dehydration:

1. ____ Thirst
2. ____ Cool, clammy skin
3. ____ Concentrated urine that has a strong odor
4. ____ Dry, cracked lips
5. ____ Listlessness, sleepiness

Reye's Syndrome

Choose the best answer.

1. ____ Due to the risk of Reye's Syndrome, which of the following should not be given to children unless specifically recommended by a health care provider?
   A. Decongestants
   B. Aspirin (salicylates)
   C. Antacids

2. ____ Reye's Syndrome commonly develops up to 2 weeks following
   A. Strep throat and scarlet fever
   B. Ear and tonsil infections
   C. Influenza, chicken pox, and upper respiratory infections

3. ____ Which of the following is a sign of Reye's Syndrome?
   A. Unexpected and continuous vomiting
   B. High fever
   C. Persistent cough

12

Child Abuse*

■ Physical Abuse ■ Emotional Abuse ■ Sexual Abuse ■ Neglect ■ The Abusive Adult ■

Child abuse and neglect are tragic problems that cause suffering and fear for thousands of children. Many children die each year from injuries received by abusive adults. Many more survive years of physical, emotional, or sexual abuse or neglect and suffer permanent damage physically, developmentally, and psychologically. An abused child often has low self-esteem and difficulty relating to others. Unfortunately, these children are likely to become abusers of their own children.

Child abuse and neglect occur at all levels of society. It is a very old problem that was quietly tolerated by society until recent times. Fortunately, significant public and professional attention has forced society to decide that it will no longer ignore a problem that jeopardizes the health and futures of so many children.

Child care providers are trusted figures to young children. Their regular interaction with a small group of children allows them to observe closely a child's conduct and appearance and notice clues that might point toward a risk to the child's health and safety at home.

Today, children have a variety of exposures to adult authority figures, such as teachers, child care providers, parents, parents' significant other, and teenage baby sitters. They need to feel safe in the company of every adult who cares for them.

Physical Abuse

Physical abuse is a willful act of cruelty or violence against a child by an adult that results in injury. It is often a chronic situation.

Signs and Symptoms

The child's appearance:

- Bruises or welts on hidden as well as visible areas of the body
- Burns from cigarettes, burns from rope, or immersion burns that look like a glove on the hand, a sock on the foot, or round like a doughnut on the buttock

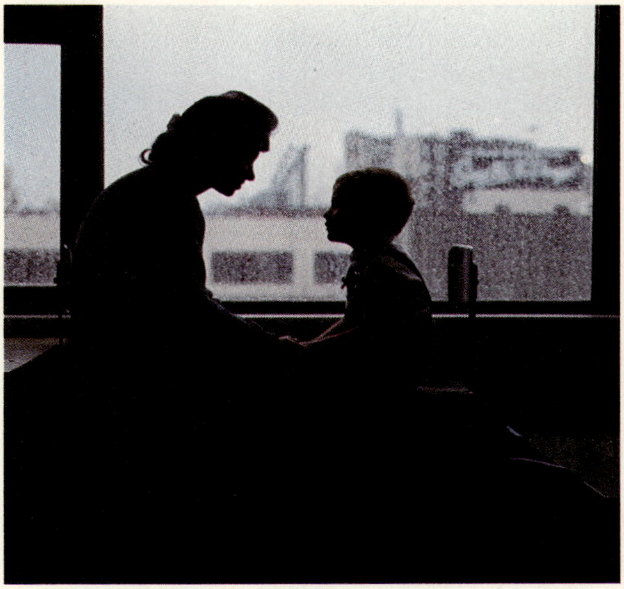

- Pattern burns that are the shape of the item used
- Broken bone injuries which might occur more than once especially those whose description of how it happened does not coincide with the appearance of the injury
- Lacerated cuts, especially on the face from the impact of a heavy object or a hand or foot

The child's behavior:

- Becomes apprehensive when other children cry
- Appears afraid and hesitant to go with abusive parent or other adult
- Not trusting of physical contact with adults in the center
- Shows extremes of behavior from aggressiveness to isolation
- Might tell the child care provider what happened

**Portions of this chapter adapted from Robert Winters,* Child Abuse Digest, *Winters Communications, Inc., Tampa, Fla., 1991.*

Emotional Abuse

Emotional abuse is continual verbal degradation and insults that cause the child to feel worthless and empty. Often it accompanies physical abuse. Clues are better indicated by behavior than appearance.

Signs and Symptoms

The child's appearance:

- Might show signs of physical abuse
- Fails to thrive

The child's behavior:

- Lags behind in intellectual, physical, and emotional development
- Fluctuates emotionally between being unusually compliant and passive, to being extremely aggressive, demanding, or violent
- Shows unusual adaptive behavior such as being inappropriately adult (for instance, parenting other children) or inappropriately infantile (for example, thumb sucking, frequent rocking, and incontinent of urine)
- Shows self-destructive behavior and might eventually attempt suicide

Sexual Abuse

Sexual abuse consists of inappropriate physical contact with a child. This covers a wide range of crimes from fondling and indecent exposure to more violent activities such as intercourse. In most cases of sexual abuse, it is recurrent and the child knows the sexual offender. The child might have been sworn to secrecy by the offender who has bribed the child or threatened with violence or death to the child or another loved one if the child tells anyone.

Signs and Symptoms

The child's appearance:

- Irritation, pain, bruises, or bleeding in the genital area
- Discharge from the vagina or penis that could be a sexually transmitted disease

The child's behavior:

- Has poor relationships with peers and withdraws from social activities
- Engages in abnormal fantasy or infantile behavior
- Has recurrent nightmares that might be shared with child care staff
- Conversation might indicate that the child has a greater knowledge of sexual matters than is age appropriate
- Fear of or hesitancy about going with a particular person
- Regressive behavior in school-age children, such as thumb sucking, crying excessively, and withdrawing into a fantasy world
- Other problem behaviors in school-age children, including aggressive or disruptive acting out, running away, delinquent activities, and failing in school work

Neglect

A neglected child suffers from chronic lack of care that can damage physical and emotional health. The child lacks consistent contact with nurturing and supportive adults.

Signs and Symptoms

The child's appearance:

- Has uncared for medical problems and rarely sees a health care provider for well child care
- Looks unkempt, is inadequately dressed, looks and smells dirty, and has chronic mouth odor
- Frequently does not attend the child care center or school, with absences unexplained
- Conversation reveals that the child is often alone or engages in activities that are dangerous or inappropriate for age

The child's behavior:

- Has little experience with rules and limit setting
- Behavior might appear delinquent compared to other children in the center or school
- Child often complains of hunger and might sneak food
- Might be constantly tired and lacks enthusiasm
- Has a poor attendance record

The Abusive Adult

The tragedy of the abusive adult is that he or she might have been abused or neglected as a child, leaving emotional scars that make being a responsible and loving adult unattainable. Some characteristics of abusive adults are that they:

- Use harsh discipline that is inappropriate to the child's age and actions

- Seem unconcerned about the child or the child's problems
- Incorrectly perceive the child's motives for actions
- Misuse alcohol or other drugs
- Attempt to conceal or make light of child's injury or blame the child for being clumsy
- Blame or belittle child in public
- Discuss and treat siblings unequally
- Can be very protective or jealous of the child, especially sexual abusers

Every adult needs to be aware of the devastation of child abuse in any form and must be willing to get involved. Reporting your concerns in good faith to professionals such as a child care center director, medical adviser, health care provider or your state's protective service office is the first step in making a diagnosis of abuse and getting help for the child and the family. You can also report suspected abuse to the National Child Abuse Hotline, 1–800–422–4453.

13

Safety

■ Playground Safety ■ Toy Safety ■ Child Passenger Safety ■ Bicycle Safety ■ Pedestrian Safety ■ Child Equipment Safety ■ Food Safety ■ Water Safety ■ Dog Safety ■ Handgun Safety ■ Child-Proofing Checklist ■

Young children have a natural drive to learn about their environment by exploring and by using their senses of taste and touch. Because they cannot make judgments about their own health and safety, this drive puts them at high risk for such injuries as choking, falls, and burns.

A child care provider's knowledge of growth and development is invaluable in creating a hazard-free environment, full of safe and age-appropriate items. It is essential to identify and remove all potential dangers. Safety is an even greater challenge in a family child care setting because there, children are likely to be of different ages and at different developmental stages.

As children grow, you need to be aware that hazards will change because of the children's expanding capabilities. Remember that a mobile child's possibilities for adventure—both horizontal and vertical—are endless.

Playground Safety

The Consumer Product Safety Commission estimates that approximately 400,000 children are injured each year on the nation's playgrounds and that 25 percent of these injuries must be treated in hospitals. An estimated 20 children die every year as the result of a playground injury.

Safety guidelines for playgrounds include the following:

- Be certain that there is sand, grass, mulch, or mats under all climbing equipment and swings.
- Place plastic caps over protruding sharp ends and screws in metal swing sets.
- Inspect wooden climbing structures and sand rough areas to prevent splinters.
- Look for swings with canvas or hard rubber sling seats. Avoid those seats made of metal and wood. This will minimize the severity of an injury to a child who is struck by an empty swing seat.
- For proper slide safety, instruct children to keep one arm's length between each other, to climb up the steps rather than the slide, to step away from the slide after they have finished their turn, and to slide feet first and one at a time.

Behavioral Characteristics of Children That Increase Their Risk of Injury

Aggressive	Obstinate, willful
Very active, restless	Poor self-control
Bold, fearless	Frequently puts small things in mouth
Overly curious	Short attention span
Easily distracted	Unable to focus
Impatient	
Impetuous	

Toy Safety

Present U.S. government regulations on newly manufactured toys continually help to improve the quality of American-made toys and reduce their potential hazards. These regulations, together with good faith compliance and conscientious testing by the industry, make toys for today's children much safer than those of the generation before them. However, not all toy-related injuries can be prevented by government regulations and the toy industry.

Toy manufacturers label toys with children's age recommendations, but this is only *their* guide. Consider the children in your care and their developmental stage; do they play vigorously and do they put toys in their mouths?

The following are guidelines for preventing toy injuries:

- Read labels. Look for manufacturers' age recommendations and for fabrics that are washable.

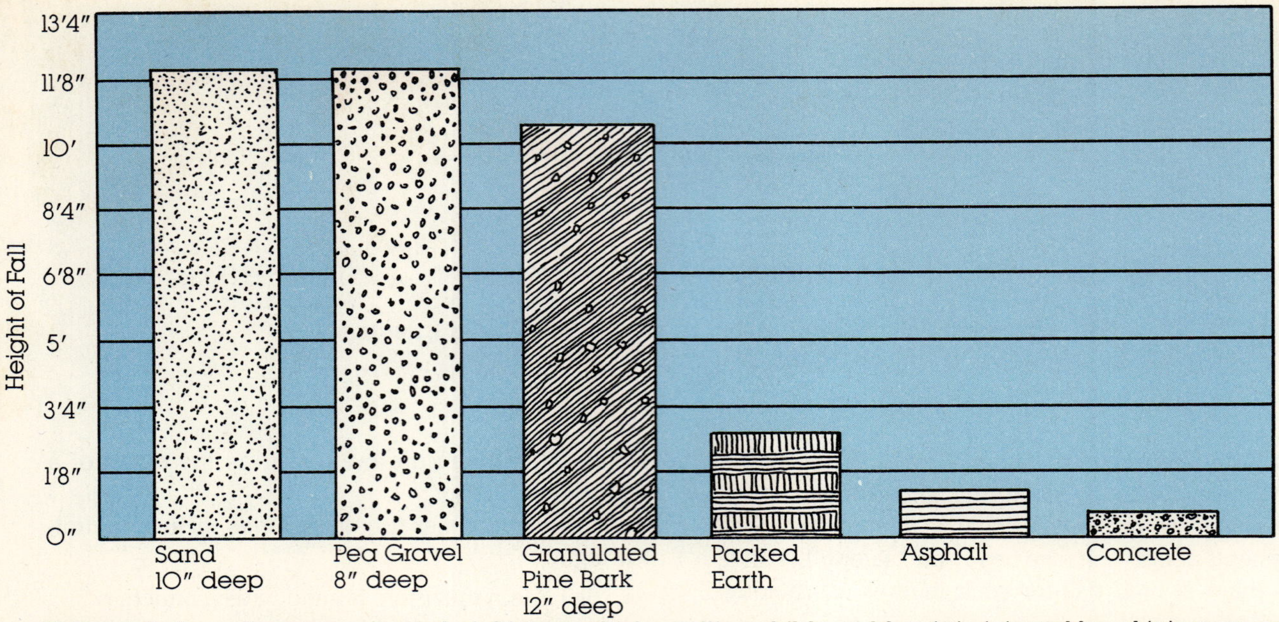

This graph shows the approximate height from which a falling child would sustain internal head injury on each playground surface.
Source: Franklin Research Center, Norristown, Pa.

- Discard plastic packaging immediately.
- Choose toys that hold up well to repetitive use.
- Discard broken toys immediately. Never repair toys for a young child who tends to throw toys or mouth them.
- Check toys carefully, making sure that no parts are small enough to be swallowed and that no small part is able to be pulled from the toy. Some children put everything in their mouths, regardless of their age.
- Check toys regularly for sharp points, exposed wires, torn seams, and sharp edges.
- Sand wooden toys if they have any rough edges.
- Never hang toys with long cords or strings in a crib or playpen due to the chance of strangulation.
- Never hang pacifiers on cords or ribbons around a child's neck. Use only pacifiers with a guard shield that is too large to fit inside the mouth, and ones that contain ventilation holes.
- Keep uninflated balloons out of reach. Discard pieces of broken balloons immediately.
- Do not allow noise-making toys, including guns, to be used near anyone's ears.
- Teach older children that their electric toys, chemistry sets, and hobby items are hazards to young siblings or children who come into their homes for child care.
- Adult toys—such as lawn darts, dart guns, and bows and arrows—have no place in a child care setting.
- Use only toy boxes with plastic lids and air holes, or store toys in plastic storage containers. Heavy lids with metal hinges are responsible for many injuries.
- Teach children at a young age to put toys away. Make a game of it with a song. This helps everyone!

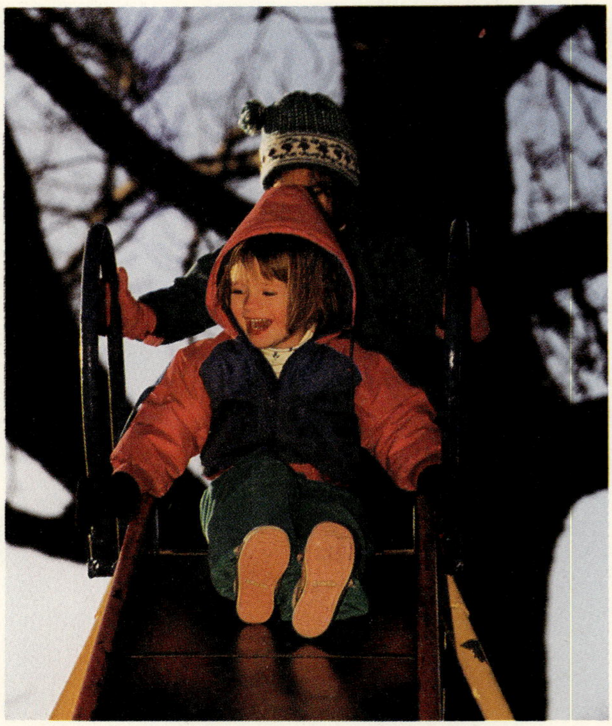

Child Passenger Safety

Car accidents are, by far, the leading cause of injury and death in children from ages 1 to 14. Most children injured or killed in motor vehicle accidents are not restrained in car seats or seat belts. All 50 states, the District of Columbia, and Puerto Rico, have child passenger safety laws making it illegal and punishable by a fine to transport a child in a vehicle without a car seat restraint or properly adjusted seat belt. Child safety seats come in a variety of sizes and styles. Choose one that is easy to use and one that fits properly in your car; use it exactly as the manufacturer instructs every time you get into the car. A car seat used part time is risky. A car seat improperly used is as dangerous as no restraint at all.

Your responsibility checklist includes the following:

- Use a car seat that meets or exceeds government safety standards. Secure infants up to 20 pounds in an infant safety seat facing backwards. Secure toddlers or children weighing between 20 and 40 pounds in a safety seat facing forward. Secure children over 40 pounds, who have outgrown safety seats but are too small for the adult lap belt and shoulder harness, in a car booster seat. This seat comes with its own shoulder harness and anchor strap or allows for the use of the adult lap belt and shoulder strap. The child should use the booster seat until he is big enough for the adult lap belt to rest on his pelvis, not his abdomen which would be injured in a collision.
- The middle of the back seat is the safest location for a child passenger.
- Never substitute houshold booster chairs for the car booster seats. Never substitute infant play seats for infant car seats.
- There must be one seat belt for every child. Do not allow children to share seat belts because the impact of a collision can crush one child against the other.
- Do not permit a child to ride on an adult's lap. An unrestrained child will be thrown from the adult's arms by the force of a crash. A child belted with an adult will be crushed between the belt and the adult.
- Never drive when a small child is standing up. A slight swerve or sudden stop could throw a child against a door window or the dashboard. Stop the car and return the child to the car safety seat.

The National Highway Safety Administration estimates that, with correct use, child safety seats could prevent 56,800 injuries and 519 fatalities per year.

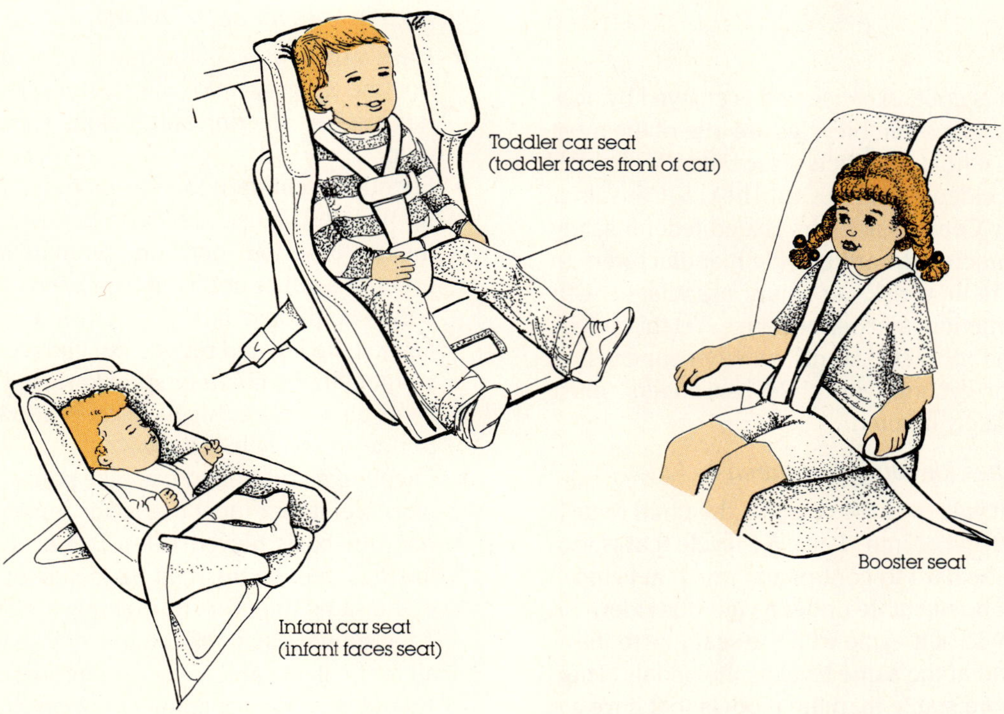

Toddler car seat (toddler faces front of car)

Infant car seat (infant faces seat)

Booster seat

- Do not allow a child to sit on a driver's lap, to pretend to drive, or to play with car controls.
- Teach children from infancy that buckling up is the first step in starting the car. As an adult, you set an example for children by your attitude and behavior in the car.
- Always lock doors securely.
- Never leave a child alone in a car.
- If your car has been in the sun in hot weather, touch the metal clasps of the child's car seat to your own arm to check the temperature. Make sure that the child's skin does not touch hot metal.
- Keep a first aid kit in your vehicle's trunk. Besides the common first aid items, it should include a blanket, flares, change for telephone calls, a flashlight, and batteries.

Restrained children are less likely to distract the driver and more likely to nap or look at books and toys. A child who uses a safety restraint from infancy will not be aware of any other way to travel and will accept car restraints with little complaint.

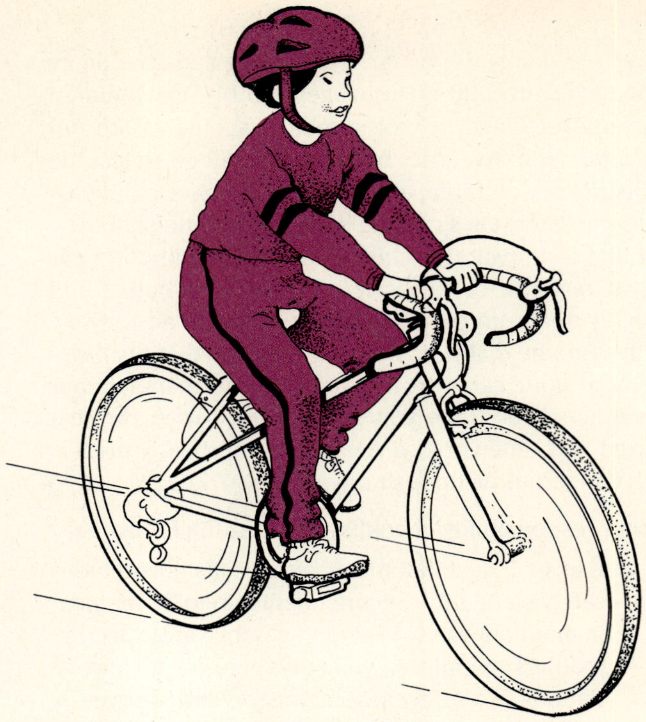

In a 30-mph car accident, an unrestrained child will hit the dashboard or windshield with the same force as falling from a third-floor window.

Bicycle Safety

Bicycle riding is good exercise and is enjoyed by people of all ages. However, bicycles are one of the most common household products associated with high numbers of accidents and injuries. The U.S. Consumer Product Safety Commission has issued federal safety regulations directed toward bicycle manufacturers to eliminate or reduce risks of injury associated with design, construction, and performance. Yet this solves only part of the problem. Adults, whether supervising child riders or cycling with child passengers, must always keep safety in mind.

Safety guidelines for younger children include:

- Have a tricycle available that fits the child today, not one to "grow into" later. A tricycle that is too large can be hard to control and one that is too small can be unstable under a vigorous rider.
- Use the style of tricycle with the seat low to the ground and at the same level as the pedals. This style is more stable than the models that have a high seat and low pedals.
- Allow only one child at a time to use a tricycle.
- Allow riding on flat surfaces only, but not on streets where motorists might have difficulty seeing the child and tricycle.
- Check tricycles for wear, sharp edges, and loose or missing parts. Store them inside overnight to prevent rust, which ages and weakens the metal.

Safety guidelines for older children include:

- Have a bicycle available that fits the child today, not one to "grow into" later. A bicycle that is too large makes steering and braking especially difficult.
- Encourage children to wear clothing designed for biking. The use of bicycle helmets reduces the risk of serious head and brain injury in the event of a fall or collision. Leg bands or rubber bands hold loose-fitting pant legs securely against the leg and reduce the chance of entanglement in the chain or sprocket. Tied shoe laces also reduce this risk. Never allow children to ride a bicycle in bare feet.
- Encourage children to use bike paths whenever possible. If they must use roads, make sure they obey the basic bicycle rules. Bikers should travel in single file, on the right hand side of the road in the same direction as motor vehicle traffic. They should use correct hand signals and obey all traffic lights and signs for motorists. Bikers should watch for opening car doors and for cars pulling out of driveways and parking spaces.

Bicycle Helmets Make Sense

- Bicycle injuries are the most common cause of sports or recreational injury in the United States.*
- More than nine hundred children are killed each year as the result of bicycle accidents, and another 500,000 are seen in emergency rooms. One study showed that three of every four children who are hospitalized for a bicycle injury do not wear helmets even after recovery.**
- The use of approved bicycle helmets reduces the risk of severe head injuries by 85 percent.***
- Seventy-five percent of all fatalities in bicycle-related accidents are due to brain injury.*
- In a bicycle accident you have a 50/50 chance of hitting your head.*
- A fall from a bicycle that is moving at 20 mph will likely result in death if the rider's head hits the pavement, rocks, or another solid object.*

*Sources: *Injury Prevention Resource and Research Center, Dartmouth Medical School. **National Head Injury Foundation. Taken from an article in* Washington Post, *Health Section, October 16, 1990. ***National Safety Council.*

- Bikes should be used only in daylight and in dry weather. In bad weather, visibility is reduced, wet tires skid, and wet handbrakes do not work effectively. Reflectors should be attached in the correct locations. Riding after sunset, even in dry weather with lights and reflectors, is dangerous.
- Discourage bike stunts, clowning, and carrying others on handlebars or fenders.

Safety guidelines for a child passenger on an adult bike include:

- Bicycle seats are for use by children beginning at the age of 1 year. When purchasing a bicycle seat, choose only a model whose seat back extends high enough to protect the child's head; the seat should also come with protective plastic that covers the spokes to prevent feet from getting caught in them. Do not buy a used bicycle seat if any of the parts are missing.
- Make certain that the child always wears a properly fitting helmet.
- Readjust the seat belt so that the closure is on the outside back of the seat instead of across the lap. Only you can then unbuckle it.
- Remember that the additional weight of the child requires more energy from the adult pedaling and makes the bicycle less stable. Braking time is increased and downhill cruising speeds can increase without your noticing.
- Pick safe routes. Do not bike in inclement weather, when visibility is reduced, wet tires skid, and wet hand brakes do not work effectively.

Pedestrian Safety

Short walks near the child care center or home or to and from a playground provide opportunities to teach safe behavior on streets and sidewalks.

For safe traveling, children should walk holding hands or holding a travel rope. This is made by tying knots or plastic bracelets a few feet apart along a length of rope. Each child holds on to a knot or bracelet and is taught not to let go while walking.

Include this safety teaching when walking outdoors with children:

- Teach children to stop just before the curb or edge of the road and wait for an adult. Never step into the street until told that it is safe to go ahead.
- Talk about traffic and pedestrian signs and symbols when walking so that the children will learn to recognize them.
- Teach how to look for vehicles when crossing an intersection.
- Teach children that people stay on the sidewalks, while cars, buses, and trucks stay on the street.
- Teach children that vehicles can injure them.
- Teach children to stay away from parked vehicles on the street and in driveways.

Child Equipment Safety

Young children are usually very active, whether they are on the floor or in one of the many pieces of equipment designed to meet their needs and yours. Because they cannot evaluate possible hazards, they can be injured in what seem to be safe places.

Standards and guidelines for juvenile equipment have been improved over the years by the U.S. Consumer Product Safety Commission. Check older equipment before using it, making certain that it conforms to current standards and guidelines.

Cribs

Current government regulations require the following:

- Standard-size cribs must have mattresses that fit snugly. If two fingers can fit between the mattress and crib, the mattress is too small.
- Crib slats must be no more than 2⅜ inches apart. This ensures that infants cannot slip through and become strangled or trapped. Avoid any decorative openings in end panels that would allow head or limb entrapment.
- Corner posts must be no more than 1⁄16 inch in height above the side rails and front/back panels. There must be no rough edges or metal hardware inside the crib.
- Locks on the side rails must not be accessible to a child who might release them.

Your responsibility checklist includes the following:

- Make sure that your crib(s) meets all of the above standards.
- Do not place crib(s) next to a window or near drapery/blind cords.
- If the crib has plastic teething rails, any that become cracked should be immediately removed and replaced.
- Use bumper pads, mobiles and crib gyms only until the child can push himself up onto hands and knees; then remove them.
- Do not use pillows for babies who cannot roll over.
- When the child can pull up to a standing position, lower the crib mattress to the lowest position.
- Do not allow cords or strings longer than 12 inches near the crib due to the risk of strangulation.
- In a crib, avoid large toys that can be stood on and can lead to a fall.
- Never use thin plastic trash bags to cover mattresses or pillows or to store bedding.
- Stop using the crib once the height of the top rails is less than three-fourths of the child's height.

Playpens

Playpens can provide a safe play environment when there are tasks or other children that require your full attention.

Your responsibility checklist includes the following:

- Make certain the playpen bars are no more than 2⅜ inches apart.
- Make certain that mesh-netting playpens have a weave tiny enough so that small items cannot be pushed into the playpen by toddlers.
- Do not place large toys in playpen. Children could stand on these and fall out.
- Do not hang toys with cords from the playpen sides due to the risk of strangulation.
- Remove the playpen once the child is able to climb over the side.
- Never leave the sides of mesh playpens down. Infants can become trapped between the mesh sides and the thin plastic mattress and suffocate.

High Chairs

High chairs allow children to explore food and feed themselves with a minimum of kitchen mess. Adult supervision is necessary to ensure against high chair injuries.

Your responsibility checklist includes the following:

- Use a high chair with both lap and crotch straps. Always fasten the straps.
- If your high chair is old or straps are missing, purchase a safety harness and leave it attached to the chair. Young children must learn early that they will be strapped in before a meal.
- If the seat seems slippery, attach rough-surfaced adhesive strips.
- Never allow children to stand on the seat.
- Keep the high chair far enough away from the table, counter, or wall to prevent a child from

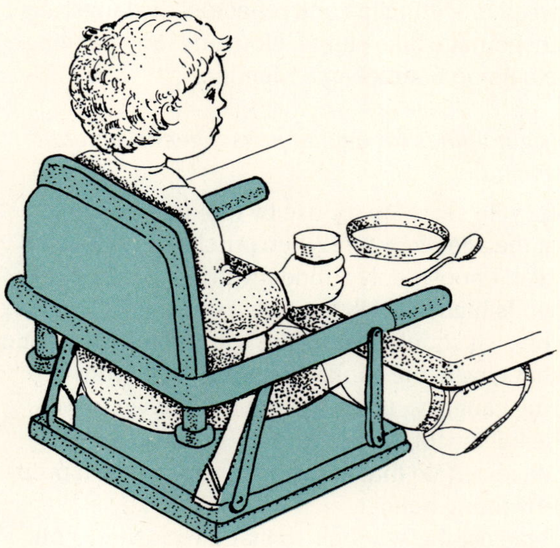

pushing the chair away from these surfaces and tipping over, or from pulling objects down.

- Do not let children climb into a high chair unassisted.
- Teach children to raise their hands over their head while you are attaching or detaching the tray to prevent pinched fingers.
- When using a chair that attaches to a table, use one that has a clamp that locks onto the table for additional security. Do not position the chair where the child's feet can reach other chairs, table supports, table legs, or anywhere the child can successfully lift weight from the chair. The weight of the child keeps the hook-on chair in position.

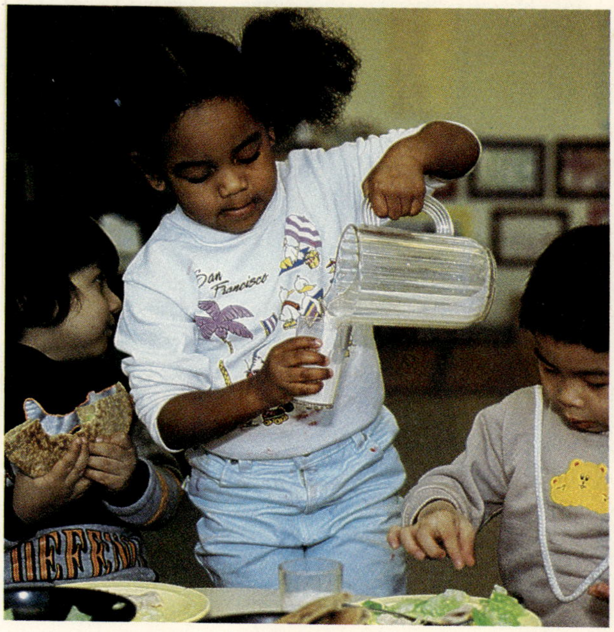

Walkers

Walkers enable older babies to walk around before they have mastered the task on their own. Because the babies are too young to understand the possible dangers, they must be supervised. Walkers can tip over if a child leans too far to one side or reaches over to pick up a toy.

Your responsibility checklist includes the following:

- Keep the walker on a smooth, flat surface. Carpets and door thresholds are uneven surfaces that increase the chance of tipping over.
- Never use a walker on grass or gravel.
- Select a walker with a wide wheelbase. This increases stability and reduces the chance of tipping.
- To prevent pinched fingers, select a walker with protective covers over the scissor component and coil springs. Avoid the older X-frame models.
- Use gates across stairways.

Food Safety

Choking is one of the leading causes of death in children. We all know that small toy parts must be kept out of the reach of babies and young children who might mouth them. But we sometimes forget that a small piece of food can choke a child as well.

Your emphasis on the methods of preventing accidental choking will help reduce the chance that you will need to use life-saving techniques. See Chapter 3.

Some safety rules regarding foods are these:

- Teach children not to speak with their mouths full of food. A laugh or sudden gasp can direct food into the airway.
- Make certain that children always sit while eating. Moving about or running while eating increases the chances of choking.
- Cut up or break food into small manageable pieces.
- Avoid giving the following foods to children under 1 year of age and give them only with supervision, if at all, to children between 1 and 3 years old:

Hotdogs	Corn kernels
Grapes	Peanut butter
Popcorn	Marshmallows
Nuts	Ice
Raisins	Bony fish
Baby food meat sticks	Raw carrots
Oranges	Raw celery
Hard candy	Apple peels
Chewing gum	

Water Safety

Water play in wading pools and tubs is always fun for children. The ever-present risk of injury in and around the water should keep the supervising adult alert to the children's activity there.

Reduce the risk of injury in the home or child care center by following these guidelines:

- Never leave children unsupervised in a tub or wading pool, no matter how shallow the water, or how short the time. Household bathtubs are a common location for infant drownings.

> Approximately 300 children drown each year in neighborhood pools.
>
> *Source: Center for Environmental Health and Injury Control, Centers for Disease Control.*

- Make certain that an adult is always present when a pool is being filled.
- Empty pools and tubs immediately after each use.
- Use caution in allowing nonswimmers to use any floating devices in deep water, including kickboards. Even a momentary loss of grip on the object can cause panic and lead to drowning.

Dog Safety

The love and loyalty of a dog make them one of the most popular pets. They can help a child learn to accept responsibility, understand about caring for others, and build self-confidence. Unfortunately, they can also be a threat to children. Each year there are nearly 1.5 million serious dog bites reported nationally. It is estimated that over 80 percent of these injuries involve preschool or school-age children. Boys are bitten more often than girls, and the majority of these bites are provoked. Most of the dog bites occur near the child's home, and the dogs belong either to a neighbor or to the child's family.

To reduce the risk of dog bites to children, these safety rules should be taught:

- It is dangerous to mistreat or tease a pet.
- Never disturb a pet that is eating or sleeping.
- Adult supervision is necessary when a child feeds a dog.
- Never break up a dog fight, even when one's own pet is involved.
- Avoid strange dogs in the neighborhood. This is especially true if the animal is sick or injured. Tell an adult, who will call for help.
- Stop, stand still, and speak softly if approached by an unfamiliar dog. Never touch a strange dog or make any threatening gestures.

Handgun Safety

It is estimated that 44 percent of American homes with children have one or more handguns. Homicides are now the second leading cause of injury-related death in children under the age of 18, followed by suicide. Approximately 66 percent of all homicides and more than half of all suicides among children are caused by handguns. In addition, approximately 16 percent of all unintentional firearm deaths occur in children under the age of 18 who were "just fooling around when it went off." The increasing availability and use of handguns can only indicate that the number of children injured and killed by handguns will continue to rise.

If you must own a handgun, store it unloaded and locked in a cabinet. Ammunition should also be locked and stored separately from the handgun. Do not let anyone under the age of 18 know where the key is kept or the gun is stored. Latchkey children with access to guns present an unknown potential for serious wounds and death.

Nonpowder firearms such as pump air guns, air rifles, air pistols, and BB guns can also cause injuries and deaths in children. Projectiles from these weapons can reach speeds comparable to some handguns and can penetrate skin and bone, in some cases, up to 4 inches.

Child-Proofing Checklist

Go through each room in your child care center or home. How well do you follow these safety precautions?

Kitchen

- Use back stove burners first.
- Teach children the meaning of "hot."
- Test foods and formula warmed in a microwave oven. Foods can be warmed unevenly creating hot spots.
- Keep the handles of pans on the stove turned inward.
- Remove stove knobs when they are not in use.
- Do not use countertops or cupboards for storing medicines, including vitamins, acetaminophen, and aspirin.
- Make sure that children cannot reach counters and tabletops from their high chairs.
- Keep poisons up high, even out of your reach. Store food and chemicals separately. See Preventing a Swallowed Poisoning, Chapter 7.
- Unplug counter appliances when they are not in use and keep cords out of the reach of children when appliances are in use.
- Use placemats, rather than tablecloths which can be pulled, causing hot liquids to spill.
- Use a sturdy step ladder for children to stand on when they are "observing."

COMMON INJURIES RELATED TO CHILD'S DEVELOPMENTAL LEVEL

Developmental Characteristics	Injuries
Infant Age 0 to 1 year	
Increasing mobility	Burns
Uses mouth to explore objects	Choking
Reaches for and pulls objects	Drowning
Unaware of dangers	Falls
Cannot understand "no"	
Toddler Age 1 to 2½ years	
Masters walking, running, climbing	Burns
Explores almost everything with mouth	Choking
Begins to imitate behaviors	Drowning
Investigates everything within reach	Falls
Curious about all never-before-seem items	Pedestrian Injuries
Unaware of most dangers	Poisoning
Impulsive	Suffocation
Preschooler Age 2½ to 5 years	
Mobility leads to increased independence	Burns
Learn to ride tricycle	Choking
Unaware of many dangers	Drowning
Might favor real, rather than toy tools, gadgets, appliances	Falls
Fascinated with fire	Pedestrian Injuries
Imitate adult behavior	Poisoning
School age Age 5 years and up	
Need to be independent	Bicycle Injuries
Need to be like peers	Burns
Need to be with peers	Falls
Need for increased physical activity	Pedestrian Injuries
Dangers do not always seem real	Firearm injuries
Increased independence can mean less closely supervised	

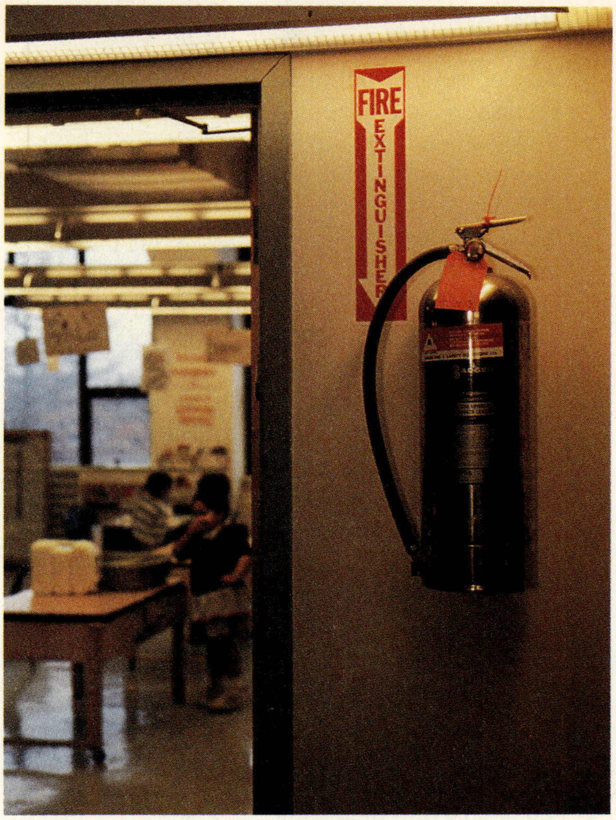

Garage, Basement, Laundry

- Keep children out of these areas. Locate a hook and eye latch above the level of the child's head on the entrance door to these areas.
- Place poisons up high in their original containers and avoid storing dangerous poisons whenever possible.
- Unplug hazardous tools and keep them out of reach.

Bathroom

- Keep poisons up high—including mouthwash, powder, and perfume. Many products kept in the bathroom, such as mouthwash and cosmetics, do not come in child-resistant containers.
- Keep the medicine cabinet locked. It should be located out of children's reach.
- Flush old medicine down the toilet and rinse out the container before discarding it.
- Keep the toilet lid down. Do not use continuous blue bowl cleaners.
- When the tub water is running, turn off the hot water first so the faucet is cool.
- Use a rubber mat or nonskid decals in bathtub.
- Never leave a baby unattended on a changing table.
- Change active babies and toddlers on the floor rather than a table to prevent falls.

Adult Bedroom

- Keep this room off limits to children unless it is used as their napping area.
- Do not keep medicines or cosmetics in bedside tables.
- Remove perfumes, powders, and heavy items from dresser tops.

General Rules

- Post emergency phone numbers at all telephones in the child care center or home.
- Check smoke detectors regularly. Have a fire escape plan posted and practice it routinely with children.
- Make certain that everyone knows the location of the fire extinguisher. Do not store it near the oven, fireplace, or wood stove.
- Place barriers around wood stoves and screens in front of fireplaces.
- Cover unused electrical outlets with plastic covers made for this purpose. Avoid brightly colored covers and those with attractively painted figures, which might attract the children's attention.
- Do not run extension cords under rugs where people walk. Regularly check for frayed or damaged electrical cords.
- Keep extension cords out of view. Children can be electrocuted by biting through a cord that has current running through it. Discourage children from playing with phone cords due to the risk of strangulation.
- Place plants up high.
- Be cautious in your use of doorway gates. Children can push through tension gates. They might catch their fingers in accordion-type gates or might climb them. Use gates only for the doorway widths suggested by the manufacturer.
- Make stairs nonskid with carpet or rubber mats. Place skid-proof padding under all small throw rugs. Teach young children to manage stairs by crawling down backward and holding onto the rail.
- Move furniture if sharp corners protrude into heavily traveled areas.
- Keep drinking alcohol out of children's reach.
- Empty ashtrays promptly. Nicotine, found in cigarette butts, is poisonous.
- Keep matches, lighters, cigarettes, cigars, and pipes out of the children's reach.
- Open windows from the top if you are on the second story or higher or if there are no window guards.
- Anchor tall and unsteady bookcases to walls.
- Set hot water heater at 110°F maximum. Measure the temperature of hot tap water with a meat or candy thermometer.
- Do not leave purses on the floor or on tables where children can reach them.
- Test paint in older houses for lead content. Call the Department of Public Health in your area to learn what procedures to follow. Remove paint immediately if lead is present. Always consider the possibility of soil contamination from lead that has been scraped off the exterior of a building. Should deleading be necessary, children must not be present.
- Do not allow children to chew on styrofoam cups and food containers. Particles can be inhaled, causing respiratory irritation.
- Small button-sized batteries for cameras and watches can cause airway blockage if inhaled and can cause tissue damage, bleeding, and poisoning if swallowed. Discard old batteries immediately.

Appendix A

Infection Prevention

Infection Prevention

Some children are the picture of health no matter what the season. Other children seem to pick up every illness to which they are exposed. On the average, toddlers and preschoolers experience six to eight episodes of illness each year. This frequency decreases to about three episodes each year by the time the child is 6 years old. Fortunately, the incidence of many of the serious and life-threatening childhood illnesses has been dramatically reduced by vaccines and antibiotics. Today in the United States common illnesses are generally mild compared to those of past generations.

Illnesses in young children are caused by several different types of organisms.

Bacterial Infections

Bacterial infections—which include illnesses such as ear infections, strep throat, scarlet fever, impetigo, and some pneumonias—must be treated by prescription antibiotics to ensure prompt and complete recovery. To help prevent an infection from recurring, it is important for a child taking an antibiotic to complete the entire course of medicine.

Viral Infections

Infections caused by viruses include such illnesses as chicken pox, colds, croup, some pneumonias, and the gastrointestinal upsets of vomiting and diarrhea. Symptoms that accompany viral infections can be treated to make the child feel more comfortable, but there are no medications available to destroy the viruses that cause these illnesses. Antibiotics have no effect on viruses, and the illnesses they cause will usually subside in time.

The viruses that cause the common cold, as well as many of the common upper respiratory infections, enter through the eyes, nose, and mouth. They are spread from one person to another as airborne particles from a cough or a sneeze or by direct contact. If children sneeze into their hands and then pick up toys without first washing their hands, they will contaminate the toys with their viruses.

Fungal Infections

Fungal infections include such conditions as ringworm, athlete's foot, and thrush; they are usually not serious. There are several effective medications for fungal infections. Antibiotics are not prescribed to treat fungal infections and, in some instances, can worsen the condition.

Parasitic Infections

Infections caused by parasites are common and include such illnesses as pinworms and giardia. They are transmitted by ingestion and need to be treated with a medication specifically for the parasite.

Infection Prevention Guidelines

Organisms that cause illness enter the body in one of four ways:

- Direct contact or touching, such as impetigo and herpes
- Ingestion, such as pinworms and hepatitis A
- Entrance of airborne microorganisms through the eyes, nose, or mouth, such as the common cold, flu, and chicken pox
- Contact with blood, such as hepatitis B and AIDS/HIV

In order to decrease the incidence of disease among children and their care givers, it is important to consistently use the good hygiene techniques described below.

1. ***Wash your hands frequently and teach children to wash their hands.*** This is the single most important measure you can take to prevent the spread of illness and infection.

How to wash your hands

- Use soap (liquid soap is most hygienic) and warm water to scrub hands vigorously for 15 to 30 seconds. The friction created by rubbing your hands together contributes as much to the cleaning as does the soap and water. Also wash the backs of the hands and under the fingernails.

- Rinse clean hands with warm running water and dry them with a clean paper towel. Then use the towel to turn off the water faucet and discard the towel.
- Fingernails should be kept short and scrubbed with a nail brush. Organisms collect more easily under long fingernails.

When to wash your hands

- Before eating or preparing foods for yourself and others.
- After toileting, helping a child with toileting, or diapering.
- After touching any body fluids (e.g., saliva, nasal discharge, blood, tears, stool, and urine) whether or not you were wearing gloves.

When to have children wash their hands

- After toileting. Young children need to be reminded and supervised. Infants and toddlers who wear diapers should have their hands washed after diaper changes. Younger children frequently put their hands in their mouths. If they do not wash their hands after touching the diaper area, they might later ingest illness-producing organisms. Even very young children should be taught how to wash their hands.
- After playing outside.
- Before participating in a cooking project.
- Before meal and snack times.
- Before playing with playdough.

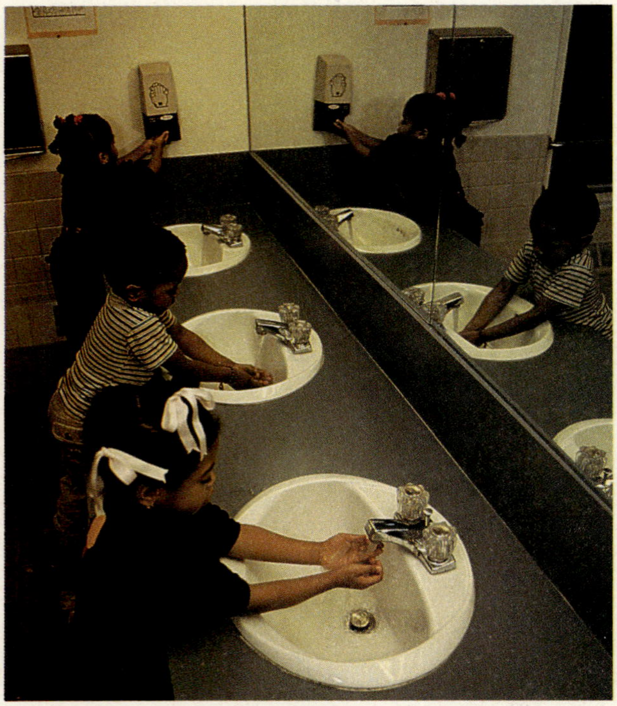

2. ***Disinfect all washable surfaces with a commercial disinfectant or a sanitizing solution of bleach and water.*** A sanitizing solution should be made of one part bleach to ten parts water and must be made fresh daily. This solution is inexpensive and is extremely effective in killing illness-producing microorganisms. Spray it on all washable surfaces and allow it to air dry. Make sure you disinfect the following areas in your center or home daily:
   - Sinks
   - Toilets
   - Potty seats
   - Diaper changing tables
   - Table tops
   - Door knobs

   Mouthed toys should be washed daily, rinsed with the sanitizing solution, rinsed with water and allowed to air dry.

   Vomitus, diarrhea, and blood should be wiped up with gloved hands, and the area should be disinfected. Soiled clothing and bedding should be placed in a plastic bag and sent home with the child.
3. ***Use disposable latex or rubber gloves.*** Gloves need not be sterile. Gloves act as a barrier between your hands and another person's body fluids, such as blood, diarrhea, urine, and vomitus. It is strongly recommended that you wear gloves when there is a chance of your touching these fluids because of the many diseases that can be spread. Gloves also protect a child with an open wound from contaminants on the child care provider's hands.

   Disposable gloves should be available in each bathroom, in the diaper-changing area, and in the first aid kit. Wash your hands thoroughly with soap and water after removing disposable gloves.

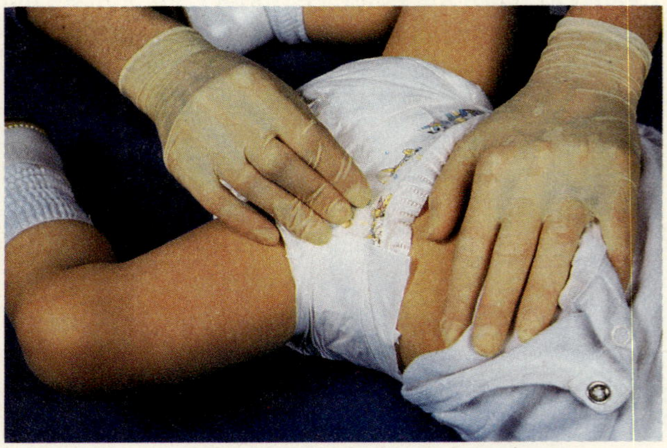

4. ***Practice good hygiene and encourage the children to follow your example.***

- Tie long hair back.
- Do not share personal items such as combs, brushes, hats, toothbrushes, cups, and drinking straws.
- Keep fingernails clean and trimmed.
- Do not bite your fingernails, rub your eyes, or otherwise touch your face without washing your hands first. This can introduce germs that will cause colds and other illnesses.
- Turn your head toward the floor or cover your mouth when coughing and sneezing.
- Use disposable tissues for coughing, sneezing, and wiping a nose. Dispose of soiled tissues promptly.
- Spend part of every day outside with the children, weather permitting.
- Leave the doors and windows open while the children are outside, weather permitting, so that fresh air can circulate through the center.
- Child care staff, parents, and visitors should not smoke in the center.
- Practice good hygiene routinely, not just when a child is ill.

5. ***Maintain clean inside and outside play areas.***

- Drain wading pools daily and as needed. Drain, clean, and disinfect water tables daily and allow to air dry. Clean and disinfect water toys.
- Cover outside sandboxes. If left uncovered, sandboxes can become litter boxes for cats and other animals. The ingestion of microscopic particles of infected animal waste can cause illness.
- Put rubber pants over diapers, even disposable diapers, when taking a young child into a swimming pool.
- Lawn sprinklers are more hygienic than wading pools for water play in the summer.

6. ***Special concerns of the adult preparing food.***

- Wash hands frequently because of the risk of passing illness-producing organisms through food.
- Tie hair back or wear a hair net.
- Do not handle food when ill.
- Avoid changing diapers if you are a food preparer. In a home care setting, where there is only one child care provider, good hand washing technique is essential.
- Keep the diaper-changing area separate from the food area.
- Do not taste the food with the utensil that is used to cook and stir.
- Wash all dishes and eating utensils in a dishwasher with the thermostat set to 170°F. If a dishwasher is unavailable, wash dishes and utensils with hot water and soap, rinse in a sanitizing solution of bleach (ten parts water to one part bleach), rinse again with clear water, and allow to air dry. If your center does not have proper cleaning facilities, disposable dishes and utensils must be used and then discarded.

7. ***Special concerns when caring for infants.***

- Wash mouthed toys daily with hot water and soap, rinse in sanitizing solution of bleach (ten parts water to one part bleach), rinse again with clear water, and allow to air dry.
- Rinse a pacifier or a toy that was dropped on the floor before handing it back to an infant.
- Wear a gown when holding an infant under 6 months of age.
- Use a separate gown for each infant.

Many states have specific written requirements concerning infection control in child care centers. In addition, many child care centers have their own written guidelines developed or approved by a health care consultant. Know your state's policies and your child care center's guidelines.

AIDS/HIV

AIDS/HIV is one of the largest health problems that the world faces today. The Centers for Disease Control estimates that in the United States alone, over 1 million people are infected with the virus that causes AIDS (acquired immune deficiency syndrome). This virus is known as HIV (human immunodeficiency virus). Initially, HIV lives within the body for months or years before the signs and symptoms of AIDS appear. In time, the virus begins to destroy the immune system, making the body susceptible to persistent, chronic infections that become increasingly difficult to fight. Illnesses that might be minor to a person with a healthy immune system, such as chicken pox and flu, can become dangerous and even life threatening to a person with AIDS/HIV.

People who have HIV in their blood but have a healthy immune system are able to fight infection but can still transmit the virus

continued

to others even though they have no symptoms of the disease and might not know they are infected. There is presently no vaccine or cure for AIDS/HIV.

HIV is spread from person to person through infected blood and certain other body fluids including semen, vaginal secretions, and breast milk. The virus is also present in other body fluids including saliva, tears, perspiration, and urine, and in stool, but not in concentrations high enough to transmit the disease. However, the virus can be spread through any of these discharges if they contain HIV-infected blood, even in microscopic amounts.

HIV is a fragile virus and is not easily transmitted from person to person through ordinary, everyday activities. Some behaviors have been identified as high risk for transmitting HIV. These include unprotected sexual activity, sharing needles and syringes for drug use, and allowing blood or any body fluid containing even microscopic amounts of blood to come in contact with an open cut or sore, no matter how small.

HIV can be transmitted from an AIDS/HIV-infected mother to her unborn child. Some children born to AIDS/HIV-infected mothers initially test positive for HIV. Many of these children, however, will lose the HIV antibody as they naturally lose other maternal antibodies during their first year of life. Therefore, a positive test for HIV shortly after birth is not a reliable indicator that the child actually is infected with HIV. In rare cases, HIV has been transmitted to a healthy infant by an AIDS/HIV-infected mother through her breast milk.

HIV can also be transmitted through a transfusion of blood or blood products contaminated with the virus. However, this risk is very small because all blood and blood products are now carefully screened for HIV. There is _no_ risk of becoming infected with HIV when donating blood.

AIDS/HIV is _not_ spread through such ordinary everyday activities as:

- Hugging
- Dry kissing
- Holding hands
- A sneeze or cough
- Cooking
- Sharing foods
- Public telephones
- Public restrooms
- Public swimming pools
- Using eating utensils
- Touching money, furniture, doorknobs, etc.
- Playground equipment and sandboxes
- Sharing books and toys
- Cats and dogs
- Mosquito bites
- Ear piercing by commercial hand-held punchers

According to the U.S. surgeon general, there are no cases of AIDS/HIV in which the virus is known to have been transmitted from one child to another in a school, child care, or foster care setting. Transmission of the virus in these settings would require the unlikely contact of one child's open cut with the blood or other body fluids of an HIV-infected child.

The number of children with AIDS/HIV in child care in the United States is small but growing. However, for every child known to have AIDS/HIV, there are many other HIV-infected children whose health care providers, parents, and child care providers do not yet know that the infection is present. It is therefore essential for all child care providers to know how to handle body fluids correctly. Child care providers must:

- Wear disposable rubber or latex gloves when giving first aid for a cut or wound, changing diapers, and handling or wiping up body fluids such as blood and vomitus. If gloves are not immediately available when first aid is necessary, use another barrier. Examples of other barriers are several thick gauze pads, a clean dish towel, or a cloth diaper. Additionally, plastic wrap or a plastic bag placed over the gauze or cloth covering increases the effectiveness of these barriers.
- Use disposable diapers. Soiled diapers should be folded with the soiled side inward and placed in a double-lined, covered diaper pail.
- Clean blood and other fluids off all surfaces with a solution of ten parts water to one part bleach. Allow this solution to air dry.
- Wash your hands vigorously with soap

and warm water after removing disposable gloves.

Handle *all* body fluids for *all* children in this manner at *all* times.

Information contained in a child's medical record is confidential. A child care center must protect the privacy of a child who is infected with HIV by limiting the number of people who have knowledge of the child's condition. Each case of a child with HIV in a child care setting must be evaluated individually to determine how the center can best provide for the needs of the child. Decisions should be made jointly by the child's parent, health care provider, and child care center director, and should be reevaluated periodically.

The problem of HIV infections and AIDS in the United States is growing at an alarming rate, and child care providers will continue to see increased numbers of children with HIV in child care in the future. Child care providers must take responsibility for keeping up with new information on AIDS/HIV. Contact your local public health department, state AIDS information office, or call the National AIDS Information Hot Line (toll free): 1-800-342-AIDS. For Spanish-speaking persons, call Linea Nacional de SIDA (toll free): 1-800-344-SIDA.

Hepatitis B in a Child Care Center

Hepatitis B is a serious illness caused by a virus that infects the liver. Like AIDS/HIV, the hepatitis B virus is found in all body fluids but can be transmitted to another person only through direct contact with blood or through sexual contact. Also, like AIDS/HIV, the hepatitis B virus cannot be spread through casual contact. See the discussion of infection prevention guidelines for AIDS/HIV.

Appendix B

Injury Report Form

Documenting an Injury

If an injury occurs to a child in your child care setting, it is important to document the nature of the injury and the care provided. This information should be kept on file in the child care center. The injury report form below is provided as a sample of a document that can help the child care provider to adequately document the injury.

INJURY REPORT FORM

Child's name: ______________________ Birth date: ______________

Date and time of injury: ______________________

Place where injury occurred: ______________________

Description of injury: ______________________

____

____

Description of how injury occurred: ______________________

____

____

Description of first aid care given: ______________________

____

____

First aid care given by: ______________________

Was EMS notified? ______________________

Was child's health care provider notified? ______________________

Adult witnesses to the injury: ______________________

____

____

Staff member supervising child at the time of the injury: ______________________

Child's parent notified: ______________________ ______________________

Date Time

______________________ ______________________

Signature of person preparing this form Date

Appendix C

Common Childhood Illnesses

COMPLAINT	WHAT YOU SHOULD KNOW	WHAT YOU CAN DO	CHILD MAY RETURN TO CHILD CARE
Headache	■ Most are minor and are caused by overexertion or stress ■ Might signal beginning of illness	■ Have child rest in a quiet area. ■ Know your center's policy about the use of acetaminophen. ■ Report recurring headache to parents.	■ When child feels better
Ear Pain	**Otitis media (middle ear infection)** ■ Can be painful ■ Signs and symptoms: • Repeated pulling of ears • Cries of pain and general irritability • Fever • Fluid draining from ear(s) ■ Ear infections are not contagious ■ Antibiotic necessary to treat ear infection ■ Never insert anything, including cotton swabs, into child's ear ■ A small object caught in child's ear can cause pain and irritation Also see *Foreign Objects*, Chapter 6	■ Take temperature and treat fever as necessary. ■ Notify parent. ■ Hold child in upright position to decrease pressure in ear and lessen pain. ■ Watch for hearing loss or speech problem in child with recurring ear infections.	■ When child feels better and temperature is normal
Eye Problems	**Conjunctivitis (pink eye)** ■ An infection of the lining of the eye ■ Signs and symptoms: • Red, itchy eyes • Yellow or watery drainage • Pain ■ Highly contagious ■ Watery drainage is most likely viral conjunctivitis and resolves without treatment ■ Pus or yellow drainage is most likely bacterial conjunctivitis and must be treated with an antibiotic	■ Clean drainage from child's eye(s) with a clean tissue and warm water as needed. ■ Encourage child not to touch eye(s). ■ Use good hand washing technique and encourage child to do the same. See Appendix A. ■ Notify parent if eye(s) has pus or yellow drainage.	■ If eye discharge contains no pus or after 24 hours of antibiotic treatment

COMPLAINT	WHAT YOU SHOULD KNOW	WHAT YOU CAN DO	CHILD MAY RETURN TO CHILD CARE
	Sty ■ An infection of a sweat gland on the eye lid ■ Appears as a painful, red pimple Also see *Eye Injuries*, Chapter 6	■ Apply warm wash cloth to eye for 5–10 minutes several times per day. ■ Encourage child not to touch eye. ■ Use good hand washing technique and encourage child to do the same. See Appendix A. ■ Notify parent at end of day.	■ When child feels better
Dental Problems 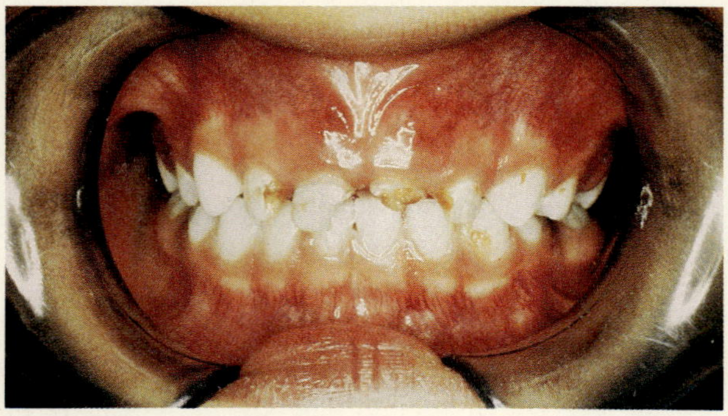 Bottlemouth	**Bottlemouth** ■ Tooth decay in very young children ■ Caused by frequent drinking of liquids containing sugar	■ Do not give child a bottle of milk or juice (or any fluid containing sugar) at nap or bedtime. ■ Avoid sticky foods that cling to teeth and cause decay, such as raisins, gummy fruit-flavored treats, caramel candy, and licorice. ■ Encourage children to brush teeth after snacks and meals.	■ Need not exclude child from child care
Source: Courtesy of William B. Chan, DMD Tufts University, School of Dental Medicine	**Teething** ■ Gum pain caused by newly erupting teeth ■ Can cause exaggerated crankiness ■ Can be very painful and cause sleepless nights	■ Provide teething toys on which child can chew. ■ Do not rub child's gums with your finger. ■ Know your center's policy about over-the-counter topical teething products.	■ Need not exclude child from child care.
Sore Throat	**General Information** ■ Most often caused by viruses and will resolve without treatment	■ Take temperature and treat fever as necessary. ■ Notify parent at end of day unless other symptoms accompany sore throat. ■ Use good handwashing technique. ■ Do not allow babies to share mouthed toys, pacifiers, or bottles.	■ When temperature is normal
	Strept Throat ■ A throat infection caused by the streptococcus bacteria	■ As above.	■ After 24 hours of antibiotic treatment and when temperature is normal

COMPLAINT	WHAT YOU SHOULD KNOW	WHAT YOU CAN DO	CHILD MAY RETURN TO CHILD CARE
	■ Occurs less frequently but is more serious than a viral throat infection ■ Contagious ■ Signs and symptoms: • Persistent, painful sore throat • White patches on throat and tonsils • Persistent fever • Swollen glands • Headache • Stomachache ■ Can be serious; if untreated, risks later damage to heart and kidneys ■ Also see *Scarlet Fever*		
	Thrush ■ A yeast infection in the mouth ■ Appears as small white patches on the mucous membranes of the mouth and on the tongue ■ Easily spread from one infant to another ■ Must be treated with antifungal medication ■ Also see *Diaper Area: Candida Rash*	■ As above.	■ Once treatment has started
Cough	■ A symptom of an irritation within the respiratory tract. ■ Often accompanies a viral infection, such as a cold ■ Also see *Croup,* Chapter 11	■ Encourage child to cover mouth and to use good handwashing technique. ■ See *Infection Prevention*, Appendix A. ■ Notify parent if cough persists.	■ Need not exclude child unless cough is accompanied by a fever
Vomiting	■ Usually caused by a virus ■ Less frequently caused by food poisoning or an emotional upset ■ Many gastrointestinal viruses that cause vomiting are contagious	■ Remove child from the group. ■ Notify parent. ■ Give no food or fluid until one hour after vomiting has stopped.	■ The following day, if child feels better and has no fever
Diarrhea	**General Information** ■ Defined as several loose or watery stools ■ Caused primarily by viruses ■ Can be caused by bacterial infection, antibiotics, and certain foods ■ Most diarrhea resolves without treatment within a few days	■ Use good handwashing technique after helping with toileting and wear disposable gloves when changing diapers. See Appendix A.	■ Need not exclude child from child care center if diarrhea can be contained in diaper or by normal toileting practices ■ Know your center's policy

COMPLAINT	WHAT YOU SHOULD KNOW	WHAT YOU CAN DO	CHILD MAY RETURN TO CHILD CARE
	■ If mild diarrhea does not resolve within a few days, the child should be seen by a health care provider	■ Eliminate foods that have a tendency to cause diarrhea, such as peaches, grapes, raisins, plums and melons. ■ Encourage child to eat foods that bind, such as bananas, apples, apple sauce (apple juice can cause diarrhea), white flour baked goods, cooked vegetables, rice and crackers. ■ Encourage child to drink clear fluids.	
	Infectious Diarrhea ■ An intestinal infection caused by bacteria (such as salmonella and shigella), a parasite (such as giardia), or a virus. ■ Signs and symptoms: • Bloody diarrhea • Cramping • Fever • Foul smelling stools • Weight loss ■ Acquired by ingestion of contaminated water or food ■ Highly contagious ■ Diagnosed by stool cultures ■ Prescription medication might be necessary to treat infectious diarrhea	■ Requires strict infection control measures in a child care center ■ Use good hand washing technique after helping with toileting and wear disposable gloves when changing diapers. ■ See *Infection Prevention,* Appendix A.	**If salmonella**: ■ After treatment with antibiotics and after 3 negative stool cultures **If shigella:** ■ After treatment with antibiotics and after severe diarrhea is under control ■ Must use strict infection control measures until 2 stool cultures are negative **If giardia:** ■ After treatment with antiparasitic medication and if diarrhea is absent ■ Must use strict infection control measures until 2 stool cultures are negative ■ Check with your health care consultant about your center's policy concerning child's return following treatment for giardia.
	Hepatitis A ■ An infection of the liver caused by a virus and spread through the intestine and stool. ■ Virus spread from person to person when contaminated hands touch food or eating utensils. ■ Mild flu-like symptoms ■ Symptoms develop 2-8 weeks after exposure ■ Illness is more serious in adults than in children	■ As above. ■ Contact your health care provider if you are exposed to hepatitis A	■ Child should remain at home while ill and may return when symptoms are no longer present and child is fever free for 24 hours. ■ Check with your health care consultant concerning child's return following hepatitis.

COMPLAINT	WHAT YOU SHOULD KNOW	WHAT YOU CAN DO	CHILD MAY RETURN TO CHILD CARE
	■ Illness should be reported to your local Department of Public Health by your health care provider. ■ No specific treatment.		
Constipation	■ Defined as hard stools that cause pain ■ Can be caused by diet low in fiber as well as inadequate fluid intake ■ Sometimes caused by postponing or resisting the urge to eliminate	■ Encourage child to drink more clear fluids. ■ Encourage eating of foods that have a tendency to soften the stool, such as peaches, prunes, grapes, raisins, plums, and melons. ■ Reduce intake of foods that bind, such as milk, cheese, cottage cheese, bananas, apples, applesauce, and white-flour baked goods. ■ Encourage regular toileting routine.	■ Need not exclude child from child care
Itching Scalp	**Pediculosis capitas (head lice)** ■ Infestation of a tiny parasitic insect on the scalp and hair ■ Signs and symptoms: • Persistent itching of scalp • Tiny red bites on scalp and on hair line at back of neck • Tiny yellow/white eggs, or nits, firmly attached to shaft of hair ■ Highly contagious ■ Not caused by uncleanliness ■ Not carried by cats or dogs ■ Requires thorough treatment ■ Lice transferred mainly from head to head and by sharing personal items, such as hats, combs, and brushes ■ Lice cannot jump or fly	■ Notify child's parent. ■ Notify all other parents of a case of lice, but maintain confidentiality. ■ Send home each child's personal items for cleaning. ■ Machine wash all washable items in hot water. ■ Use high heat setting on dryer. ■ Place pillows and stuffed animals in a dryer on high heat setting for 30 minutes. ■ Vacuum all rugs, upholstered furniture and items that cannot be washed. ■ Also see Rashes: *Ringworm* ■ Do not use lice sprays. ■ Do daily head checks on all children. ■ Check with health care consultant if more than one child is infested. ■ Lice killing products are pesticides, use cautiously	■ After treatment with a lice killing product and thorough nit removal. ■ Know your center's policy.
Diaper Area Irritation and Itching	**Pinworms** ■ An intestinal parasitic (worm) infection causing intense anal itching	■ Encourage children to wash hands after outdoor play. ■ Notify parent.	■ After initial treatment.

COMPLAINT	WHAT YOU SHOULD KNOW	WHAT YOU CAN DO	CHILD MAY RETURN TO CHILD CARE
	■ Acquired by ingesting microscopic pinworm eggs after outdoor play in dirt or sand ■ Common among young children who frequently have their hands in their mouths and are poor handwashers ■ Contagious ■ Diagnosed with special pinworm kit used by parents to collect parasite specimen from anal skin		
	Diaper Rash ■ Commonly occurs when bacteria in the bowel react with urine to form ammonia which irritates and burns the skin ■ Prolonged exposure and friction against diaper worsens the rash ■ Can be painful	■ Change diaper frequently. ■ Wash diaper area with soap and warm water; allow complete drying. ■ Protect diaper area with over-the-counter ointment. ■ Do not use baby powder on diaper area because the child might inhale it.	■ Need not exclude child from child care
	Candida Rash (yeast) ■ Caused by a yeast infection within the intestines ■ Appears as a fiery red rash in diaper area ■ Infection can also be present in mouth—see *Thrush* under Sore Throat ■ Easily spread from child to child by adult who does not wash hands well ■ Needs treatment with prescription medication	■ Use good hand washing technique after each diaper change.	■ Once medication is started
Fever	See *Fevers,* Chapter 11		
Rashes	**Fifth Disease** ■ Signs and symptoms: • Solid, bright red rash on cheeks giving face a "slapped cheek" appearance • Lacey red rash on arms, legs, and trunk; usually gone in 10 days • Other symptoms include: low grade fever, fatigue, headache, stomachache	■ Notify all parents if a child develops Fifth Disease because of possible health risks to unborn babies and children with serious illnesses. ■ Use good hand washing technique.	■ Need not exclude child from child care if temperature normal and child otherwise fine

COMPLAINT	WHAT YOU SHOULD KNOW	WHAT YOU CAN DO	CHILD MAY RETURN TO CHILD CARE
	■ Incubation period 4–14 days before rash breaks out ■ Contagious several days before appearance of rash ■ Rash might recur periodically over the following 3–4 months, but the child will not be contagious ■ A mild, viral illness, harmless for most children ■ Can be serious for children with leukemia, sickle cell anemia, and Thalessemia ■ A pregnant woman exposed to Fifth Disease should consult her health care provider ■ No vaccine available ■ One infection is believed to provide lifelong immunity	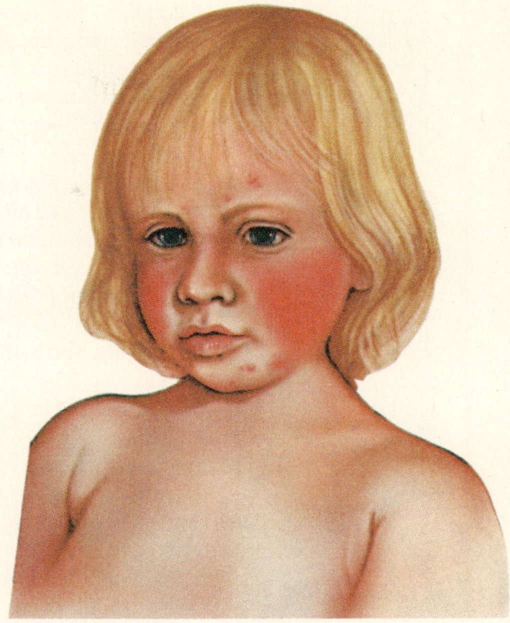 Fifth Disease *Drawing courtesy of Merck, Sharp, and Dohme, West Point, Pa.*	
	Scarlet Fever ■ A bacterial (strept) infection that causes a generalized illness ■ More serious than simple strept throat ■ Contagious ■ Rash appears primarily on trunk and is most intense at underarms, groin, behind knees, and on inner thighs ■ Rash resembles a sunburn covered with tiny goose bumps ■ Rash starts on chest and spreads downward ■ Sore throat ■ High fever ■ Tongue has white coating which changes to strawberry color after 4–5 days ■ Nausea and vomiting ■ Skin peels after one week ■ Must be treated with an antibiotic ■ Untreated, Scarlet Fever puts child at risk of developing rheumatic fever	■ Take temperature and treat for fever as necessary. ■ Notify parent. 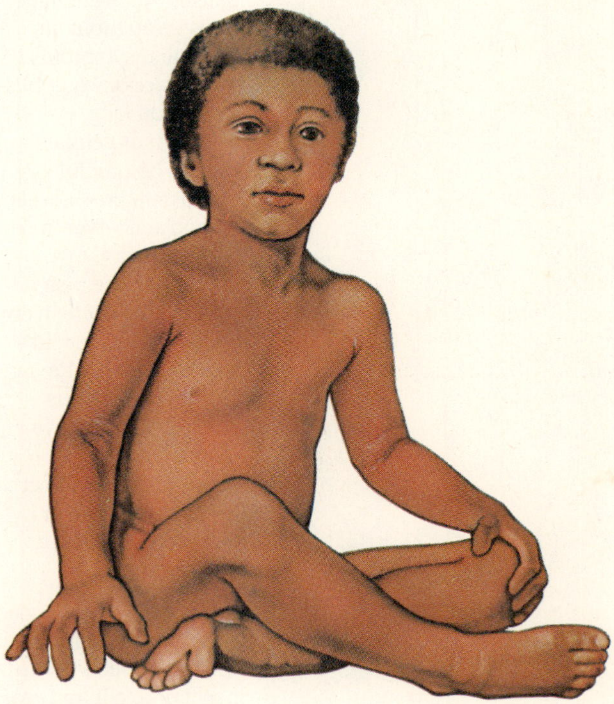 Scarlet Fever *Drawing courtesy of Merck, Sharp, and Dohme, West Point, Pa.*	■ 24 hours after antibiotic treatment has started, 24 hours fever-free, and child is otherwise fine

COMPLAINT	WHAT YOU SHOULD KNOW	WHAT YOU CAN DO	CHILD MAY RETURN TO CHILD CARE
	Chicken Pox ■ A common viral illness ■ Rash primarily appears on face and trunk as fluid-filled bubbles which break, weep, and scab over ■ Rash can also appear on arms, legs, or any mucous membrane surface, such as inside the mouth, throat, eyes, and vagina ■ Other signs and symptoms: • Fever • Itching ■ Incubation period 10–21 days ■ Contagious from 1–2 days before rash appears until all blisters have scabbed over ■ Dry scabs are not contagious ■ One bout gives immunity ■ Vaccine not yet available	■ Take temperature and treat for fever as necessary. ■ Notify parent. 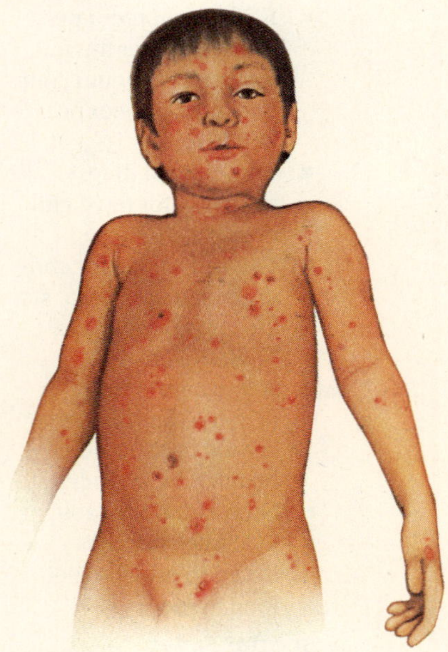 Chicken Pox *Drawing courtesy of Merck, Sharp, and Dohme, West Point, Pa.*	■ When all blisters have scabbed over
	Herpes Simplex ■ A viral disease that causes recurrent infections throughout life ■ Signs and symptoms: • Cluster of water blisters on face, eye, hand, or genitals • Can be painful • Blisters break, weep, and scab over in several days ■ In children the rash occurs almost exclusively on the face as a cold sore or fever blister ■ Child is contagious until all blisters have scabbed over ■ Virus spread by direct contact with sore or by secretions from sore ■ No cure available	■ Alert parent to developing infection. ■ Also see *Infection Prevention,* Appendix A.	■ Once an open sore has completely scabbed over or open sore can be completely covered
	Impetigo ■ A bacterial skin infection often following an insect bite, cut, or break in the skin	■ Alert parent to the presence of the rash. ■ Observe rash and note any improvement or worsening.	■ 24 hours after treatment started

COMPLAINT	WHAT YOU SHOULD KNOW	WHAT YOU CAN DO	CHILD MAY RETURN TO CHILD CARE
	■ Most commonly seen on the face ■ Signs and symptoms: • Fine, honey-colored scab • Pain and itching ■ Can spread to other parts of the child's body if child scratches ■ Can spread to others in close contact ■ Requires topical antibiotic treatment	■ Discourage scratching. ■ Do not permit the sharing of towels and wash cloths. ■ Use good handwashing technique. Encourage child to do so.	
	Scabies		
	■ A parasitic infection caused by mites which burrow under the skin ■ Causes intense itching ■ Frequently seen in moist areas of the body, such as the groin, buttocks, webbed spaces of fingers and toes, and under the arms ■ Burrows first appear as fine, gray lines under the skin; area of infection enlarges as adult mites burrow and lay eggs under the skin ■ Incubation period up to 30 days ■ Transferred by close body contact and shared clothing ■ Mites cannot jump or fly ■ Child must be treated at home with a prescription mite-killing lotion. ■ Itching can last 2–4 weeks after treatment	■ Notify child's parent. ■ Notify all other parents of a case of scabies, but maintain confidentiality. ■ Send home each child's personal items for cleaning. ■ Machine wash all washable items. ■ Use high heat setting on dryer. ■ Place pillows and stuffed animals in the dryer on high heat setting for 30 minutes. ■ Vacuum all rugs, upholstered furniture and items that can not be washed. ■ Do not use spray pesticides. ■ Check with health care consultant if several children are infected. ■ Discourage the child from scratching.	■ One day after treatment applied
	Ringworm		
	■ A superficial fungal infection of the skin, affecting young children primarily on the scalp and trunk ■ Mildly contagious ■ Scalp infection causes temporary bald patches 1½ to 2 inches in diameter ■ Trunk infection causes round or oval, red, scaly patches that spread out-	■ Notify parent at end of day.	■ Immediately after treatment started

COMPLAINT	WHAT YOU SHOULD KNOW	WHAT YOU CAN DO	CHILD MAY RETURN TO CHILD CARE
	ward and heal in the center, resembling a doughnut Infection cannot penetrate skin, but sits on the surface Treated with antifungal topical cream that must be used for several weeks after rash disappears		
	Roseola ■ A viral illness occurring in young children primarily under the age of two ■ Causes a persistent high fever (103°F or higher) for 3–4 days without other symptoms ■ Fever drops suddenly on 4th day and generalized red rash appears over the entire body ■ Rash is gone in 24 hours ■ Incubation period 5–15 days ■ Mildly contagious ■ One bout gives immunity	■ Take temperature and treat fever as necessary. ■ Notify parent. ■ Encourage clear fluids.	■ When child feels better and temperature is normal for 24 hours

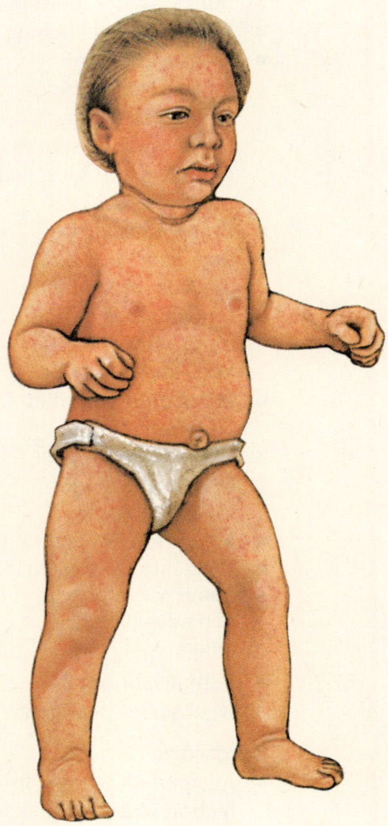

Roseola
Drawing courtesy of Merck, Sharp, and Dohme, West Point, Pa.

Appendix D

First Aid Kit

Although you hope an emergency never occurs, you need to be prepared. Part of being prepared for an emergency means keeping a well stocked first aid kit. With all necessary supplies on hand, you will be better able to act quickly and effectively should an emergency arise.

Store all supplies in a sturdy, locked container out of the reach of children. Plastic tool or tackle boxes make good containers for first aid supplies because they are light weight and portable. Keep the first aid kit in a cool, dry location. Make sure all staff members know where the kit is stored.

Antibiotics and other medicines prescribed by a health care provider for children's periodic illnesses should not be stored in a first aid kit. Many of these medicines should be refrigerated and all should be kept out of the reach of children.

Check the first aid kit regularly for items that have been used and not replaced. Discard expired items.

Items for a Child Care Center First Aid Kit

- Adhesive bandages (assorted sizes)
- Blanket
- CPR mouth barrier
- Coins for a pay phone
- Commercial cold pack
- Cotton balls
- Cotton swabs
- Disposable latex or rubber gloves
- Flashlight and spare batteries
- Measuring spoons
- Nonstick sterile pads in all sizes
- Paper cups
- Pencil and paper
- Petroleum jelly
- Rolled elastic bandages
- Rolled gauze bandage (3" size)
- Soap
- Sterile gauze pads (4" size)
- Sterile eye pads
- Syrup of ipecac
- Scissors
- Thermometer
- Tongue depressor
- Tape
- Tweezers
- White cotton handkerchief

An allergic emergency self-treatment kit, if prescribed for a child in your center, should be kept in your first aid kit. In addition, you might want to include these items. Know your center's policies regarding the use of these products.

- Acetaminophen
- Antibacterial topical ointments
- Baking soda
- Calamine lotion
- Hydrogen peroxide
- Oil of cloves

Appendix E

Basic Life Support Proficiency Checklist

S = self check **P = partner check** **I = instructor check**

CHILD RESCUE BREATHING	S	P	I
■ Check responsiveness	☐	☐	☐
■ Send someone to activate EMS system.	☐	☐	☐
■ Position child on back	☐	☐	☐
■ Open airway (to the above-neutral position)	☐	☐	☐
■ Check for breathing (allow 5 seconds)	☐	☐	☐
■ Give two slow breaths (1–1-1/2 seconds each)	☐	☐	☐
■ Check for carotid pulse (allow 10 seconds)	☐	☐	☐
■ Perform rescue breathing (1 breath every 3 seconds)	☐	☐	☐
■ Recheck pulse and breathing after about 1 minute or 20 breaths (allow 5 seconds)	☐	☐	☐
■ Continue rescue breathing (rechecking pulse and breathing every minute or every 20 breaths)	☐	☐	☐

CHILD CPR	S	P	I
■ Check responsiveness	☐	☐	☐
■ Send someone to activate EMS system.	☐	☐	☐
■ Position child on back	☐	☐	☐
■ Open airway (to the above-neutral position)	☐	☐	☐
■ Check for breathing (allow 5 seconds)	☐	☐	☐
■ Give two slow breaths (1–1-1/2 seconds each)	☐	☐	☐
■ Check for carotid pulse (allow 10 seconds)	☐	☐	☐
■ Find compression location	☐	☐	☐
■ Perform CPR (5 compressions to 1 breath)	☐	☐	☐
■ Recheck pulse after about 1 minute or 12 cycles (allow 5 seconds)	☐	☐	☐
■ Continue CPR (rechecking pulse every few minutes)	☐	☐	☐

CONSCIOUS CHOKING CHILD	S	P	I
■ Determine if child is choking	☐	☐	☐
■ Shout for help	☐	☐	☐
■ Give abdominal thrusts	☐	☐	☐

UNCONSCIOUS CHOKING CHILD	S	P	I
■ Check responsiveness	☐	☐	☐
■ Send someone to activate EMS system	☐	☐	☐
■ Position child on back	☐	☐	☐
■ Open airway	☐	☐	☐
■ Check for breathing (allow 5 seconds)	☐	☐	☐
■ Give two slow breaths (1–1-1/2 seconds each)	☐	☐	☐
■ Retilt head and try another 2 breaths	☐	☐	☐
■ Give 5 abdominal thrusts	☐	☐	☐
■ Check for foreign object	☐	☐	☐
■ Give 2 breaths	☐	☐	☐
■ Repeat thrusts, check, and breaths until successful	☐	☐	☐

INFANT RESCUE BREATHING	S	P	I
■ Check responsiveness	☐	☐	☐
■ Send someone to activate EMS system	☐	☐	☐
■ Position infant on back	☐	☐	☐
■ Open airway to the neutral position	☐	☐	☐
■ Check for breathing (allow 5 seconds)	☐	☐	☐
■ Give two slow breaths (1–1-1/2 seconds each)	☐	☐	☐
■ Check for brachial pulse (allow 10 seconds)	☐	☐	☐
■ Perform rescue breathing (1 breath every 3 seconds)	☐	☐	☐
■ Recheck pulse and breathing after about 1 minute or 20 breaths (allow 5 seconds)	☐	☐	☐
■ Continue rescue breathing (rechecking pulse and breathing every minute or every 20 breaths)	☐	☐	☐

INFANT CPR	S	P	I
■ Check responsiveness	☐	☐	☐
■ Send someone to activate EMS system.	☐	☐	☐
■ Position infant on back	☐	☐	☐
■ Open airway (to the neutral position)	☐	☐	☐
■ Check for breathing (allow 5 seconds)	☐	☐	☐
■ Give two slow breaths (1–1-1/2 seconds each)	☐	☐	☐
■ Check for brachial pulse (allow 10 seconds)	☐	☐	☐
■ Find compression location	☐	☐	☐
■ Perform CPR (5 compressions to 1 breath)	☐	☐	☐
■ Recheck pulse after about 1 minute or 12 cycles (allow 5 seconds)	☐	☐	☐
■ Continue CPR (rechecking pulse every few minutes)	☐	☐	☐

CONSCIOUS CHOKING INFANT	S	P	I
■ Determine if infant is choking	☐	☐	☐
■ Shout for help	☐	☐	☐
■ Give 5 back blows and 5 chest thrusts until successful or infant becomes unconscious	☐	☐	☐

UNCONSCIOUS CHOKING INFANT	S	P	I
■ Check responsiveness	☐	☐	☐
■ Send someone to activate EMS system	☐	☐	☐
■ Position infant on back	☐	☐	☐
■ Open airway to neutral position	☐	☐	☐
■ Check for breathing (allow 5 seconds)	☐	☐	☐
■ Give two slow breaths (1–1-1/2 seconds each)	☐	☐	☐
■ Retilt head and try another 2 breaths	☐	☐	☐
■ Give 5 back blows	☐	☐	☐
■ Give 5 chest thrusts	☐	☐	☐
■ Check for foreign objects	☐	☐	☐
■ Give 2 breaths	☐	☐	☐
■ Repeat back blows, chest thrusts, check, and breaths until successful	☐	☐	☐

Quick Emergency Index